Ethics and Epidemiology

Ethics and Epidemiology

Second Edition

Edited by

Steven S. Coughlin

Tom L. Beauchamp

Douglas L. Weed

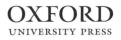

OXFORD
UNIVERSITY PRESS

2009

OXFORD
UNIVERSITY PRESS

Oxford University Press, Inc., publishes works that further
Oxford University's objective of excellence
in research, scholarship, and education.

Oxford New York
Auckland Cape Town Dar es Salaam Hong Kong Karachi
Kuala Lumpur Madrid Melbourne Mexico City Nairobi
New Delhi Shanghai Taipei Toronto

With offices in
Argentina Austria Brazil Chile Czech Republic France Greece
Guatemala Hungary Italy Japan Poland Portugal Singapore
South Korea Switzerland Thailand Turkey Ukraine Vietnam

Published by Oxford University Press, Inc.
198 Madison Avenue, New York, New York 10016
www.oup.com

Oxford is a registered trademark of Oxford University Press

Library of Congress Cataloging-in-Publication Data
Ethics and epidemiology / edited by Steven S. Coughlin, Tom L. Beauchamp,
Douglas L. Weed. — 2nd ed.
    p. ; cm.
    Includes bibliographical references and index.
    ISBN 978-0-19-532293-4
1. Epidemiology—Moral and ethical aspects. I. Coughlin, Steven S. (Steven Scott), 1957-
    II. Beauchamp, Tom L.   III. Weed, Douglas L., 1952-
    [DNLM: 1. Epidemiology—ethics. 2. Codes of Ethics. 3. Epidemiologic
Methods.   4. Ethics, Medical.   5. Health Services Research—ethics.
6. Social Medicine—ethics. WA 105 E84 2009]
RA652.E84 2009
174.2'944—dc22   2008030611

9 8 7 6 5 4 3 2 1
Printed in the United States of America
on acid-free paper

Preface

In the 10 years since the first edition of *Ethics and Epidemiology* was published, there have been many important ethical developments in epidemiology and related fields in public health and medicine. These developments include implementation of the HIPAA privacy rules, the completion of the American College of Epidemiology (ACE) ethics guidelines and ACE policy statement on sharing data from epidemiologic studies, and the drafting of a public health code of ethics, to name a few.

This revised edition of the book includes selected chapters from the first edition, which have been substantially updated and revised, along with several new chapters on issues concerning the ethics of public health practice, international health research, and genetic epidemiology. The chapters are organized topically and divided into four parts. The first part is titled "Foundations" because the chapters introduce basic and recurring concepts and principles. The subsequent parts deal with "Informed Consent, Privacy, and Confidentiality," "Balancing Risks and Benefits," and "The Regulatory Context and Professional Education." The latter subject includes discussion of the institutional review board (IRB) system and issues surrounding scientific misconduct in epidemiologic research.

The objective of this work is to make students, epidemiologists, and health professionals aware of situations that require moral reflection, judgment, or decision, while pointing to ways in which justified moral conclusions can be reached. We hope the book will also be of use to persons interested more broadly in bioethics and health policy. The text is most suited to the situation in North America, whose history, institutions, and studies represent the bulk of the material covered. However, several chapters examine international issues, and much of the book's content can easily be construed beyond the North American context.

S.S.C.

T.L.B.

D.L.W.

Contents

PART IV   THE REGULATORY CONTEXT AND PROFESSIONAL EDUCATION

Contributors

PETER H. ABBRECHT
Medical Expert
Division of Investigative
  Oversight
Office of Research Integrity
Department of Health and
  Human Services
Rockville, MD

TOM L. BEAUCHAMP
Professor of Philosophy
Senior Research Scholar
Kennedy Institute of Ethics
Georgetown University
Washington, DC

LAURA M. BESKOW
Assistant Professor
Duke Institute for Genome Sciences
  and Policy
Center for Genome Ethics, Law,
  and Policy
Duke University
Durham, NC

WYLIE BURKE
Professor and Chair
Department of Bioethics
  and Humanities
University of Washington School
  of Medicine
Seattle, WA

ELLEN WRIGHT CLAYTON
Rosalind E. Franklin Professor of
  Genetics and Health Policy
Professor of Pediatrics and Law
Director of the Center for Biomedical
  Ethics and Society
Vanderbilt University
Nashville, TN

STEVEN S. COUGHLIN
Current affiliations: Environmental
  Epidemiology Service
Department of Veterans Affairs
Washington, DC
and
Adjunct Professor of Epidemiology
Rollins School of Public Health
Emory University
Atlanta, GA

NANCY M. DAVIDIAN
Deputy Director
Division of Investigative Oversight
Office of Research Integrity
Department of Health and Human
  Services
Rockville, MD

KAREN GLANZ
Georgia Cancer Coalition Distinguished
  Research Scholar
Professor of Behavioral Sciences and
  Health Education

Rollins School of Public Health
Director, Emory Prevention Research
  Center
Emory University
Atlanta, GA

KENNETH W. GOODMAN
Professor and Director
Bioethics Program
University of Miami
Miami, FL

JEFFREY P. KAHN
Maas Family Endowed Chair in Bioethics
Director and Professor
Center for Bioethics
University of Minnesota
Minneapolis, MN

MICHELLE C. KEGLER
Associate Professor
Department of Behavioral Sciences
  and Health Education
Rollins School of Public Health
Emory University
Atlanta, GA

ANTHONY KESSEL
Director of Public Health
Camden Primary Care Trust, and
  Honorary Professor
Department of Public Health and Policy
London School of Hygiene and
  Tropical Medicine
London, United Kingdom

R. MAX LEARNER
Director
Office of Public Health Preparedness
South Carolina Department of Health
  and Environmental Control
Columbia, SC

CAROL LEVINE
Director, Families and Health Care
  Project
United Hospital Fund
New York, NY

ROBERT J. LEVINE
Co-director, Yale University
  Interdisciplinary Center for Bioethics
Director, Law, Policy, and Ethics Core,
Center for Interdisciplinary Research on
  AIDS, and
Professor of Medicine and Lecturer in
  Pharmacology
Yale University
New Haven, CT

ANNA C. MASTROIANNI
Associate Professor
School of Law
University of Washington
Seattle, WA

ROBERT E. MCKEOWN
Professor and Chair
Department of Epidemiology &
  Biostatistics
Arnold School of Public Health
Director, Health Sciences Research Core
University of South Carolina
Columbia, SC

JOHN D. H. PORTER
Reader in International Health
Departments of Infectious and Tropical
  Diseases and Public Health and Policy
London School of Hygiene and Tropical
  Medicine
London, United Kingdom

ALAN R. PRICE
Price Research Integrity Consultant
  Experts
Lago Vista, TX

RONALD J. PRINEAS
Professor
Director EPICARE
Department of Epidemiology and
  Prevention
Division of Public Health Sciences
Wake Forest University School of
  Medicine
Winston-Salem, NC

BARBARA K. RIMER
Dean and Alumni Distinguished
    Professor
School of Public Health
University of North Carolina
Chapel Hill, NC

PAUL A. SCHULTE
National Institute for Occupational
    Safety and Health
Centers for Disease Control and
    Prevention
Cincinnati, OH

ANDREA SMITH
Centre for Health Economics and Policy
    Analysis
Health Policy PhD Program
McMaster University
Hamilton, Ontario, Canada

COLIN L. SOSKOLNE
Professor
Department of Public Health Sciences
School of Public Health
University of Alberta
Edmonton, Alberta, Canada

CAROLYN STEPHENS
Senior Lecturer in Environment and
    Health
London School of Hygiene and Tropical
    Medicine
London, United Kingdom

DOUGLAS L. WEED
Founder and Managing Member
DLW Consulting Service, LLC
Kensington, MD

I

FOUNDATIONS

1

Historical Foundations

STEVEN S. COUGHLIN

In this chapter, we consider the history of the rise of ethical concerns in the public health movement and epidemiology, which is the study of the distribution and determinants of disease in human populations. Epidemiology is clearly a basic science in public health. We offer an overview of early developments in public health and ethics and discuss more recent developments, including the origins of bioethics, regulatory safeguards for human subjects research, and contemporary epidemiologic ethics.

Early Developments in Public Health and Ethics

Until the end of the Middle Ages, few advances were made in public health except for the control of a very limited number of communicable diseases achieved through the segregation and quarantine of persons thought to be infectious.[1, 2] Around the 16th century in Europe, hypotheses began to emerge regarding the social genesis of disease and some proposals were advanced concerning the role of government in public health. At the outset, these ideas had little practical impact, but they ultimately contributed to the emerging realization that government has an obligation to improve unsanitary conditions that threatened the health of rich and poor alike.[1]

The early writings relied on speculative hypotheses and were based more in the humanities than the sciences. For example, Thomas More (1478–1535) wrote about a fictitious story set in the land of *Utopia* (1516) in which hygiene protected health and insurance was provided against sickness and unemployment. Jean-Jacques Rousseau (1712–1778) also speculated in *Discourse on the Origins and*

Foundations of Inequality Among Men (1755)[2-4] that in the context of a prolonged criticism of "civil society," disease developed from social circumstances and ill health resulted from many factors, most of which were beyond the power of medicine to heal.

> With regard to illnesses, [I note] the extreme inequality in our lifestyle: excessive idleness among some, excessive labor among others; the ease with which we arouse and satisfy our appetites and our sensuality; the overly refined foods of the wealthy, which nourish them with irritating juices and overwhelm them with indigestion; the bad food of the poor, who most of the time do not have even that, and who, for want of food, are inclined to stuff their stomachs greedily whenever possible; staying up until all hours, excesses of all kinds, immoderate outbursts of every passion, bouts of fatigue and mental exhaustion; countless sorrows and afflictions which are felt in all levels of society and which perpetually gnaw away at souls; these are the fatal proofs that most of our ills are of our own making, and that we could have avoided nearly all of them by preserving the simple, regular and solitary lifestyle prescribed to us by nature.[4]

Rousseau subsequently influenced writers in ethical theory during the Enlightenment. Rousseau's theories also had an impact on later public health writers, such as the influential German physician Johann Peter Frank (1745–1821), who held high positions in both government and academia in Germany, Austria, Italy, and Russia and was an early proponent of social medicine controlled by the state. Frank promoted the idea of "medical police," or physicians with a public health role of sufficient authority to protect people against the health consequences of squalid urban living conditions. He argued that the physician's primary obligations were not owed merely to patients or the local community, but to the state and the monarch. Public health responsibilities were thereby reconceived as physicians' primary responsibilities.[1,5]

Pathogenic microorganisms were still unknown during the Enlightenment. With the exception of a few diseases such as smallpox, disease was regarded as the result of unhealthy lifestyles and environments rather than of contagion. Poor air, water, and living conditions were thought to foster miasmas (poisonous vapors) that caused illness. Hence, many Enlightenment physicians undertook public health campaigns emphasizing both personal and environmental hygiene. They understood that prevention methods were more effective than curative techniques and believed that people were responsible for maintaining their own health. The success of their efforts was not surprising because then-standard therapies such as laxatives, bloodletting, and induced vomiting yielded less impressive results than did public health efforts.[6,7]

A small number of Enlightenment figures, including American physician Benjamin Rush (1745–1813) and Scottish physician John Gregory (1724–1773), focused on professional medical ethics. They were among the first writers to lecture and publish extensively on this subject. Both Rush and Gregory believed that physicians had a moral obligation to educate the public and disclose relevant information to patients. However, neither believed that physicians had a moral obligation to obtain informed consent from patients for the care they provided. Rush and Gregory only wanted patients and the general public to be sufficiently educated to understand physicians' recommendations and be motivated to comply.

Rush and Gregory doubted that nonphysicians could intelligently form their own opinions about medical issues and make appropriate choices about care. For example, Rush advised physicians to "yield to [patients] in matters of little consequence, but maintain an inflexible authority over them in matters that are essential to life." Gregory was quick to underscore that the physician must be keenly aware of the harms that untimely disclosures might cause to patients or to the public. Rush, Gregory, and other Enlightenment figures did not discuss the need to respect the patient's right to self-determination or to obtain consent for any purpose other than a medically successful outcome. Gregory and Rush appreciated the value of providing information, but ideas of informed consent in health care did not originate in their writings. The language of "informed consent" was not used during the Enlightenment, and indeed not until the 1950s.[8,9]

An organized system to protect public health was not developed until the 19th century in England.[10] England was the first country to experience the social costs of the Industrial Revolution.[2] Due to the efforts of Edwin Chadwick (1800–1890) and other English reformers, laws were enacted that provided relief to the poor, made it illegal to employ children under the age of nine in factories, and promoted the health and welfare of industrial workers.[1,10] Chadwick was largely responsible for the passage of the Public Health Act of 1848, which created a board of health to oversee sanitary improvements at about the time that British physician John Snow began his classic series of investigations on cholera in London.[1,3,10] A royal commission headed by Chadwick recommended improvements in drainage systems in large towns, where a lack of sanitation had resulted in the spread of typhoid, cholera, and other diseases.[1] Legislation of this type quickly spread to other countries and had a major impact on public health and life expectancy.

The primary motivation for reform was the realization that poverty and unsanitary conditions had adverse economic and social consequences.[1,10] Chadwick maintained an association with English philosopher Jeremy Bentham (1748–1832), whose progressive social reforms for children employed in the factories, the poor, and women had a major impact in Victorian England and caused repercussions throughout Europe and India. As a young man, Chadwick was Bentham's assistant and later applied Bentham's utilitarian theories[11] to practical public health problems. Chadwick came to see poverty as a major cause of ill health through increased exposures to toxic substances, poor diet, and so forth.

Chadwick was a contemporary of John Stuart Mill (1806–1873), a Benthamite and the foremost utilitarian writer of the 19th century. Mill was elected to the British Parliament in 1865 and supported such unpopular measures as increased protection for the more vulnerable members of society, especially women, the poor, and persons condemned to capital punishment. Mill described his views on how to control disease in the following passage from his book *Utilitarianism*, which is still the most widely read account of utilitarian ethics:

Even that most intractable of enemies, disease, may be indefinitely reduced in dimensions by good physical and moral education, and proper control of noxious influences; while the progress of science holds out a promise for the future of still more direct conquests over this detestable foe. And every advance in that direction relieves us from some, not only of the chances which cut short our own lives, but, what concerns us still more, which deprive us of those in whom our happiness is wrapt up.[12]

Many of the founders of the public health movement in 19th-century England were guided by the utilitarian moral philosophy of Bentham, Mill, and other philosophers. The leaders of the sanitary movement attempted to use epidemiologic methods of observation to prevent or control diseases that afflicted those who were the worse off in society. For example, Chadwick led an inquiry into the diseases and unsanitary living conditions that were prevalent among England's impoverished working-class population. The resulting *General Report on the Sanitary Conditions of the Labouring Population of Great Britain* (1842) was a powerful indictment of the appalling living conditions of industrial workers and their families.[1,10,13] A similar sanitary survey was undertaken subsequently by legislator Lemuel Shattuck (1793–1859) in Massachusetts. Shattuck's influential *Report of the Sanitary Commission of Massachusetts 1850* outlined the basis for an organized system of public health.[14]

By the end of the 19th century, the germ theory of disease causation gained widespread acceptance because of influential bacteriological discoveries by German physician and Nobel Prize winner Robert Koch, French chemist and biologist Louis Pasteur, and others.[15,16] Microbiology and bacteriology became the most important medical sciences of both the United States and Europe, while epidemiology focused on the prevention of infectious diseases.[16,17] With major breakthroughs in bacteriology and immunology, disease prevention in the individual moved to the forefront.[10]

20th-Century Developments in Epidemiology and Ethics

Since the start of the public health movement in the mid-1800s—roughly the period in which epidemiology originated—the goal of epidemiology and public health has been to prevent premature death and disease by applying scientific and technical knowledge.[18] However, as events in the 20th century attest, the rights of individuals have not always been respected in pursuing these important societal and scientific objectives.

At the beginning of the 20th century, epidemiology in the United States was developed primarily in federal, state, and local health departments. In 1891, the Marine Hospital Service, later the U.S. Public Health Service, was a major center for epidemiologic research in the United States. It was organized by the Hygienic Laboratory. Investigators at the Hygienic Laboratory, renamed the National Institute of Health in 1930, studied both infectious and nutritional deficiency diseases, such as pellagra. Joseph Goldberger, Wade Hampton Frost, and other prominent epidemiologists received their training at the Hygienic Laboratory.[17]

Epidemiology developed separately in England, where leading epidemiologists in the 1930s, such as Major Greenwood of the London School of Hygiene, were concerned about both infectious and noninfectious epidemiology.[16,17] Greenwood was an active member of the Socialist Medical Association and an early advocate of socialized medicine. Like other British epidemiologists of the era, he was concerned about the social causes of disease and the health of all groups in society.[10,16]

The leading epidemiologists during this period rarely mentioned ethical issues in their publications. Experts in medicine, public health, and moral philosophy showed little interest in the major issues of biomedical ethics that we focus closely on today. A noteworthy exception was U.S. Army surgeon Walter Reed, who developed formal procedures for obtaining the consent of potential subjects in his yellow fever experiments using a written contract that set forth Reed's understanding of the ethical duties of medical researchers.[19] Although deficient by contemporary standards of disclosure and consent (discussed by Jeffrey Kahn and Anna Mastroianni in Chapter 4), these procedures recognized the right of patients to refuse or agree to participate in research.

By the mid-20th century, the focus in epidemiology had shifted in both Europe and the United States in response to the increasing spread of chronic diseases such as cardiovascular disease, cancer, and diabetes. These diseases were believed to have multiple environmental and genetic etiologies. The late 1940s was notable for both the founding of the World Health Organization and the initiation of the Framingham Study, a well-known cohort study of heart disease that has been ongoing since 1949.[20] The Nuremberg Code and the Declaration of Geneva were also developed during this period (as discussed in the next section). In 1956, Sir Richard Doll and Sir Austin Bradford Hill released the results of their cohort study of cigarette smoking and lung cancer among British doctors.[21] A few years later, in 1960, Brian MacMahon and his colleagues published *Epidemiological Methods*, the first text to provide a clear description of case-control and cohort study designs.[20,22]

In the years immediately following World War II, references to ethical issues in the epidemiologic literature were limited to narrowly focused discussions of the ethics of randomized controlled trials.[23,24] Epidemiologic researchers, primarily physicians, undertook studies with little or no public scrutiny of their methods or professional obligations. In addition, they were unencumbered by what would later become regulatory safeguards for the protection of human subjects such as the shift to review by institutional review boards.

Since that time, major regulatory changes have been made in the United States and many other countries (see discussion below and in Chapter 12). These changes have substantially improved the safeguards for the welfare and rights of human research subjects. These improvements have largely been driven by the widespread belief that people possess fundamental rights that should not be violated in the pursuit of scientific and medical progress.[25–27]

The Origins of Regulatory Safeguards for Human Subjects Research

In 1908, Sir William Osler, a physician who revolutionized the U.S. medical school curriculum, appeared before the British Royal Commission on Vivisection. He used the occasion to discuss Reed's research on yellow fever. When asked by the commission whether risky research on humans is morally permissible, a view Osler attributed to Reed, Osler answered: "It is always immoral without a definite, specific statement from the individual himself, with a *full knowledge* of the circumstances. Under these circumstances, any man, I think is *at liberty to submit himself to experiments*" (emphasis added). When then asked if "voluntary consent…entirely changes the question of morality," Osler replied "Entirely."[28] Some writers on the history of this period describe Osler's testimony as reflecting the usual and customary ethics of research at the turn of the century,[29] but this sweeping historical claim has little supporting evidence. The extent to which any principle of research obligation scrutiny and any consent requirement was then ingrained in the ethics of research, or would become ingrained in the next half century, is still a matter of historical controversy.

One reason for the relatively late emergence of interest in research ethics is that scientifically rigorous research involving human subjects did not become common in the United States or Europe until the middle of the 20th century. Only shortly before the outbreak of World War II had research evolved into an established and thriving concern.[30–32] Research ethics prior to World War II had approximately the same influence on research practices as medical ethics had on clinical practices.[33]

The major events that pushed research ethics to the forefront occurred at the Nuremberg trials, when prominent leaders of Nazi Germany were prosecuted for crimes committed during the Holocaust. The Nuremberg military tribunal developed the Nuremberg Code of 1947, which was a set of 10 principles for human experimentation. According to the famous Principle 1, the primary consideration in research is the subject's voluntary consent, which is "absolutely essential."[34] The Nuremberg Code was not an attempt to formulate new rules of professional conduct.[35] Rather, it delineated principles of medical and research ethics in the context of a trial for war crimes. Although it had little immediate impact on the conduct of biomedical research, the Nuremberg Code served as a model for many professional and governmental codes formulated in the 1950s and 1960s, and its provision requiring *voluntary* consent was a forerunner of informed consent practices in biomedical research.[33,36]

The General Assembly of the World Medical Association (WMA), an international organization of physicians founded in 1947, drafted the Declaration of Geneva in 1948. Subsequently, the WMA began to formulate a more comprehensive code to distinguish ethical from unethical clinical research. A draft was produced in 1961, but the WMA did not adopt the code until its 1964 meeting in Helsinki.[37] This three-year delay was not caused by vacillation or indifference, but rather by international political processes and a determination to produce a universally applicable and useful document.[38]

The Declaration of Helsinki made consent a central requirement of ethical research and introduced an important distinction between therapeutic and nontherapeutic research. The former is defined in the declaration as research "combined with patient care" and is permitted as a means of acquiring new medical knowledge only insofar as it "is justified as purely scientific research without therapeutic value or purpose for the specific subjects studied." The declaration requires consent for all instances of nontherapeutic research, unless a subject is incompetent, in which case guardian consent is necessary. According to paragraph I.9 of the declaration, "In any research on human beings, each potential subject must be adequately informed of the aims, methods, anticipated benefits and potential hazards of the study and the discomfort it may entail [and] that he is at liberty to abstain...The doctor should then obtain the subject's freely given informed consent."[25,35]

The American Medical Association, the American Society for Clinical Investigation, the American Federation for Clinical Research, and many other medical groups either endorsed the Declaration of Helsinki or established their own ethical requirements consistent with the Declaration's provisions.[39] Officials at federal agencies in the United States also developed provisions based on the declaration, some of which were almost verbatim reformulations of the declaration. Regardless of its shortcomings, the Helsinki Code is a foundational document in the history of research ethics and the first significant attempt at self-regulation by the medical research community. The Nuremberg Code was the first code of medical research developed externally by a court system, and the Declaration of Helsinki was the first code of medical research developed internally by a professional medical body.

More comprehensive guidelines formulated in 1982 by the World Health Organization (WHO) and the Council of International Organizations of Medical Sciences (CIOMS) used the Declaration of Helsinki (1975 revision) as a starting point.[25,35] According to these guidelines, all human subjects research should be reviewed by an independent committee.[35] However, the WHO/CIOMS guidelines also contain special provisions for protecting vulnerable persons in medical experiments, such as pregnant women, children, people who are mentally ill, and people in developing countries.[35] Many of these issues are discussed by Robert Levine in Chapter 12.

In the United States, Congress passed the Drug Amendments of 1962 to make fundamental changes in federal regulation of the drug industry.[40] These Amendments were passed in response to large numbers of prescriptions of the drug thalidomide, which had not been adequately tested for pregnant women. Thalidomide caused severe birth defects in many children of such pregnant women. The amendments required researchers to inform research subjects of a drug's experimental nature and receive their consent before starting an investigation, except when the researchers "deem it not feasible or, in their professional judgment, contrary to the best interests of such human beings."[41]

On January 17, 1966, James Lee Goddard, a former assistant surgeon general, became U.S. Food and Drug Administration (FDA) Commissioner. Beset by numerous reports of medical experimentation without consent of subjects as well as the swirl of controversy caused by the injection of live human cancer cells into 22 chronically ill patients without their consent at the Jewish Chronic Disease Hospital, Goddard was determined to resolve the ambiguities surrounding informed consent. He appointed several FDA officials to study the issue and make recommendations. In August 1966, the FDA published new provisions in its "Consent for Use of Investigational New Drugs on Humans: Statement of Policy."[42,43]

This publication took place two months after the appearance of an influential article in the *New England Journal of Medicine* by Henry Beecher, M.D., an anesthesiologist credited with establishing the peer-review system for experimental protocols in medicine. In his article,[44] Beecher charged that many patients involved in clinical research experiments had never had the risks of participating satisfactorily explained to them or were unaware that they were the subjects and was noticed by leaders of the National Institutes of Health (NIH). In late 1963, James Shannon, Director of NIH from 1955 to 1968, asked the NIH division that supported research centers to investigate these problems and make recommendations.[45] An associate chief for program development, Robert B. Livingston, led this study.[46] His report, in November 1964, noted the absence of an applicable code of conduct for research, as well as an uncertain legal context.[47]

According to the Livingston report, it would be difficult for NIH to assume responsibility for ethics and research practices without striking an unduly authoritarian posture on requirements for research. The authors also noted that ethical problems were raised by policies "inhibiting the pursuit of research on man" and added that "NIH is not in a position to shape the educational foundations of medical ethics, or even the clinical indoctrination of young investigators."[45]

NIH Director Shannon was disappointed with this part of the report because he believed that NIH should command a position of increased responsibility. However, he accepted the report and regarded some of its recommendations as urgent. In early 1965, Shannon asked the U.S. Surgeon General to give "highest priority" to "rapid accomplishment of the objectives" of the basic recommendations. He suggested more consultation with members of the legal profession and clergy as well as the medical profession and endorsed the idea of "review [of research protections] by the investigator's peers." [48]

Shannon and Surgeon General Luther Terry jointly decided to present the problems discussed in the report to the National Advisory Health Council (NAHC) in September 1965. At this decisive meeting, Shannon argued that NIH should assume responsibility for placing formal controls on the independent judgment of investigators to remove conflicts of interest and biases. Specifically, he argued in favor of subjecting research protocols to impartial peer review of the research risks and the adequacy of protections of subjects' rights.[49] Shannon knew that "consent" could easily be manipulated by physicians using their authority to persuade otherwise-unwilling patients to participate and prompted a discussion of how the consent process could also become impartial. The NAHC members agreed that all of these concerns were valid, but they did not believe that the many fields involved in government-supported research, including epidemiology and the social sciences, could be governed by a single set of procedures or regulations. Nevertheless, within three months, NAHC supported a resolution at its December 3, 1965 meeting that followed the broad outlines of Shannon's recommendations and proposed guidelines for federal research ethics.[50]

The resolution was accepted by newly installed Surgeon General William H. Stewart, who issued a policy statement in February 1966 that became a landmark in the history of research ethics in the United States. This policy statement on "Clinical Investigations Using Human Subjects" compelled institutions receiving grant support from the Public Health Service to provide prior review by a committee for proposed research with human subjects. The new Institutional Review Boards (IRBs) would be responsible for reviewing (1) the rights and welfare of subjects, (2) the appropriateness of methods used to obtain informed consent, and (3) the balance of risks and benefits for research subjects.[51] The subjective judgment by a principal investigator or program director that human subjects' rights would be adequately protected in a proposed study was no longer sufficient for federal funding eligibility.

These developments, along with parallel developments in other countries such as Australia and Great Britain, began the "movement to ethics committees." [52] Peer review served as the basis for several federal policies governing research ethics. The federal initiatives were endorsed by much of the biomedical community [53] and were adopted in modified form by the Association of American Medical Colleges as "a requirement" for medical school accreditation.[54] Over the next decade, they served as a crude model that was gradually refined and finally became accepted in institutional practices for the protection of human research subjects throughout the United States.

Shortly after these developments, the U.S. Department of Health, Education, and Welfare (now the Department of Health and Human Services) issued a series of guidebooks and regulations for the protection of human research subjects. The National Research Act of 1974 established the National Commission for the Protection of Human Subjects of Biomedical and Behavioral Research, which made a number of important recommendations by 1978, many having the effect of federal law.[25,33,55] Subsequent federal regulations for the protection of human research subjects in the United States, including those of the FDA and the Department of Health and Human Services, have resulted in a complex IRB system (to ensure the rights and welfare of research subjects as well as justice in the selection of subjects) and other regulatory safeguards.[25,26,33]

The Origins of Contemporary Epidemiologic Ethics

Ethics in contemporary epidemiology have their origin in the historical developments that led to regulatory safeguards for human subjects research and in parallel developments in the history of bioethics that are beyond the scope of this chapter. Nevertheless, as discussed by Tom Beauchamp in Chapter 2, the foundational concepts and principles of bioethics are an important part of ethics in epidemiology.

The 1970s. By the early 1970s, the Tuskegee Syphilis Study (an observational study of 400 black men with syphilis who were not given curative treatment), the Jewish Chronic Disease Hospital case, and Beecher's article had fostered a growing awareness of the potential for ethical problems and dilemmas in epidemiology and clinical research.[25,33,56–58] Some ethical issues in epidemiologic research and practice drew widespread attention in the 1970s when U.S. legislators responded to public concern and began drafting stringent laws, including the Privacy Act of 1974 to protect the privacy and confidentiality of medical records.[59] (Privacy and confidentiality are discussed by Ellen Wright Clayton in Chapter 5. Similar data protection legislation was enacted in the Federal Republic of Germany in 1970, and Great Britain followed suit in 1984.

Because of this legislative trend, some forms of epidemiologic research and routine surveillance activities, including study designs that had provided important insights into the environmental causes of disease, were at risk of becoming unjustifiably restricted. Leading epidemiologists responded to the threat of growing limitations on the use of routinely collected medical records by explaining the usefulness of the endangered research to society and future patients and by outlining the confidentiality safeguards that should be employed by epidemiologists.[60] An influential article by Leon Gordis, Ellen Gold, and Raymond

Seltser on privacy protection in epidemiologic research appeared in the *American Journal of Epidemiology* in 1977, the same year that the Privacy Protection Study Commission report was released in the United States.[60,61] Mervyn Susser, Zena Stein, and Jennie Kline published a far-ranging paper on ethical issues in epidemiology in 1978.[62]

In the late 1970s, epidemiologists had no ethics guidelines or professional codes of conduct specific to their field. Unlike many other professional groups, they had no acknowledged means of self-regulation.[59] As a result of the growth of epidemiology graduate programs for nonphysicians, epidemiologists were being trained without direct exposure to the ethical traditions of medicine.[20,60]

The 1980s. New public health problems, such as the global spread of AIDS, brought new ethical questions, as discussed by Carol Levine in Chapter 10. In the mid-1980s, Colin Soskolne and others proposed the development of ethics guidelines for epidemiologists.[63,64] In "Epidemiology: Questions of Science, Ethics, Morality, and Law," published in the *American Journal of Epidemiology* in 1989, Soskolne argued that ethics guidelines could be useful for teaching purposes and as a framework for the debate of ethical issues.[59]

By 1987, the Society for Epidemiologic Research had formed committees to examine the ethical problems of conflict of interest and access to data by third parties. Also in 1987, the International Epidemiological Association held a major session on ethics at its annual conference in Helsinki, Finland. The Industrial Epidemiology Forum organized a conference on ethics in epidemiology in Birmingham, Alabama in 1989, in conjunction with the annual meeting of the Society for Epidemiologic Research. The papers presented at this conference were published in 1991 with proposed ethics guidelines for epidemiologists.[65,66]

The 1990s. In 1990, the International Epidemiological Association circulated draft ethics guidelines for epidemiologists at an ethics workshop in Los Angeles,[67] and the International Society of Pharmacoepidemiology established an ethics committee. The next year, the American College of Epidemiology established its Committee on Ethics and Standards of Practice and CIOMS published the *CIOMS International Guidelines for Ethical Review of Epidemiological Studies.*[59,68]

By this time, most major groups of epidemiologists had seen the importance of a number of ethical issues. Epidemiologists in Italy, Canada, the United States, and many other countries had discussed the development of ethics guidelines for epidemiologists. A symposium on Ethics and Law in Environmental Epidemiology was held in Mexico City in 1992 in conjunction with the annual meeting of the International Society for Environmental Epidemiology (ISEE),[69] and WHO and the ISEE jointly convened an International Workshop on Ethical and Philosophical Issues in Environmental Epidemiology in North Carolina in 1994, where findings of an international ethics survey were presented.[70,71] The International Clinical Epidemiology Network Ethics Group also met during 1994 to discuss the recently published CIOMS ethics guidelines and to determine which participating clinical epidemiology units around the world were adequately protecting human subjects.

In the mid-1990s, many epidemiology graduate programs began incorporating an ethics curriculum (see Kenneth Goodman and Ronald Prineas in Chapter 14).[72] During this period, the Society for Epidemiologic Research, the American College of Epidemiology, and other international professional organizations for epidemiologists began including ethics workshops in their annual meetings. By July 1994, membership in the American Public Health Association (APHA) Forum on Bioethics, which organizes sessions on bioethics and public health during the APHA annual meeting, had risen to 145 bioethicists, legal experts, epidemiologists, and other public health professionals. These developments in professional ethics in epidemiology occurred against a background of social and political movements in the early 1990s that included vigorous efforts to ensure that women and minorities were adequately represented in research projects funded by NIH.[73,74] NIH launched the Women's Health Initiative in 1991, and other epidemiologic investigations of understudied women's health problems began during this period.[75] Women's health advocates testified on Capitol Hill in support of increased federal spending for breast cancer research and improved procedures for recruiting and obtaining the informed consent of patients in breast cancer chemoprevention trials. Other important developments during this period included increased public concern about the integrity of scientific research,[69,76] as discussed by Colin Soskolne and colleagues in Chapter 13.

Another recent development in Europe and North America has been renewed concern among legislators, data protection advocates, and members of the general public about the privacy and confidentiality of information in health information systems. In light of pending legislation in the European Community that would severely restrict the use of routinely collected medical data for epidemiologic research,[77] both the International Society of Pharmacoepidemiology Ethics Committee and the joint WHO-ISEE International Workshop on Ethical and Philosophical Issues in Environmental Epidemiology have made recommendations to policy makers and legislative bodies that underscore the societal value of epidemiologic research (for example, the contribution of epidemiologic studies to scientific knowledge about the etiologies of birth defects and cancer).[70]

From 1995 to the present, there has been an increased recognition of the societal importance of epidemiologic research and practice. The ethical duties of epidemiologists have also been clarified.[78] In addition, the number of publications on ethical issues in epidemiology has continued to increase.[78-90] Many of these articles have dealt with professional responsibilities of epidemiologists.[88,90] Ethical issues in public health practice have also increasingly been addressed,[84,91] as discussed by Robert McKeown and Max Learner in Chapter 8. Interest in ethical issues in epidemiology has extended beyond North America and Europe to include researchers in many other parts of the world, including developing countries, as discussed by John Porter and colleagues in Chapter 11.[92]

One sign of the increased attention to ethics in epidemiology in recent years is the development of refined ethics guidelines for epidemiologists and policy statements on data sharing, privacy and confidentiality protection, DNA testing for disease susceptibility, and other issues.[86,87,93,94] Ethical issues in genetic epidemiology are discussed by Laura Beskow and Wylie Burke in Chapter 9. The International Society for Environmental Epidemiology adopted ethics guidelines for environmental epidemiologists in 1999.[95] The American College of Epidemiology adopted a set of ethics guidelines for epidemiologists in North America in 1999.[96]

Ethics surveys of epidemiologists and other public health professionals, public health students, and institutions that train epidemiologists and other public health professionals have provided information about the ethical interests and concerns of epidemiologists. [97–101] Several institutions that train public health professionals have created new courses on ethics in epidemiology and public health.[99,102] Other institutions have created curricula on public health ethics for epidemiology graduate students, and the Association of Schools of Public Health has developed model curricula in public health ethics, as discussed by Kenneth Goodman and Ronald Prineas in Chapter 14. In the United States, these efforts have been strengthened by training on ethical principles and IRB procedures recommended by the Office for Human Research Protections of the U.S. Department of Health and Human Services.[103]

2000 to the present. The Health Insurance Portability and Accountability Act (HIPAA) of 1996 privacy rules took effect in the United States early in 2004 after years of planning and discussion.[104] As discussed by Ellen Wright Clayton in Chapter 5, the new regulations protect the privacy of certain individually identifiable health data, referred to as protected health information. The privacy rules permit disclosures without individual authorization to public health authorities authorized by law to collect or receive the information to prevent or control disease, injury, or disability, including public health practice activities such as surveillance.[105] In 2004, the American College of Epidemiology circulated a request to its members to identify problems implementing the new rules when conducting research. A policy forum on the impact of the new HIPAA privacy rules was held at the American College of Epidemiology meeting in Boston in 2004. The forum suggested that epidemiologists were encountering new obstacles to the performance of their research (for example, more hospitals were refusing to release medical records for research purposes).

These developments in ethics in epidemiology occurred in conjunction with a number of important biomedical research policy developments in the late 1990s and early 21st century, including implementation of new NIH guidance on sharing research data from NIH grants and contracts and updated institutional policies following controversies involving conflicts of interest in research.

Summary and Conclusions

The upsurge of interest in the ethics of epidemiologic research and practice in recent decades could be regarded as a sign of both the maturation of epidemiology as a profession and the important role that epidemiology plays in contemporary society. In the spirit of William Farr and other founders of the public health movement, today's epidemiologists are addressing a wide range of public health problems. Their research could give rise to new ethical problems, many of which are anticipated in this volume.

ACKNOWLEDGMENT

The findings and conclusions in this chapter are those of the author and do not necessarily represent the official position of the Centers for Disease Control and Prevention, or the Department of Veterans Affairs.

References

1. Brockington, C. F. "The History of Public Health." In *The Theory and Practice of Public Health*, ed. W. Hobson. London: Oxford University Press, 1971: 1–7.
2. Kerkhoff, A. H. M. "Origin of Modern Public Health and Preventive Medicine." In *Ethical Dilemmas in Health Promotion,* ed. S. Doxiadis. New York: John Wiley & Sons, 1987: 35–45.
3. Lilienfeld, A. M. and Lilienfeld, D. E. "Threads of Epidemiologic History." In *Foundations of Epidemiology.* New York: Oxford University Press, 1980: 23–45.
4. Rousseau, Jean-Jacques. *The Basic Political Writings*, trans. and ed. Donald A. Cress. Indianapolis: Hackett Publishing Co., 1987.
5. Frank, Johann Peter. *A System of Complete Medical Police*, trans. Erna Lesky. Baltimore: Johns Hopkins University Press, 1976.
6. Porter, R. *Disease, Medicine and Society in England, 1550–1860.* London: Macmillan, 1987.
7. Temkin, O. "Health and Disease." In *The Double Face of Janus and Other Essays in the History of Medicine*, ed. Owsei Temkin. Baltimore: Johns Hopkins University Press, 1977.
8. Gregory, J. *Lectures on the Duties and Qualifications of a Physician.* London: W. Strahan and T. Cadell, 1772.
9. Rush, B. *Medical Inquiries and Observations.* Vol. 2, ch. 1. Published as a single essay titled *An Oration...An Enquiry into the Influence of Physical Causes upon the Moral Faculty.* Philadelphia: Charles Cist, 1786.

10. Chave, S. P. W. "The Origins and Development of Public Health." In *Oxford Textbook of Public Health,* ed. W. W. Holland, R. Detels, and G. Knox. New York: Oxford University Press, 1984: 3–19.
11. Bentham, J. *An Introduction to the Principles of Morals and Legislation*, ed. J. H. Burns and H. L. A. Hart. Oxford: Clarendon Press, 1970.
12. Mill, J. S. *Utilitarianism*. In *Collected Works of John Stuart Mill*, vol. 10. Toronto: University of Toronto Press, 1969.
13. Chadwick, E. *Report on the Sanitary Condition of the Labouring Population of Great Britain*, ed. M. W. Flinn. Edinburgh: University Press, 1964.
14. Shattuck, L. *Report of the Sanitary Commission of Massachusetts 1850*. Cambridge, MA:,1948.
15. Greison, G. L. "Pasteur's Work on Rabies: Reexamining the Ethical Issues," *Hastings Center Report* 8 (1978): 26–33.
16. Terris, M. "The Changing Relationships of Epidemiology and Society: The Robert Cruikshank Lecture," *Journal of Public Health Policy* 6 (1985): 15–36.
17. Terris, M. "Epidemiology and the Public Health Movement," *Journal of Public Health Policy* 8 (1987): 315–29.
18. Hanlon, J. J. and Pickett, G. E. "Philosophy and Purpose of Public Health." In *Public Health Administration and Practice*, 7th ed. St. Louis: C.V. Mosby Company, 1979: 2–12.
19. Bean, W.B. "Walter Reed and the Ordeal of Human Experiments," *Bulletin of the History of Medicine* 51 (1977): 75–92.
20. Susser, M. "Epidemiology in the United States After World War II: The Evolution of Technique," *Epidemiologic Reviews* 7 (1985): 147–77.
21. Doll, R. and Hill, A. B. "Lung Cancer and Other Causes of Death in Relation to Smoking," *British Medical Journal* 2 (1956): 1071–81.
22. MacMahon, B., Pugh, T. G., and Ipsen, J. *Epidemiological Methods*. Boston: Little, Brown & Co., 1960.
23. Hill, A. B. "The Clinical Trial," *British Medical Journal* 7 (1951): 278–82.
24. Mainland, D. "The Clinical Trial: Some Difficulties and Suggestions," *Journal of Chronic Diseases* 11 (1959): 484–96.
25. Levine, R. J. *Ethics and Regulation of Clinical Research*. New Haven: Yale University Press, 1986.
26. Katz, J. "The Regulation of Human Experimentation in the United States—A Personal Odyssey," *IRB: A Review of Human Subjects Research* 9 (1987): 1–6.
27. Katz, J. "Ethics and Clinical Research Revisited. A Tribute to Henry K. Beecher," *Hastings Center Report* 23 (1993): 31–39.
28. Cushing, H. *The Life of Sir William Osler*. London: Oxford University Press, 1940.
29. Brady, J. V. and Jonsen, A. R. "The Evolution of Regulatory Influences on Research with Human Subjects," In *Human Subjects Research*, ed. R. Greenwald, M. K. Ryan, and J. E. Mulvihill. New York: Plenum Press, 1982.
30. Ivy, A. C. "The History and Ethics of the Use of Human Subjects in Medical Experiments," *Science* 108 (1948): 1–5.
31. Beecher, H. *Experimentation in Man*. Springfield: Charles C Thomas, 1959.
32. Brieger, G. H. "Human Experimentation: History." In *Encyclopedia of Bioethics*, 4 vols., ed. W.T. Reich. New York: Free Press, 1978: 684–92.
33. Faden, R. R. and Beauchamp, T. L. *A History and Theory of Informed Consent*. New York: Oxford University Press, 1986.

34. *United States v. Karl Brandt, Trials of War Criminals Before the Nuremberg Military Tribunals under Control Council Law No. 10,* vols. 1 and 2. "The Medical Case" (Military Tribunal I, 1947). Washington, DC: U.S. Government Printing Office, 1948–1949.

35. Howard-Jones, N. "Human Experimentation in Historical and Ethical Perspectives," *Social Sciences and Medicine* 16 (1982): 1429–48.

36. Katz, J. *The Silent World of Doctor and Patient.* New York: Free Press, 1984.

37. World Medical Association. "Declaration of Helsinki: Recommendations Guiding Medical Doctors in Biomedical Research Involving Human Subjects," *New England Journal of Medicine* 271 (1964): 473.

38. Winton, R. R. "The Significance of the Declaration of Helsinki: An Interpretative Documentary," *World Medical Journal* 25 (1978): 58–59.

39. World Medical Association. "Human Experimentation: Declaration of Helsinki," *Annals of Internal Medicine* 65 (1966): 367–68.

40. Public Law 87–781, U.S.C. 355, 76 Stat. 780; amending Federal Food, Drug, and Cosmetic Act.

41. Federal Food, Drug, and Cosmetic Act, Sec. 505(i), 21 U.S.C. 355(i).

42. Curran, W. J. "Governmental Regulation of the Use of Human Subjects in Medical Research: The Approach of Two Federal Agencies," *Daedalus* 98 (Spring 1969).

43. Curran, W. J. "1938–1968: The FDA, the Drug Industry, the Medical Profession, and the Public." In *Safeguarding the Public: Historical Aspects of Medicinal Drug Control,* ed. J. Blake. Baltimore: The Johns Hopkins University Press, 1970.

44. Beecher, H. K. "Ethics and Clinical Research," *New England Journal of Medicine* 274 (1966): 1355–60.

45. Livingston, R. B. Memorandum to Director J. A. Shannon on "Moral and Ethical Aspects of Clinical Investigation" (February 20, 1964).

46. Memorandum from Clinical Director, NCI (Nathaniel I. Berlin) to Director of Laboratories and Clinics, OD-DIR, on "Comments on Memorandum of November 4, 1964 from the Associate Chief of Program Development DRFR, to the Director, NIH" (August 30, 1965).

47. Livingston, R. B. Memorandum to Director J. A. Shannon on "Progress Report on Survey of Moral and Ethical Aspects of Clinical Investigation" (November 4, 1964).

48. Shannon, J. A. Memorandum and Transmittal Letter to the U.S. Surgeon General on "Moral and Ethical Aspects of Clinical Investigations" (January 7, 1965).

49. Transcript of the NAHC meeting. Washington, DC, September 28, 1965.

50. "Resolution Concerning Clinical Research on Humans" (December 3, 1965), transmitted in a Memorandum from Dr. S. John Reisman, Executive Secretary, NAHC, to Dr. J. A. Shannon ("Resolution of Council") on December 6, 1965. Reported in a Draft Statement of Policy on January 20, 1966.

51. U.S. Public Health Service, Division of Research Grants. Policy and Procedure Order (PPO) 129, February 8, 1966, "Clinical Investigations Using Human Subjects," signed by Ernest M. Allen, Grants Policy Officer.

52. Curran, W. "Evolution of Formal Mechanisms for Ethical Review of Clinical Research." In *Medical Experimentation and the Protection of Human Rights,* ed. N. Howard-Jones and Z. Bankowski. Geneva: Council for International Organizations of Medical Sciences, 1978.

53. Editorial, "Friendly Adversaries and Human Experimentation," *New England Journal of Medicine* 275 (1966): 786.

54. Marston, R. Q. "Medical Science, the Clinical Trial, and Society," a speech delivered at the University of Virginia on November 10, 1972 [typescript].

55. National Commission for the Protection of Human Subjects of Biomedical and Behavioral Research. *The Belmont Report: Ethical Principles and Guidelines for the Protection of Human Subjects of Research*. Washington, DC: U.S. Government Printing Office, 1978.

56. Brandt, A. M. "Racism and Research: The Case of the Tuskegee Syphilis Study," *Hastings Center Report* 8 (1978): 21–29.

57. *Final Report of the Tuskegee Syphilis Study Ad Hoc Panel*. Public Health Service, April 28, 1973.

58. Hearings before the Subcommittee on Health of the Committee on Labor and Public Welfare, U.S. Senate. "Quality of Health Care—Human Experimentation" (1973).

59. Soskolne, C. L. "Epidemiology: Questions of Science, Ethics, Morality, and Law," *American Journal of Epidemiology* 129 (1989): 1–18.

60. Gordis, L., Gold, E., and Seltser, R. "Privacy Protection in Epidemiologic and Medical Research: A Challenge and a Responsibility," *American Journal of Epidemiology* 105 (1977): 163–68.

61. Privacy Protection Study Commission. *Personal Privacy in an Information Society*. Washington, DC: US Government Printing Office, 1977.

62. Susser, M., Stein, Z., and Kline, J. "Ethics in Epidemiology," *Annals of the American Academy of Political and Social Sciences* 437 (1978): 128–41.

63. Soskolne, C. L. and Zeighami, E. A. "Research, Interest Groups, and the Review Process." Paper presented at the 10th Scientific Meeting of the International Epidemiological Association, Vancouver, British Columbia, Canada, August 19–25, 1984.

64. Soskolne, C. L. "Epidemiological Research, Interest Groups and the Review Process," *Journal of Public Health Policy* 7 (1985): 173–84.

65. Fayerweather, W. E., Higginson, J., and Beauchamp, T. L., eds. "Industrial Epidemiology Forum's Conference on Ethics in Epidemiology," *Journal of Clinical Epidemiology* 44 (Suppl. I) (1991): 1S–169S.

66. Beauchamp, T. L., Cook, R. R., Fayerweather, W. E., et al. "Ethical Guidelines for Epidemiologists," *Journal of Clinical Epidemiology* 44 (1991): 151S–169S.

67. American Public Health Association. 1991 Section Newsletter Epidemiology. Winter, 1990.

68. Council for International Organizations of Medical Sciences. "International Guidelines for Ethical Review of Epidemiological Studies," *Law, Medicine and Health Care* 19 (1991): 247–58.

69. Soskolne, C. L., ed. "Proceedings of the Symposium on Ethics and Law in Environmental Epidemiology," *Journal of Exposure Analysis and Environmental Epidemiology* 3 (Suppl. 1) (1993).

70. World Health Organization Meeting Report. "Joint WHO-ISEE International Workshop on Ethical and Philosophical Issues in Environmental Epidemiology, Research Triangle Park, North Carolina, U.S.A., September 16–18, 1994," *Science of the Total Environment* 184 (1996): 131–36.

71. Soskolne, C. L., Jhangri, G. S., Hunter, B., and Close, M. "Interim Report on the International Society for Environmental Epidemiology/Global Environmental Epidemiology Network Ethics Survey." Working paper presented at the joint WHO/ISEE International Workshop on Ethical and Philosophical Issues in

Environmental Epidemiology, Research Triangle Park, North Carolina, U.S.A., September 16–18, 1994.

72. Coughlin, S. S., Etheredge, G. D., Metayer, C., and Martin, S. A., Jr. "Curriculum Development in Epidemiology and Ethics at the Tulane School of Public Health and Tropical Medicine. Results of a Needs Assessment and Plans for the Future." Paper presented to the Association of Schools of Public Health Council on Epidemiology, Washington, DC, October 30, 1994.

73. Coughlin, S. S. and Beauchamp, T. L. "Ethics, Scientific Validity, and the Design of Epidemiologic Studies," *Epidemiology* 3 (1992): 343–47.

74. U.S. House of Representatives, Committee on Energy and Commerce. *National Institutes of Health Revitalization Amendments of 1990 (report 101–869).* Washington, DC: U.S. Government Printing Office, 1990.

75. Cummings, N. B. "Women's Health and Nutrition Research: US Governmental Concerns," *Journal of the American College of Nutrition* 12 (1993): 329–36.

76. Weed, D.W. "Preventing Scientific Misconduct," *American Journal of Public Health* 88 (1998):125–29.

77. James, R. C. "Consent and the Electronic Person." Working paper presented at the joint WHO/ISEE International Workshop on Ethical and Philosophical Issues in Environmental Epidemiology, Research Triangle Park, North Carolina, U.S.A., September 16–18, 1994.

78. Coughlin, S. S. "Ethics in Epidemiology at the End of the 20th Century: Ethics, Values, and Mission Statements," *Epidemiologic Reviews* 22 (2000):169–75.

79. Soskolne, C. L. and Sieswerda, L. E. "Implementing Ethics in the Professions: Examples from Environmental Epidemiology," *Science and Engineering Ethics* 9 (2003): 181–90.

80. Soskolne, C. L. and Bertollini, R., eds. *Ethical and Philosophical Issues in Environmental Epidemiology.* Proceedings of a WHO/ISEE International Workshop, September 16–18, 1994, Research Triangle Park, North Carolina, USA, *Science of the Total Environment* 184 (1996).

81. Coughlin S. S., ed. *Ethics in Epidemiology and Clinical Research: Annotated Readings.* Newton, MA: Epidemiology Resources Inc., 1995.

82. Weed, D. L. and McKeown, R. E. "Epidemiology and Virtue Ethics," *International Journal of Epidemiology* 27 (1998): 343–49.

83. Weed, D. L. and Coughlin, S. S. "New Ethics Guidelines for Epidemiology: Background and Rationale," *Annals of Epidemiology* 9 (1999): 277–80.

84. Coughlin, S. S., Soskolne, C. L., and Goodman, K. W. *Case Studies in Public Health Ethics.* Washington, DC: American Public Health Association, 1997.

85. Coughlin, S. S. *Epidemiology and Public Health Practice: Collected Works.* Columbus, GA: Quill Publications, 1997: 9–26.

86. Hunter, D. and Caporaso, N. "Informed Consent in Epidemiologic Studies Involving Genetic Markers," *Epidemiology* 8 (1997): 596–99.

87. American College of Epidemiology. "Draft Policy Statement on Privacy of Medical Records." *Epidemiology Monitor* 19 (1998): 9–11.

88. Weed, D. L. and Mink, P. J. "Roles and Responsibilities of Epidemiologists," *Annals of Epidemiology* 12 (2002): 67–72.

89. Soskolne, C. L. and Sieswerda, L. E. "Implementing Ethics in the Professions: Examples from Environmental Epidemiologists," *Science and Engineering Ethics* 9 (2003): 181–90.

90. Weed, D. L. and McKeown, R. E. "Science and Social Responsibility in Public Health," *Environmental Health Perspectives* 111 (2003): 1804–48.
91. Fairchild, A. L. and Bayer, R. "Ethics and the Conduct of Public Health Surveillance," *Science* 303 (2004): 631–32.
92. Kahn, K. S. "Epidemiology and Ethics: The Perspective of the Third World," *Journal of Public Health Policy* 15 (1994): 218–25.
93. Clayton, E. W., Steinberg, K. K., Khoury, M. J., et al. "Informed Consent for Genetic Research on Stored Tissue Samples," *Journal of the American Medical Association* 274 (1995): 1786–92.
94. Beskow, L. M., Burke, W., Merz, J. F., et al. "Informed Consent for Population-based Research Involving Genetics," *Journal of the American Medical Association* 286 (2003): 2315–21.
95. Soskolne, C. L. and Light, A. "Toward Ethics Guidelines for Environmental Epidemiologists," *Science of the Total Environment* 184 (1996): 137–47.
96. American College of Epidemiology. "Ethics Guidelines," *Annals of Epidemiology* 10 (2000): 487–97.
97. Soskolne, C. L., Jhangri, G. S., Hunter, B., et al. "Interim Report on the Joint International Society for Environmental Epidemiology (ISEE)—Global Environmental Epidemiology Network (GEENET) Ethics Survey," *Science of the Total Environment* 184 (1996): 5–11.
98. Prineas, R. J., Goodman, K., Soskolne, C. L., et al. "Findings from the American College of Epidemiology Ethics Survey on the Need for Ethics Guidelines for Epidemiologists," *Annals of Epidemiology* 8 (1998): 482–89.
99. Rossignol, A. M. and Goodmonson, S. "Are Ethical Topics in Epidemiology Included in the Graduate Epidemiology Curricula?" *American Journal of Epidemiology* 142 (1996): 1265–68.
100. Coughlin, S. S., Etheredge, G. D., Metayer, C., et al. "Remember Tuskegee: Public Health Student Knowledge of the Ethical Significance of the Tuskegee Syphilis Study," *American Journal of Preventive Medicine* 12 (1996): 242–46.
101. Coughlin, S. S., Katz, W. H., and Mattison, D. R. "Ethics Instruction at Schools of Public Health in the United States," *American Journal of Public Health* 89 (1999): 768–70.
102. Coughlin, S. S. "Model Curricula in Public Health Ethics," *American Journal of Preventive Medicine* 12 (1996): 247–51.
103. Office for Human Research Protections, U.S. Department of Health and Human Services. Federalwide Assurance (FWA) for the Protection of Human Subjects. Available at: http://www.hhs.gov/ohrp/humansubjects/assurance/filasurt.htm., accessed on September 1, 2008.
104. "Health Insurance Portability and Accountability Act of 1996." Public Law No. 104–191, 110 Stat. 1936 (1996).
105. Epidemiology Program Office, U.S. Department of Health and Human Services. "HIPAA Privacy Rule and Public Health. Guidance from CDC and the U.S. Department of Health and Human Services." *Morbidity and Mortality Weekly Report* 52 (2003): 1–12.

2

Moral Foundations

TOM L. BEAUCHAMP

The issues discussed in this book have emerged from professional practice in epidemiology. In later chapters, we consider specific moral problems that confront epidemiologists. The goal of this chapter is to provide an understanding of philosophical ethics sufficient for reading other chapters and for appreciating the relevance of philosophical investigations for epidemiologic ethics. Some central concepts and methods of biomedical ethics are explained. While philosophical reflection is not by itself an adequate basis for professional ethics of any sort, it does facilitate impartial examination of assumptions that are commonly made in the professions.

The terms "ethical" and "moral" are treated in this introduction as identical in meaning, but "morality" and "moral philosophy" (as well as "ethical theory") have very different meanings. The term "morality" refers to norms about right and wrong human conduct that are so widely shared that they form a stable (although usually incomplete) social agreement. Morality encompasses many standards of conduct, including moral principles, rules, rights, and virtues. "Moral philosophy," "ethical theory," and "philosophical ethics" are reserved for philosophical theories.

In the section on Social Morality and Professional Morality, several questions about the nature of morality and moral responsibility are discussed, including, "What morality is already embedded in epidemiologic practice?" Then, in the Section on Problems and Methods in Moral Philosophy, several problems and methods in moral philosophy are discussed, and, in the final section, some ethical theories of importance for biomedical ethics are investigated.

Social Morality and Professional Morality

The term *morality* refers to a social institution with a code of learnable norms. Morality comprehends many forms of social protection that we acknowledge through language such as "moral rules" and "human rights." Like natural languages and political constitutions, morality exists before we are instructed in its demands. As we grow up, we learn moral responsibilities along with other social responsibilities, such as those imposed by laws. Eventually we learn to distinguish general social rules of both law and morals from particular social rules fashioned for and binding on the members of special groups, such as the members of a profession. Hence, we learn to distinguish general or social morality from professional morality. But how sharp is this distinction?

The Common Morality and Professional Moralities

The morality that is shared by all morally committed persons in all societies is not one morality among others; it is simply morality, or what is sometimes called the common morality. This morality is universal, because it contains a body of fundamental ethical precepts constituting morality wherever it is found. Morality encompasses many standards of conduct, including moral principles, rules, rights, and virtues. In recent years the favored category in international discourse has been universal or basic human rights,[1,2] but we can also capture large parts of our common morality through the language of obligations and virtues. All persons living a moral life grasp the core dimensions of this morality. The following are examples of universal precepts that all morally committed persons share in common: Tell the truth; Respect the privacy of others; Protect confidential information; Obtain consent before invading another person's body; Do not kill; Do not cause pain; Do not steal or otherwise deprive of goods; Prevent harm from occurring to others. All persons committed to morality do not doubt the relevance and importance of these rules.

Many attempts have been made in the history of philosophy, political theory, and law to formulate the precepts of morality (in the narrow sense) in order to show that these precepts do not depend, as do mere customs and law, on local codifications. As the Dutch jurisprudential thinker Hugo Grotius put it, basic moral rules are obligatory and binding on everyone, kings not excepted.[3] However, many problems are present in such philosophical formulations of the basic demands of morality found in these writings, in part because these formulations presuppose controversial ethical theories (see the Section on Ethical Theories).

PROFESSIONAL MORALITY Whereas the common morality contains general moral norms that are abstract and universal, *particular* moralities such as professional codes present concrete and nonuniversal. These specific moralities include the many responsibilities, aspirations, ideals, sympathies, attitudes, and sensitivities found in diverse cultural traditions, religious traditions, professional practice standards, institutional expectations, and the like. Professional moralities are one—but only one—form of particular morality. Religious moralities are another form.

Most professions have, at least implicitly, an indigenous professional morality whose precepts are widely shared in them. Particular codes written for groups such as physicians, nurses, and psychologists are sometimes explicitly defended by appeal to general norms in the common morality, such as the rules listed above. Usually, however, professional codes are attempts to discover, formulate, and develop an inchoate morality widely accepted in the profession. Professions often control entry into occupational roles by formally certifying that candidates have acquired the necessary knowledge and skills. Authorities may require some forms of instruction in ethics, or at least some evidence verifying good moral character. Professions typically specify and enforce responsibilities, seeking to ensure that persons who enter into relationships with their members will find them competent and of good moral character. Many moral responsibilities that professions attempt to enforce are role obligations that are correlative to the rights of persons they serve. A professional code commonly emphasizes these role obligations, but it may also be broader in scope.

PROFESSIONAL MORALITY IN EPIDEMIOLOGIC RESEARCH AND PRACTICE In recent years, codes of ethics for epidemiologists have been the subject of numerous meetings and commentaries[4,5,6,7]—as discussed in other chapters of this volume. Attempts to devise codes have been difficult because of the diversity of professional backgrounds found in epidemiology, which draws its practitioners and consultants from a number of different disciplines, including medicine, statistics, public health, demography, sociology, genetics, anthropology, psychology, and industrial hygiene. Ethics for epidemiologists involves an interplay between the model of public health (protecting the public welfare) and the model of medicine (protecting the welfare of the individual), and must also take account of ethical issues arising from the social sciences.

Despite the diversity of training brought into epidemiologic practice and its continuing evolution and change, we can meaningfully speak of a morality internal to epidemiologic practice and research.[8,9,10] The remainder of this section will be devoted to explaining these professional moral commitments. That is, I will attempt to formulate a framework of rules that draws primarily on the internal morality already accepted by epidemiologists. However, I do not assume that acceptable moral standards for epidemiologists are entirely a matter of rules and beliefs that already have an embedded and well-articulated position in epidemiologic practice. The formulations I provide occasionally develop and extend the professional morality in epidemiology. However, I will remain faithful to the fundamental moral commitments in epidemiology even when proposing revisions.

The following types of responsibility, with major topics under each type, is a brief listing of the professional moral commitments in epidemiology, some of which are discussed in the remainder of this chapter:[11]

Responsibilities to Research Subjects
    Welfare Protection
    Informed Consent
    Privacy
    Confidentiality
    Committee Review

Responsibilities to Society
    Providing Benefits
    Public Trust
    Avoiding Conflict of Interest
    Impartiality

Responsibilities to Employers and Funding Sources
    Formulating Responsibilities
    Protecting Privileged Information

Responsibilities to Professional Colleagues
    Reporting Methods and Results
    Reporting Unacceptable Behavior and Conditions

This outline lists the major topics in the professional morality of epidemiology. These topics will be treated hereafter as rules that specify responsibilities (or obligations). These rules are not mechanical or definitive procedures for decision making. Experience and sound judgment are indispensable allies for any system of rules. I will now develop this framework by explaining its basic commitments.

Responsibilities to Subjects of Research. Research involving human subjects is an ancient practice, but serious concern about its consequences and about the protection of human subjects is a relatively recent phenomenon. Mechanisms of control such as the Declaration of Helsinki, government commissions, regulatory agencies, and professional societies have become prominent parts of the historical landscape of research ethics (see Chapter 1). However, epidemiology needs more specific and detailed guidelines.

Protecting the welfare of subjects. The mid-20th century developments in protecting human subjects were primarily directed at eliminating dangerous research that exploited subjects' confidence in a physician–patient therapeutic relationship.[12] Although risks are usually lower in epidemiology than in most other areas of biomedicine, epidemiologists should always strive to minimize discomfort, disturbances, inconveniences, and risks caused to subjects, and they should be aware of any intrusive or harmful potential present in their investigations. A fundamental responsibility exists to avoid harming subjects and, insofar as conditions permit, a responsibility exists to prevent or remove possible harms.

The idea that professionals are obligated to avoid inflicting harm has been associated for centuries with the maxim *primum non nocere*—"above all (or first) do no harm." This general obligation is a complex responsibility that includes obligations not to cause, prevent, and remove harm.[13] In epidemiology, risks of harm presented by studies must constantly be weighed against possible benefits for patients, subjects, or the public. The epidemiologist who professes to "do no harm" is not pledging never to cause harm, but only to strive to create a positive balance of goods over inflicted harms. Whenever risk of harm is imposed on subjects, law and morality alike recognize a standard of "due care." Negligence is a departure from the standard of due care owed to others and includes not only deliberately imposed risks that are unreasonable, but also carelessly imposed ones.

The epidemiologist should gather, store, and use data in a fashion that minimizes risk to subjects. Even in situations in which the data have been gathered for purposes other than epidemiologic research (e.g., personnel records, death certificates, tax rolls, and the like), epidemiologists should recognize that with these data goes a trust to protect persons from harm. For example, failures to disclose hazards in work environments or risks in medical procedures are violations of this trust. In some cases harm can be caused by overemphasizing a risk or by suggesting a risk where none truly exists. The epidemiologist should also guard against circumstances in which information gathered for health research might be used for unjustifiable purposes such as determining employability, promotion, or insurability.

Finally, epidemiologic research may inadvertently pose potential risks to groups of individuals and communities. For example, populations defined by race, ethnicity, or lifestyle may suffer stigmatization or lowered self-esteem following the publication and dissemination of research findings that create or reinforce negative cultural stereotypes. Disparaging information about a group can result in harms such as discrimination in employment, housing, or insurance, and lowered self-esteem or racial or cultural pride.[14,15,16]

Obtaining informed consent. When problems of the autonomy rights of subjects gradually grew more insistent in 20th-century research, the idea of respecting autonomy gained equal recognition with protecting against risk. At this point informed consent began to play a central role in research ethics. The justification of requirements of informed consent is the principle of respect for autonomy. However, the goal of *enabling* a subject to make an "autonomous choice" is difficult to articulate with precision. What does it take to enable the subject? Is it only to disclose information? Is it to engage in teaching? Is it to engage in dialogue to be sure that the subject understands?

In studies requiring the active participation of human subjects, explicit informed consent must be obtained. Disclosures should be made regarding the aims, methods, anticipated benefits and risks of the research, any inconvenience or discomfort that may be involved, and the right to withdraw from the research. If participation in the research is voluntary, subjects should understand that they are not required to participate and that they may refuse participation initially or at any stage in it.[17,18]

An informed consent is, by definition, an *autonomous authorization* given by individual patients or subjects. Thus, a patient or subject must understand the relevant circumstances, decide in substantial absence of control by others, and intentionally authorize a professional to proceed with a medical or research intervention. The person does more than merely acquiesce in or comply with an arrangement or a proposal. He or she actively authorizes a proposal in the act of consent. A truthful disclosure therefore does not by itself warrant inferences about the moral acceptability of consent solicitations or practices, because it says nothing about the basis on which the subject consented.[19]

It is neither feasible nor necessary to obtain informed consent in certain types of research. For example, some research in epidemiology could not be conducted if consent were needed in order to obtain access to records. Use of records without consent is not necessarily an ethical violation. Research may be the first stage of an investigation to determine whether one needs to trace and contact particular individuals and obtain their permission for further participation in a study. In other cases, third-party consent is sometimes acceptable when access to a subject is impractical or the subject is incompetent.[20,21]

Epidemiologists often analyze data initially gathered by others for purposes beyond health research. Application of informed consent requirements may under these conditions be overly burdensome, and in some cases subjects of research will not need to be contacted at all. In other cases it will suffice if persons are notified in advance of how data will be used and given the opportunity not to participate in the research. Thus, disclosures and warnings may sometimes be substituted for informed consents. (See further needed qualifications and examples in Chapter 4.)

Finally, significant issues occur in epidemiology regarding surveillance activities, cohort studies, and sequential study designs. In some cases, the processes of data collection and analyses are continuous, and some analyses that might take place in the future cannot be anticipated. The investigator should periodically consider whether informed consent is needed and should place any judgments about bypassing informed consent before a review panel. In some circumstances written informed consent will be needed, whereas in others ongoing communication of study results and continuing review may be the best policy.

Protecting privacy. Privacy, the condition of limited access to a person, should be aggressively protected by epidemiologists. Disclosure of confidential information to third parties is a threat to privacy and a special concern for epidemiologists since massive bodies of data involve the disclosure of medical and other records to third parties. Here questions can be raised about to whom the disclosures may be made, whether the entire record should be open to inspection (including, for example, a psychiatric record), whether the subject is to be informed of the disclosure, and whether the subject must authorize the disclosure.[22,23,24,25]

Infringements of privacy are at times justified, but only under exceptional circumstances such as contact tracing for sexually transmitted diseases mandated by law. When under a legal responsibility to make disclosures that invade privacy, an epidemiologist should carefully weigh an obligation to the law against the moral importance of preserving the privacy of subjects. Breaking the law or ignoring a court order may be required in rare cases. If an epidemiologist must infringe privacy, those involved should be informed of the reasons and of their rights in the circumstances. For epidemiologic research that invades privacy to be justified, several conditions must be satisfied. First, the invasion of privacy must be necessary for the conduct of the research. Second, there must be no reason to believe that risks of harm to subjects that are created by the invasion of privacy will be substantial risks (e.g., a risk that a person might be fired or divorced by a spouse). Third, the research must show promise of societal benefit by contributing to the protection of health or survival.

Those zealous in the defense of medical and other stored records have sometimes argued that a further condition must be present, namely, that these records cannot be examined without the authorization of the patient.[26,27,28,29] Guidelines requiring such authorization would, however, threaten epidemiologic and other legitimate forms of medical and social research, which often depend on a condition of unauthorized disclosure to third parties. A requirement of authorization would be overprotective of a person's interests and inconsistent with the objectives of public health.

Maintaining confidentiality. Privacy and confidentiality are often blended in professional guidelines on ethics, as if protecting a person's privacy is essentially a matter of protecting confidential information about the person. However, privacy and confidentiality are distinct concepts. An infringement of confidentiality occurs only if a person to whom information was disclosed *in confidence* fails to protect that information or deliberately discloses it to someone without proper consent. Confidentiality can be violated or infringed in several ways, including deliberate and accidental disclosure.

As discussed elsewhere in this volume, measures that may and should be taken to protect the confidentiality of health information include securing records with personal identifiers, limiting access to records to a small set of members of the research team, eliminating personal identifiers whenever possible, strengthening the understanding of the importance of confidentiality at training sessions for study personnel, and preventing information from release in a form that would allow identifications to occur.[30,31]

A breach of confidentiality cannot be justified unless it is necessary to meet a strong conflicting obligation, such as a court order, but this rule does not restrain epidemiologists from obtaining and using confidential information. The obligation to protect confidential information is neither an obligation never to obtain confidential information, nor an obligation never to share the information with appropriate parties. Confidential medical and other vital records that identify individuals are essential to epidemiologic research, and identification of persons whose records have been obtained is often needed to prevent those individuals or others associated with them from developing disease or to identify the disease at an early stage. Although confidential data may be passed between responsible professionals, just as clinical data are passed between physicians, care must be paid to how and under what protections it is transmitted.

Whenever an epidemiologist publicly disseminates information collected from confidential data, all information that might point to individuals should be removed. In some unusual circumstances, usually involving a threat to the public health or to the safety of other persons, the epidemiologist may be justified in infringing confidentiality by communicating personally identifying information to public health officials, family members, or other involved parties. Nevertheless, in almost all cases the individuals who have been identified should be notified of the action taken.[32,33,34,35,36,37]

Epidemiologists have often obtained access to medical records, school records, social agency records, employment records, and some federal records. Credit, Census, and Internal Revenue records have been far less accessible. These restraints on access are socially important, but from a moral perspective the type of record is usually irrelevant.

Reviewing research protocols. Since roughly the late 1960s and early 1970s, a massive, increasingly international system of prior review of research with human subjects has developed. Epidemiologists are obligated to submit their research protocols for review and to provide a justification of their procedures. Review committees and (if appropriate) administrative review are often structured so that officials work closely with investigators in improving the ethical quality of research. However, investigators have a personal responsibility to evaluate the ethics of a study and to ensure its ethical adequacy throughout its term. Responsibility for ethical evaluation cannot be justifiably transferred to the review committee or to administrative review.

In order for epidemiologic research with human subjects to be approved, at least the following conditions should be satisfied: (1) consent procedures are adequate for procuring consent from each individual subject; (2) the privacy of subjects and the confidentiality of information have been adequately protected; (3) risks to subjects have been minimized and have been shown to be justifiable by reference to anticipated benefits of the research; (4) subjects who might be especially vulnerable to influence or harm have been protected by stringent measures; (5) the selection of subjects is fair and the research does not place an undue burden on a particular class of subjects; (6) provisions have been made to monitor the research as it continues in order to deepen the protection of human subjects; (7) plans have been included for the communication of study results.

Research conducted by epidemiologists occasionally need not meet these conditions, because some research is legitimately exempted from ethical review. But regardless of the judgments and demands of particular committees, every study in epidemiology involving human subjects should have an approved, written protocol.

Responsibilities to Society. The main argument justifying epidemiologic research is that its societal benefits are substantial and that various risks are reduced or eliminated. Because of the commitment to better the public's health and improve survival rates epidemiologists often have dual professional obligations to advance scientific knowledge and to enhance, protect, and restore public health through the application of this knowledge.[38,39] The freedom to perform epidemiologic research also entails a correlative responsibility to perform it with due care, competence, and objectivity.

Providing benefits. Obligations to confer benefits, to prevent and remove harms, and to weigh and balance possible goods against possible harms of an action are central to the health professions. By the very nature of epidemiology and its implicit contract with the members of society, risks to rights or welfare must be justified by potential benefits. The benefits of epidemiologic research can be substantial in providing knowledge about areas such as cancer, cardiovascular disease, infectious disease, psychiatric disorders, injuries, and child health.[40] Consequently, epidemiologists have role obligations to provide such benefits when the opportunity arises, and obligations to advance the profession as well.

Epidemiologists should employ the means available to them to enlarge the reach of sound epidemiologic inquiry and to disseminate their findings, so that the widest possible community benefits from the research. When properly carried out, the review of protocols also requires a justification of research through an honest and comprehensive comparison of anticipated benefits and anticipated risks.

Sustaining public trust. Epidemiologists should attempt to promote and preserve public confidence by properly presenting the methods, results, and public health significance of their epidemiologic inquiries. All information vital to public health should be communicated in a timely, comprehensive, understandable, and responsible manner so that the widest possible community benefits from the research. Difficult judgments sometimes have to be made about whether some problem of security, confidentiality, or trade secrets justifies withholding information, and, if so, whether some more restricted dissemination of findings might outweigh any larger need for the information. Information that is believed to be correct may also be difficult to verify. Withholding information can be justified in unusual cases. However, to withhold information for personal or institutional reasons is almost always a violation of the epidemiologist's responsibility. Failure to provide full information (except in highly unusual situations) is morally no better than failure to provide any information at all, and may be worse if the presentation is distorted in the interests of a party at risk.

Avoiding conflict of interest. A conflict of interest occurs when a personal interest or a role obligation of an investigator conflicts with an obligation to uphold another party's interest, thereby compromising normal expectations of objectivity and impartiality in regard to the other party. Conflicts of interest typically arise when a person must make a judgment in a context in which others should be able to rely on the person to remain free of interests or influences that jeopardize the person's objectivity and professionalism. An epidemiologist on the payroll of a corporation, a university, or a government does not encounter a conflict of interest merely by the condition of employment. A conflict exists whenever an epidemiologist's role obligation or personal interest in accommodating the institution, in job security, or in personal goals compromises responsibilities to others who have a right to expect impartial treatment and objective judgment.

The "conflict" in conflict of interest is a confrontation between professional judgment and an influence that potentially could distort or critically impair that judgment. Some influences clearly distort judgment, others have some reasonable probability of doing so, and others have only some distant possibility of doing so. Thus, a difference exists between having a conflict of interest and potentially having a conflict of interest. There is also a difference between having a real conflict of interest and a perceived conflict of interest. In the latter, there is no conflict of interest, only the appearance of one. It is not obvious that an epidemiologist must avoid either *potential* or *perceived* conflicts of interest. It would be morally dubious to ask someone to avoid a circumstance in which others suspect the person of a conflict of interest while there is no substance to the claim. Perceived conflicts can erode trust, but mere perceptions of conflict may be little more than unjustified suspicions. Nonetheless, a perceived conflict usually provides reasonable grounds for suspicion of an actual conflict, because the perception usually has some basis in fact. Conflicts of interest are often too easily dismissed on grounds that they are merely potential or perceived conflicts.

Obviously it is best to avoid such circumstances altogether, but, when conflicts arise, there is no a priori reason to suppose that loyalty to an employer, agency, or academic institution is always the foremost consideration. Personal integrity, moral responsibilities to other parties, or responsibilities to professional colleagues may also turn out to be weightier considerations. Epidemiologists can and have confronted many forms of conflict of interest involving sources of support (including grants and contracts) and in their work as consultants, witnesses, and the like. Widely discussed problems of conflict of interest concern gifts, favors, potential gains from products with commercial value, and lucrative side contracts.[41,42,43]

Maintaining impartiality. Closely related to issues of conflict of interest are failures of impartiality that occur when a value-directed departure from accuracy, objectivity, and balance takes place. Partiality can be a factor in research design, critical analysis, the publication of results, and peer review. It is a reasonable presumption that the deeper the commitment to sound principles of scientific method, the less a risk of partiality threatens results and conclusions. There is no reason to assume, however, that epidemiologists who employ observational study designs are more susceptible to partiality than experimental scientists. Perhaps most importantly, the presence of a value judgment does not entail that partiality taints the judgment. Epidemiologists are often called upon to reach legitimate value judgments about the conclusions and implications of their research. Epidemiologic research and the reporting of its results also necessarily involve selection among facts for emphasis and the taking of points of view, which often are openly stated in the conclusions of the study. We therefore should distinguish partiality from legitimate forms of appraisal.

Failures of impartiality do not occur unless there is a *value-directed* departure from accuracy, objectivity, and balance. If, for example, an epidemiologist fails to notice that an accidental omission has distorted a crucial part of a study, the distortion results from error, not from partiality. Failures of impartiality in scientific research may result from specific sources, for example, an ideology, an employer-controlled framework of beliefs, or affiliation with special-interest groups. Failures to maintain impartiality may also derive from sources such as career ambition, institutional goals, irrationality, prejudice, greed, and even religious fervor.

In scientific research, charges of partiality often stem from the belief that an epidemiologist might adopt an inappropriate advocacy role or be hired as a consultant or employee to represent narrow institutional views or special interests, for example, taking public stands on policies to protect the health of vulnerable children they have studied. The concern is that this relationship may lead an investigator to report results in a fragmentary or imbalanced fashion that promotes the desired values and conclusions (or at least will report conclusions so as to limit dangers to those values), causing a loss of scientific objectivity.[44,45] However, value-directed roles do not themselves necessarily produce partiality. A partisan or institutionally loyal epidemiologist may restrain or even completely eliminate his or her beliefs in conducting a study or reporting its findings.

Responsibilities to Employers and Funding Sources. Valid interests and rights are retained by funders and employers. The epidemiologist's responsibilities to them sometimes conflict with responsibilities to subjects, society, or colleagues.[46,47]

Formulating responsibilities. Epidemiologists should inform employers and funders, preferably in contractual form, how research is to be conducted and how it might involve moral and legal responsibilities. The respective responsibilities of employer, funder, and epidemiologist, including responsibilities to report findings, should be clearly articulated in documents such as program manuals or protocols. All parties should be cognizant of any moral or other professional codes to which an epidemiologist should adhere. No valid agreement exists among the parties unless the arrangements have been thoroughly disclosed and all parties understand their specific responsibilities. Epidemiologists should not accept any such contractual responsibilities if particular conclusions must be reached from a proposed study or if one must refrain from publishing any conclusions that might be reached.

Protecting privileged information. Epidemiologists may use privileged information furnished by a funder or employer under a requirement that the information remain confidential. The privileged information may include intellectual property, such as trade secrets. However, epidemiologic methods, procedures, and results should not, in addition, be retained as confidential and should be included in any final report(s). Conflicts between the various parties sometimes arise over proprietary or other privileged information. An epidemiologist who possesses confidential information that could damage the economic interests of an employer or the privacy interests of a subject is under an obligation of confidentiality that should not be broken except in highly unusual circumstances (when a more demanding moral obligation requires that it be broken). This responsibility remains in force when the epidemiologist leaves a firm or completes a project.

Responsibilities to Professional Colleagues. Codes of professional ethics typically assert that colleagues should be dealt with honestly and should be criticized when deficient in character, competence, or action. These demands are sensitive in professional practice, and codes and guidelines have typically said little about how to handle these responsibilities. Less problematic, but no less important, are professional responsibilities to report methods and results publicly, and to communicate ethical requirements to colleagues and associates in institutions.

Reporting methods and results. Upon completion of their studies, epidemiologists should provide adequate information to colleagues in order to permit the methods, procedures, techniques, and findings of their research to be critically assessed. The communication should occur within a reasonable period after completion of the research (that is, within the standard amount of time it takes to write, critique, and polish such work) and should address all results, including those that do not fit the investigators' preferences or preconceptions. It is unacceptable to fail to communicate the results of a study because the results turned out differently than expected.

Epidemiologists should likewise avoid being placed in a situation in which their results might be unduly suppressed or edited by other persons. For example, academic epidemiologists and their universities should not accept grants or contracts in which a funding source retains the right to edit or suppress results; government and corporate epidemiologists should avoid circumstances in which their superiors can unduly edit, suppress, or delay publication; and epidemiologic reviewers should only attempt to deter publication of work by other epidemiologists for reasons of inferior science or some critical unclarities in reporting results.

Quality assurance and internal review procedures may legitimately cause short delays in publication in many institutions. Some responsible institutions and departments believe that the reputation of the institution, the development of younger colleagues, and related considerations justify manuscript-clearance procedures prior to submission for publication. There may be sound informational and educational reasons for such policies, resulting in constructive critique of studies and manuscripts. However, the constructive side of the process can be subverted, which suggests the need for oversight of these review procedures.

Reporting unacceptable behavior and conditions. Epidemiologists at times encounter fraud, illegal behavior, unethical conduct, and incompetence. When such behavior is discovered in colleagues or in other associates, an epidemiologist has a responsibility to confront the problem and to encourage the repudiation of improper activities. In some cases there may be a responsibility to take specific action to correct the behavior, though protection against unjust accusations should also be maintained. Fraud and misrepresentation in research are instructive examples. Even a single act of misrepresentation or tampering with data is a morally serious matter.

Disclosures about colleagues and others found to be engaging in unacceptable conduct are essential in order to preserve trust with the public, an employing institution, and professional colleagues. In exposing unacceptable behavior or conditions, the epidemiologist sometimes must assume the role of advocate for the public, colleagues, and perhaps the institution at which the research is conducted, although institutions often have a vested interest in not having such problems brought to light. It is inexcusable for epidemiologists to capitulate to such vested interests. For example, if an institution seeks publicly to promote the view that "no health effects" are shown by a study, when it is quite reasonable to interpret the study as having shown some health effects, it is unethical to remain silent in the face of press releases and the like that distort the study's findings.

These observations conclude this overview of the professional morality of epidemiologic endeavors. Several issues deriving from this morality are discussed in subsequent chapters, and we can now move to a study of some problems and methods in moral philosophy.

Problems and Methods in Moral Philosophy

Professionals are typically not trained in or exposed to moral philosophy even when they receive formal instruction in professional ethics. Moral philosophy involves disciplined reflection on the nature, function, and justification of moral beliefs. The purpose is to confront fundamental problems and to introduce clarity, substance, and precision of argument into moral thinking. This section on Problems and Methods in Moral Philosophy is devoted to a few questions and methods in moral philosophy that should improve the quality of moral thinking in epidemiology.

Moral Justification

Because we all have a good grasp of the common morality, we generally have no difficulty in deciding how to act morally. We make moral judgments through appeals to rules, cases, moral exemplars, and the like. These moral beacons work well as long as we are not asked to justify our judgments. However, when we experience moral problems, we begin moral deliberation. In reaching a moral judgment, any agent should be prepared to defend the judgment by a process of giving reasons—often referred to as moral justification. The reasons we offer express the conditions under which we believe some course of action is warranted.

The objective of justification is to establish one's case by presenting sufficient grounds for action or belief. One might attempt a justification by appealing to preexisting rules, such as those listed above or those in codes of ethics. One might also appeal to authoritative institutional agreements and practices or to the moral convictions in which we have the highest confidence in the common morality. In each case, appeals are made to the best moral reasons for the proposed course of action. Justification also requires that all relevant and obtainable information be acquired and that one be impartial in the process of moral deliberation. One's reasons must be impartially selected and impartially applied, while remaining sensitive to moral conflicts as well as conflicts with legal obligations, religious traditions, and the like.

THE MORAL BASIS OF PROFESSIONAL ETHICS Many scholars of professional ethics believe that morality should be justified in terms of fundamental norms or principles. One hint to this effect was found in my earlier proposal that the justification of requirements of informed consent is the principle of respect for autonomy.

We also noted that many codes have traditionally relied upon the implications of the general principle "Do no harm." Ideally, a set of general principles, such as the two just mentioned, could be developed as an analytical framework of basic principles that expresses the values underlying specific guidelines, such as rules of confidentiality, disclosure, impartiality, and conflict of interest. Elsewhere I have defended the view that four clusters of moral principles can serve this function by mapping our most general values.[12]

1. Respect for autonomy (respecting the decision-making capacities of autonomous persons),
2. Nonmaleficence (avoiding the causation of harm),
3. Beneficence (providing benefits and balancing benefits, burdens, and risks),
4. Justice (fairness in the distribution of benefits and risks).

These principles do not form a moral system or theory, but they do provide a framework through which we can identify and reflect on moral problems. The framework is abstract and spare, and moral thinking and judgment must take account of other considerations. Abstract principles do not contain sufficient content to address the nuances of moral circumstances—as professional guidelines, such as those governing epidemiology. Accordingly, I will not here attempt to show how these four groups of principles are related to more particular rules, such as the rules of professional ethics discussed previously.

Instead, I will focus on a related problem that is directly pertinent to constructing practical moral guidelines, which is the following: Principles (and all general moral norms) are abstract instruments that dispense vague, nonspecific advice open to competing interpretations. Morality in the narrow sense is comprised entirely of general precepts and has little power to demand particular actions until the precepts are given more content that will render them suitably specific for particular contexts. Across time, the basic precepts of morality become implemented in many different ways in cultures, groups, and even by individual decision makers, thereby creating morality in the broad sense. To see how this process of growth in moral belief occurs and how it should occur, I begin with the need for specification.

SPECIFICATION AND REFORM Practical moral problems typically require that we make our general norms suitably specific (whether principles, rules, or more particular maxims).[48] General precepts have insufficient resources to resolve deep or complex moral problems, and even specific norms are often too indeterminate and need further specification. Progressive specification will be needed on an ongoing basis as new problems arise. Such specification is the heart of what happens in biomedical ethics as a means to the formulation of institutional and public policy. None of this should be surprising. We all lack a complete understanding of the range of commitments made in accepting a moral precept such as a rule of confidentiality, and we find ourselves unable to specify it all the way down to concrete cases.

In managing difficult cases, the first line of attack should be to specify general norms and thereby to reduce or eradicate conflicts. The following is a typical example of the kind of problem an epidemiologist might confront, together with a possible solution: Research data and conclusions generated by private corporations that produce commercial health-care products and services are often valuable to the health community at large. Yet the information is proprietary to the corporation, and the interests of stockholders must be protected. Publishing research that is valuable to the public's health is a moral responsibility, but so is protecting the stockholder's interests. Corporate officers therefore must carefully balance duties to stockholders with duties to society and professional colleagues. A corporation attempting to devise an adequate set of guidelines to govern these responsibilities must state the conditions under which the methods, techniques, and findings of its research and product development will be shared and the conditions under which the data will remain confidential. In so acting, corporate officers will be engaged in a process of specifying abstract norms and rendering them coherent.

For example, the corporate officers in this health information example might specify as follows: (1) "Disclose *all* available information about (a) *epidemiologic research* regarding workplace safety and (b) *research on product risks and safety*; disseminate all findings, so that the widest possible community benefits from the research." (2) "Disseminate *no* findings of research pertaining to (a) product development and (b) consumer preferences." Although contingent conflicts are still possible among even these rules (for example, between rule 1b and rule 2a), incoherence, the possibilities for contingent conflict, and subjective balancing are reduced by these specifications of general norms. In the process, the corporation has developed a policy to handle contingent conflicts.

Because we inventively create rather than simply discover these more specific rules and policies, John Mackie argues that ethics is "invented."[49] Mackie does not mean that individuals create personal moral policies, but that specific standards are built up over time through communal agreements and decision making. What is morally demanded, enforced, and condemned is not merely what we discover in already available basic precepts, but what we decide in the development of those precepts. We constantly invent rules and policies that clarify and specify both the commitments of morality in the narrow sense and our previous specifications. For example, since approximately 1966 we have been inventing many of the rules and policies in the United States to protect human subjects of biomedical and behavioral research that were mentioned previously. These rules extend well beyond the content of any pre-1966 guidelines and practices relevant to the development of these rules (see Chapter 1).

We cannot reasonably expect that these strategies of specification will function as a cure-all for our deepest problems of moral conflict. Specification will not always eliminate competing proposals for the resolution of contingent conflicts, and in problematic or dilemmatic cases, several specifications will emerge that are well-defended proposals for resolution. Nonetheless, specification is often helpful in professional ethics.

MORAL DILEMMAS AND THE RESOLUTION OF MORAL DISAGREEMENTS Many problems in professional practice are moral dilemmas in which strong moral reasons support the rival conclusions of at least two well-supported points of view. If any one set of reasons is acted upon, events will result that are desirable in some respects but undesirable in others. Here an agent morally ought to do one thing and also morally ought to do another, but the agent is precluded by circumstances from doing both. Parties on both sides of dilemmatic disagreements can correctly present good moral reasons in support of their competing conclusions. Most moral dilemmas therefore present a need to balance rival claims.

However, some dilemmas and disputes can be relieved or even eliminated. The following six methods for dealing constructively with moral disagreements have been employed in the past, and each deserves recognition as a method of easing dilemmas and addressing controversies.

1. *Specification.* The first, and most important, is the method of specification discussed above. The need for specification is often particularly evident when dilemmas arise.
2. *Adopting a code or policy.* Second, resolution of moral problems can be facilitated if disputing parties can come to agreement on a common set of moral guidelines, such as rules that define "conflict of interest" and then state obligations to avoid such conflicts. If this method requires a complete shift from one starkly different moral point of view to another, agreement will rarely be achieved. Differences that divide persons at the level of their most cherished views are deep divisions, and conversions are infrequent. Nonetheless, carefully articulated codes reached by discussion and negotiation can lead to the adoption of a new or changed moral framework that can serve as a common basis for evaluation of conduct. Specification will likely play a critical role in this process, which often eventuates in a code of ethics or institutional policy.
3. *Obtaining information.* Many moral disagreements can be reduced by obtaining factual information about central matters in the moral controversy. It has often been assumed that moral disputes are produced solely by differences over moral principles or their interpretation and application, rather than by a lack of information. However, disputes over what morally ought or ought not to be done often have nonmoral elements as central ingredients. For example, debates about the justice of government allocation of health dollars to

preventive and educational strategies have often bogged down over factual issues of whether these strategies actually do function to prevent illness and promote health. New information often facilitates negotiation and compromise. Additional epidemiologic information about the alleged dangers involved in certain industries, for instance, have often affected controversies about risks in science. Controversies about sweetening agents for drinks, toxic substances in the workplace, pesticides in agriculture, and radiation therapies among others have all involved issues of both values and facts. Controversies over compulsory or voluntary screening for HIV often turn critically on factual claims about how the virus is transmitted, which benefits can be gained by screening, how many persons are threatened and the magnitude of their risks, whether testing and counseling reduces HIV risk, and the like.[50,51,52,53,54]

4. *Providing definitional clarity.* Third, controversies have been settled by reaching agreement over the meaning of the language used by disputing parties. In some cases stipulation of a definition or a clear explanation of a term may prove sufficient, but in other cases agreement will involve negotiation over a meaning. Controversies over the ethics of obtaining informed consent, for example, are often needlessly entangled because disputing parties use different senses of the term "informed consent" and have invested heavily in their particular definitions. One party may equate "informed consent" with *disclosure* by a physician or investigator, while another party equates it with *mutual decision making* between patient and physician or investigator. These notions are different and any resulting moral controversy over obligations of informed consent will be ensnared in terminological problems, rendering it doubtful that disputants are discussing the same problem.

5. *Using examples and counterexamples.* Fifth, resolution of moral controversies can be aided by a constructive use of an example and opposed counterexample. Cases or examples favorable to one point of view are brought forward, and counterexamples are proposed against them. This form of debate occurred when a national bioethics commission once considered the level of risk that can justifiably be permitted in scientific research involving children as subjects, where no therapeutic benefit is offered to the child. Commissioners were at first inclined to accept the view that only "minimal" risk procedures could be justified for children (where "minimal risk" refers to the level of risk present in standard medical examinations of patients). Many examples were put forward of unnecessary risk that had been presented to children in research. Examples from the history of medicine were then cited that revealed how significant diagnostic, therapeutic, and preventive advances in medicine would have been retarded or prevented unless procedures that posed a higher level of risk had been employed. Counterexamples of overzealous researchers who placed children at too much risk were then thrown up against these examples, and the debate continued in this way for several months.[55] Eventually a

majority of commissioners abandoned their original view that nontherapeutic research involving more than minimal risk was unjustified. Instead, the majority accepted the position that a higher level of risk can be justified by the potential benefits provided to other children, as when a group of terminally ill children is studied in the hope that something will be learned about their disease that can be applied to help other children. Resolution was thereby achieved on the primary moral controversy.

6. *Analyzing arguments.* Finally, one of the most important methods of philosophical inquiry—that of exposing the inadequacies, gaps, and fallacies in an argument—can also be brought to bear on moral disagreements. For example, if an argument rests on two incoherent positions, then pointing out the incoherence will require a change in the argument. Again, if a moral argument leads to conclusions that a proponent is not prepared to defend and did not previously anticipate, part of the argument will have to be changed, and this process may reduce the distance between the parties who are disagreeing. This style of argument is often supplemented by one or more of the above five ways of reducing moral disagreement.

Much of the work published in journals of ethics takes the form of attacking arguments, using counterexamples, and proposing alternatives. To use these methods is not to assume, of course, that conflicts can always be eliminated. The moral life will always be plagued by some conflict or ambiguity that cannot easily be eradicated without producing some other problem. Our pragmatic goal should be a method that helps push the discussion forward through refinements, not a method that will always resolve the problems.

RELATIVISM AND OBJECTIVITY IN ETHICS Problems of moral disagreement raise questions about whether there can be correct or objective moral judgments. Tensions between the belief that morality is purely personal or a matter of social convention and the belief that it has an objective grounding lead to issues of relativism in morals. Cultural differences raise these questions in profound ways.

A widespread view challenges the validity of moral precepts that are accepted in one culture when these precepts are applied to a different culture. Some figures in contemporary biomedical ethics cite "American values" such as requiring informed consent as a representative example of the problem. Because they fear "medical-ethical imperialism," they defend notions such as "culturally sensitive" standards, thereby rejecting a transcultural applicability for standards of informed consent, confidentiality, peer review, and the like.[56,57,58]

The most obvious thesis to counter this relativist position is the one presented above: Obligations such as those of obtaining informed consent express universally applicable moral values that cannot be compromised without compromising morality itself.[59] Morality *in the narrow sense* is not relative to cultures or individuals, and any norms closely associated with these fundamental moral values can never be validly compromised. At the same time, morality *in the broad sense* does show considerable diversity, and we can expect many valid cultural and philosophical differences to appear. For roughly this reason, other writers have proposed a partial relativism (of morality in the broad sense) that retains a core of universalistic components.[60,61,62,63]

Relativism can also be criticized by showing the *inapplicability* of leading relativistic views on factual grounds, without showing their *unjustifiability* on moral grounds.[64] Relativists often start with and defend their position by appealing to anthropological data indicating that moral rightness and wrongness vary from place to place and that no absolute or universal moral standards apply to all persons at all times. They add that rightness is contingent on cultural beliefs and that rightness and wrongness are meaningless apart from the specific contexts in which they arise.

Relativist arguments pertaining to epidemiology have been used largely when researchers from developed countries are engaged in research in developing countries. Informed consent has been a particularly important topic. Relativists who challenge the importation of informed consent from one culture to another question the appropriateness of first-person informed consent in nations with no history of its use, on three grounds. They argue that (1) informed consent is culturally insensitive, (2) potential patients and subjects are of questionable competence, and (3) the critical importance of clinical interventions or research investigations renders informed consent requirements dangerous for certain cultures. The first is the most important of the three.

In many countries, relativists say, persons view their social roles in terms of close relationships rather than in terms of individual rights or personal ambitions. Culture is multiform, and every culture contains values, beliefs, and rituals that are of overriding importance. These should not be nullified by values imported from external cultures, such as informed consent. But how adequate are the data on which these claims rest? In many societies it is easy to misrepresent or overstate widespread beliefs, social structures, and changing circumstances. There is often a time-lag in our evidence about many cultures, and before we can claim a lack of interest in (or preparation for) informed consent in a culture we have a responsibility to obtain solid and recent evidence. In many cultures we know that major groups have diverse moral and political commitments, which necessitate a threshold line of guaranteed international rights (drawn from morality in the narrow sense) that cannot be overturned even by the most culturally sensitive analysis.

Relativists also sometimes point to a lack of competence to consent in many cultures. This proposal is difficult to assess, because such claims sometimes rely for their credibility on inadequate resources for obtaining valid consent from persons in developing countries. But questions about *resources* should be kept separate from questions of *competence*. The idea that normal patients and research subjects in countries other than one's own are psychologically incompetent to give an informed consent is likely to be offensive, and perhaps abusive. It can demean people and fail to respect them in ways persons in one's own culture are respected.[65]

Finally, relativists have argued that the need for interventions or data is so critical in many countries that the time required to obtain bona fide informed consent should not be taken. Everyone can, of course, agree that interventions may permissibly occur without consent under emergency circumstances. The emergency situation is a long-established exception to many moral requirements, including informed consent. But is there any justification for the claim that the gravity of medical, public health, or research interventions *generally* warrants an exception to informed consent?

No one would deny that we should be "culturally sensitive" in exporting moral requirements to other cultures, but whether we can validly dispense with the responsibility to obtain first-person informed consent or with any other norm required by morality in the narrow sense is a difficult claim to sustain. Except in the aberrant case, such acts may simply be failures to treat one human being as he or she ought to be treated. At the same time, we can recall the distinction between morality in the narrow sense and morality in the broad sense and put it to a new use by distinguishing between a *relativism of judgments* and a *relativism of standards*: A relativism of judgment (involving morality in the broad sense) is so pervasive in human social life that it would be foolish to deny it. For example, when individuals and committees differ about whether one policy for keeping health information confidential is more acceptable than another, they differ in their moral judgments about alternative policies, but it does not follow that they have different moral standards of confidentiality. Many divergent *particular* judgments can call upon the same *general* standards (those of morality in the narrow sense) for their justification.

Ethical Theories

Many figures in the history of philosophical ethics have attempted more than an examination of problems and methods of the sort addressed in the section on Problems and Methods in Moral Philosophy. They have attempted to develop general, systematically organized ethical theories. These theories are complicated and only the most general features of a few influential types of ethical theory will be examined here: utilitarian theories, Kantian theories, and virtue theories. Casuistry, which is not an ethical theory in the usual sense, will also be discussed. Some knowledge of these theories is indispensable for reflective study in biomedical ethics, because a sizable part of the field's literature draws on the terminology, arguments, methods, and conclusions in these theories. The objective in this section and the next is not to defend an ethical theory or to argue that it has the capacity to resolve practical problems in epidemiology, but rather to explicate types of theory that are often helpful in thinking about moral justification.

Utilitarian Theories

To utilitarians, the object of morality is to promote human welfare by minimizing harms and maximizing benefits. They regard an action or practice as right if it leads to the greatest possible balance of good consequences or to the least possible balance of bad consequences. Utilitarians defend one and only one basic principle of ethics: the principle of utility. This principle asserts that we ought always to produce the maximal balance of positive value over disvalue (or the least possible disvalue, if only undesirable results can be achieved). Utilitarians see moral rules as the means to the fulfillment of individual needs as well as to the achievement of broad social goals.

The most influential exposition of utilitarianism is John Stuart Mill's book *Utilitarianism*.[66] In this work Mill refers to the principle of utility as the Greatest Happiness Principle: "Actions are right in proportion as they tend to promote happiness, wrong as they tend to produce the reverse of happiness, i.e., pleasure or absence of pain." Four essential features of utilitarianism may be extracted from the reasoning of Mill and other utilitarians.

1. *The principle of utility: Maximize the good.* First, as noted above actors are obliged to maximize the good: We ought always to produce the greatest possible balance of value over disvalue (or the least possible balance of disvalue). But what is the good or the valuable? This question takes us to the second condition.
2. *The standard of goodness.* The goodness or badness of consequences is to be measured by items that count as the primary goods or utilities. Many utilitarians agree that ultimately we ought to look to the production of intrinsic values, those that do not vary from person to person. But many utilitarians interpret the good as that which is subjectively desired or wanted, and in this account the satisfaction of desires or wants is the goal of our moral actions.
3. *Consequentialism.* All utilitarian theories decide which actions are recommended entirely by reference to the consequences of the actions, rather than by virtue of any intrinsic moral features they may have, such as truthfulness or fidelity. The utilitarian need not demand that all future consequences be anticipated, but only that we take account of what can reasonably be expected to produce the greatest balance of good or least balance of harm.[67]
4. *Impartiality.* Finally, in a utilitarian theory all parties affected must receive equal and impartial consideration. Utilitarianism thus aligns good and mature moral judgment with personal distance from the choices to be made.

A significant dispute has arisen among utilitarians over whether the principle of utility is to be applied to particular acts in particular circumstances or to rules of conduct that determine which acts are right and wrong. For the rule utilitarian, actions are justified by appeal to rules such as "Don't deceive" and "Don't break promises." These rules are themselves justified by appeal to the principle of utility. An act utilitarian simply justifies actions directly by appeal to the principle of utility.

Kantian Theories

A second type of theory departs significantly from utilitarianism. Sometimes called *deontological*, it is now increasingly called *Kantian*, because of its origins in the theory of Immanuel Kant (1734–1804).

Duty from rules of reason. Kant believes that an act is morally praiseworthy only if done neither for self-interested reasons nor as the result of a natural disposition; the person's motive for acting must be a recognition of the act as resting on duty. It is not good enough that one performs the morally correct action, because one could perform one's duty for self-interested reasons having nothing to do with morality. For example, if an employer discloses a health hazard such as a chemical with known health effects to an employee only because he or she fears a lawsuit, and not because of a belief in the importance of truth telling, then the employer acts rightly but deserves no moral credit for the action.

Kant regards all considerations of utility and self-interest as secondary, because the moral worth of an agent's action depends exclusively on the moral acceptability of the rule on which the person is acting. An action has moral worth only when performed by an agent who possesses a good will, and a person has a good will only if moral duty based on a universally valid rule is the sole motive for the action. Morality, then, provides a rational framework of universal principles and rules that constrain and guide everyone.

Kant's supreme principle, called "the moral law" or "the categorical imperative," is expressed in several ways in his writings. In what appears to be his favored formulation, the principle is stated as follows: "I ought never to act except in such a way that I can also will that my maxim should become a universal law."[68] This moral law offers worthwhile lessons for biomedical ethics. Many clear cases of immoral behavior involve a person trying to make a unique exception for himself or herself for personal reasons. This conduct could not be made universal, or else the rules presupposed by the idea of "being an exception" would be destroyed. If carried out consistently by others, this conduct would violate the rules presupposed by the system of morality.

Kant's view is that wrongful practices, including invasion of privacy, theft, cheating, and bribes, are "contradictory"; that is, they result in some form of inconsistency. When we examine the maxim of a person who deceitfully promises, we discover, Kant says, that this maxim is incapable of being conceived and willed universally without yielding a contradiction. It is inconsistent with what it presupposes and is like saying, "Though promising is not deceitful, this promise of mine is deceitful." The universalized maxim is inconsistent with the very point of the proposed maxim of action—a maxim that would be undermined if everyone were to act on it. Lying, too, works only if the person being lied to expects or presupposes that people are truthful, but in a world in which everyone lied, a maxim approving lying would make the purpose of truth telling impossible, and no one would believe the person who told a lie. Many examples from everyday life illustrate this thesis. For instance, maxims permitting cheating on tests are inconsistent with the practices of honesty on tests that they presuppose.[69,70]

The requirement never to treat persons as means. Kant states his categorical imperative in another and distinctly different formulation (which many interpreters take to be a wholly different principle). This form is probably more widely quoted and endorsed in contemporary philosophy than the first form, and certainly it is more frequently invoked in biomedical ethics. This formulation stipulates that "One must act to treat every person as an end and never as a means only."[69,71] Thus, one must treat persons as having their own autonomously established goals.

It has been widely reported in contemporary textbooks that Kant is arguing categorically that we can never treat another as a means to our ends. This interpretation, however, misrepresents his views. He argues only that we must not treat another *exclusively* as a means to our own ends. When adult human research subjects are asked to volunteer to test new drugs, for example, they are treated as a means to a researcher's ends (and perhaps society's ends). However, they are not exclusively used for others' purposes, because they do not become mere servants or objects. Their consent justifies using them as means to the end of research. Kant's imperative demands only that persons in such situations be treated with the respect and moral dignity to which all persons are always entitled, including the times when they are used as means to the ends of others.

Virtue Ethics

In discussing utilitarian and Kantian theories, we have looked chiefly at theories erected on obligations and rights, but we often reflect on the *agents* who perform actions, have motives, and follow principles. In recent years, several philosophers have proposed that ethics should redirect its preoccupation with principles of obligation and look to decision making by persons of good character, that is, virtuous persons.

Virtue ethics descends historically from the classical Greek tradition of ethics represented by Plato and Aristotle. Here the cultivation of virtuous traits of character is viewed as morality's primary function. Aristotle held that virtue is neither a feeling nor an innate capacity, but a disposition bred from a properly trained innate capacity.

For example, epidemiology students acquire virtues much as they do skills such as learning to develop a questionnaire or perform statistical tests. They become just by performing just actions and become temperate by performing temperate actions.[72]

Here are ten examples of moral character traits, or virtues, that are in the common morality: (1) nonmalevolence; (2) honesty; (3) integrity; (4) conscientiousness; (5) trustworthiness; (6) fidelity; (7) gratitude; (8) truthfulness; (9) lovingness; and (10) kindness. These virtues are universally admired traits of character. A person is everywhere recognized as deficient in moral character if he or she lacks such traits.[73] Negative traits that are the opposite of these virtues are *vices* (malevolence, dishonesty, lack of integrity, cruelty, etc.). They are moral defects, universally so recognized.

Virtue ethics investigates the role of a person's characteristic motivational structure. A conscientious person, for example, not only has a disposition to act conscientiously, but a morally appropriate desire to be conscientious. Likewise, a just person not only has a disposition to act fairly, but has a morally appropriate desire to do so. Such persons characteristically have a moral concern and reservation about acting in a way that would be unfair and lack conscientiousness. Having only the motive to act in accordance with a rule of obligation is not morally sufficient for virtue.

Consider persons who always perform obligations because they are obligations, but who intensely dislike having to allow the interests of others to be taken into account. These individuals do not cherish, feel congenial toward, or think fondly of others, and treat them as they should only because obligation requires it. Suppose this person is a physician who always meets his moral responsibilities, but his underlying motives and desires are morally inappropriate. This physician detests his job and hates having to spend time with every patient who comes through the door. He cares not at all about being of service to people or creating a better environment in the office. All he wants to do is make money and avoid malpractice suits. Although this man meets his moral responsibilities, something in his character is defective morally. The admirable compassion guiding the lives of many dedicated health professionals is absent in this person, who merely engages in rule-following behavior.

The merit of an action does not reside entirely in motive or character, of course. The action must be gauged to bring about the desired results and must conform to relevant principles and rules. For example, the epidemiologist who is appropriately motivated to help discover the causes of health effects, but who acts incompetently in seeking the desired result, does not act in a praiseworthy or acceptable manner, whatever the motive of the action. In professional life the traits that warrant encouragement and admiration often derive from role responsibilities. Roles internalize conventions, customs, and procedures of teaching, doctoring, and the like. The virtues in professional contexts are thus often established by practices and tradition.

Virtue ethics has practical value for biomedical ethics because a morally good person with right desires or motives is more likely to understand what should be done, more likely to perform required acts, and more likely to form and act on moral ideals than a morally bad person. A person who is ordinarily trusted is one who has an ingrained motivation and desire to perform right actions and who characteristically cares about morally appropriate responses. A person who simply follows rules of obligation and who otherwise exhibits no special moral character may not be trustworthy. A proponent of virtue ethics need not claim that analysis of the virtues subverts or discredits ethical principles and rules. It is enough to argue that ethical theory is more complete if the virtues are included and that moral motives deserve to be at center stage.[74,75]

Casuistry

Casuistry is an alternative to the abovementioned classical theories. It focuses on decision making in particular cases, where new judgments rely on judgments reached in relevantly similar prior cases. Casuists are skeptical of the power of principles and theory to resolve problems in specific cases. They think that many forms of moral thinking and judgment do not involve appeals to general guidelines, but to narratives, paradigm cases, and precedents.[76] One can make successful moral judgments of agents, actions, and policies, casuists say, only when one has an intimate understanding of particular situations and an appreciation of treating similar cases similarly.

How exactly is a moral judgment made? The casuist believes it cannot come through traditional appeals to general principles and rules, because many forms of moral thinking and judgment do not involve appeals to rules, rights, or virtues. The casuist holds that we sometimes appeal to narratives or paradigm cases, to classification schemes, and to the precedents established by previous cases.[77,78]

An analogy to law is helpful: The normative judgments of courts of law become authoritative through the assessment of cases, and it is reasonable to hold that these judgments are primary for later judges who assess other cases, even though the particular features of each new case will be different. Matters are similar in ethics. Normative judgments about certain cases emerge through case comparisons: A new case is placed in the context of a set of cases that show a family resemblance, and the similarities and differences are assessed. The relative weight of competing values is presumably determined by the comparisons to analogous cases. Moral guidance is provided by an accumulated mass of influential cases, which represent a consensus in society and its influential institutions.[79]

At first sight, casuistry seems strongly opposed to the frameworks of principles and rules at work in traditional moral theory. However, closer inspection of casuistry shows that its primary concern is only with an *excessive* reliance in recent philosophy on impartial, universal action-guides. Some casuists hold that casuistry often applies well-understood general principles to particular cases.

An account with general norms is therefore not necessarily a rival of casuistry. The casuist can consistently hold that as a history of similar cases and similar judgments mounts, we legitimately become confident in our general judgments. As confidence in these generalizations increases, they can be accepted less tentatively and moral knowledge develops. Just as case law (legal rules) develops incrementally from legal decisions in actual cases, so the moral law (moral rules) develops incrementally. So understood, casuistry is not inconsistent with classical ethical theory; it simply places an emphasis on practical decision making, rather than on formulating a general theory.[80]

From the casuists' perspective, moral reasoning is also similar to that of a physician in clinical diagnosis: Paradigms of proper treatment function as sources of comparison when new problem-cases arise. Recommendations are made by analogy to the paradigm. If the analogy is proper, a resolution of the problem and a recommendation will be achieved; but uncertainty may remain if there is no close analogy. Casuists thus remind us of the importance of analogical reasoning, paradigm cases, and practical judgment. They also emphasize that generalizations and new knowledge are often learned, accommodated, and implemented by using case discussion and methods of case analysis.

Conclusion

In conclusion, some perspective is needed on the limitations of moral philosophy and ethical theory as sources for our judgments in practical ethics. Philosophical theory is abstract and contains within its fabric a sustained body of controversies that render it unsuitable for generating specific, applied rules for practical ethics. Just as theoretical epidemiology concentrates on mathematical-statistical models to explain disease occurrences, so ethical theory concentrates on abstract models that attempt to explain and justify general principles and features of the moral life. These fields serve us well, but usually cannot be directly applied in our thinking about particular cases and policies.

ACKNOWLEDGMENT

The author wishes to thank Ralph Cook and Bill Fayerweather for stimulating conversations and suggestions.

References

1. Macklin, R. "Universality of the Nuremberg Code." In *The Nazi Doctors and the Nuremberg Code*, ed. G. J. Annas and M. Grodin. New York: Oxford University Press, 1992: 240–57.

2. Gostin, L. "Human Rights in Mental Health: A Proposal for Five International Standards Based upon the Japanese Experience," *International Journal of Law and Psychiatry* 10 (1987): 353–68.

3. Grotius, H. *De jure belli ac pacis*, ed. J. B. Scott, trans. Francis W. Kelsey. Oxford: Clarendon Press, 1925.

4. Last, J. M. Association News. "Guidelines on Ethics for Epidemiologists," *International Journal of Epidemiology* 19 (1990): 226–29.

5. Fayerweather, W., Beauchamp, T. L., and Higginson, W., eds. *Ethics and Epidemiology*. Amsterdam: Pergamon Press/Elsevier, 1991.

6. Beauchamp, T. L., Cook, R. R., Fayerweather, W. E., et al. "Ethical Guidelines for Epidemiologists," *Journal of Clinical Epidemiology* 44 (1991): 151S–69S.

7. Bankowski, Z., Bryant, J. H., and Last, J. M., eds. *Ethics and Epidemiology: International Guidelines*. Proceedings of the XXVth Council for International Organizations of Medical Sciences Conference, November 7–9, 1990 (Summary of Discussions). Geneva: CIOMS 1991.

8. Susser, M., Stein, Z., and Kline, J. "Ethics in Epidemiology," *Annals of the American Academy of Political and Social Science* 437 (1978): 128–41.

9. Gordis, L. "Ethical and Professional Issues in the Changing Practice of Epidemiology," *Journal of Clinical Epidemiology* 44 (1991): 9S–13S.

10. Capron, A. M. "Protection of Research Subjects: Do Special Rules Apply in Epidemiology?," *Law, Medicine and Health Care* 19, no. 3–4 (Fall–Winter 1991): 184–90.

11. Beauchamp T. L., Cook R. R., Fayerweather W. E., et al. "Ethical guidelines for epidemiologists." *Journal of Clinical Epidemiology* 44 (1991): 151S–69S.

12. National Commission for the Protection of Human Subjects of Biomedical and Behavioral Research. *The Belmont Report: Ethical Principles and Guidelines for the Protection of Human Subjects of Research*. Washington, DC: U.S. Government Printing Office, 1978.

13. Beauchamp, T. L. and Childress, J. F. *Principles of Biomedical Ethics*. 6th ed. New York: Oxford University Press, 2009.

14. Gostin, L. "Ethical Principles for the Conduct of Human Subject Research: Population-Based Research and Ethics," *Law, Medicine and Health Care* 19 (1991): 191–201.

15. Dickens, B. M. "Issues in Preparing Ethical Guidelines for Epidemiological Studies," *Law, Medicine and Health Care* 19 (1991): 175–83.

16. Dickens, B. M., Gostin, L., and Levine, R. J. "Research on Human Populations: National and International Ethical Guidelines," *Law, Medicine and Health Care* 19 (1991): 157–61.

17. Levine, R. J. *Ethics and Regulation of Clinical Research*. 2nd ed. New Haven: Yale University Press, 1988.

18. President's Commission for the Study of Ethical Problems in Medicine and Biomedical and Behavioral Research. *Making Health Care Decisions*. Vols. 1–3. Washington, DC: Government Printing Office, 1982.

19. Faden, R. R. and Beauchamp, T. L. *A History and Theory of Informed Consent*. New York: Oxford University Press, 1986.

20. Meisel, A. "The 'Exceptions' to the Informed Consent Doctrine: Striking a Balance Between Competing Values in Medical Decision Making," *Wisconsin Law Review* 1979 (1979): 413–88.

21. Buchanan, A. E. and Brock, D. W. *Deciding for Others: The Ethics of Surrogate Decision Making*. Cambridge: Cambridge University Press, 1989.

22. Gordis, L., Gold, E., and Seltser, R. "Privacy Protection in Epidemiologic and Medical Research: A Challenge and a Responsibility," *American Journal of Epidemiology* 105 (1977): 163–68.
23. Last, J. M. "Individual Privacy and Health Information: An Ethical Dilemma?," *Canadian Journal of Public Health* 77 (1986): 168–70.
24. Privacy Protection Study Commission. *Personal Privacy in an Information Society.* Washington, DC: Government Printing Office, 1977.
25. Schoeman, F. D., ed. *Philosophical Dimensions of Privacy: An Anthology.* New York: Cambridge University Press, 1984.
26. Kelsey, J. L. "Privacy and Confidentiality in Epidemiological Research Involving Patients," *IRB* 3 (1981): 1–4.
27. Kmentt, K. A. "Private Medical Records: Are They Public Property? A Survey of Privacy, Confidentiality and Privilege," *Medical Trial Technique Quarterly* 33, no. 3 (1987): 274–307.
28. Cleaver, C. M. "Privacy Rights in Medical Records," *Fordham Urban Law Journal* 13, no. 1 (1984–85): 165–204.
29. Parmet, W. "Public Health Protection and The Privacy of Medical Records," *Harvard Civil Rights-Civil Liberties Law Review* 16, no. 1 (Summer 1981): 265–304.
30. NCHS Staff Manual on Confidentiality. Hyattsville, MD: National Center for Health Statistics, 1984. DHHS Publ. No. (PHS) 84–1244.
31. McCarthy, C. R. and Porter, J. P. "Confidentiality: The Protection of Personal Data in Epidemiological and Clinical Research Trials," *Law, Medicine and Health Care* 19 (1991): 238–41.
32. Rennert, S. American Bar Association. Commission on the Mentally Disabled [and] Center on Children and the Law. *AIDS/HIV and Confidentiality: Model Policy and Procedures.* Washington, DC: American Bar Association, 1991.
33. Maney, A. and Wells, S., eds. *Professional Responsibilities in Protecting Children: A Public Health Approach to Child Sexual Abuse.* New York: Praeger, 1988.
34. Lako, C. J. and Lindenthal, J. J. "The Management of Confidentiality in General Medical Practice: A Comparative Study in The U.S.A. and The Netherlands," *Social Science and Medicine* 32, no. 2 (1991): 153–57.
35. Appelbaum, P. S. and Rosenbaum, A. "Tarasoff and The Researcher: Does The Duty to Protect Apply in The Research Setting?," *American Psychologist* 44, no. 6 (June 1989): 885–94.
36. Price, D. P. T. "Between Scylla and Charybdis: Charting a Course to Reconcile The Duty of Confidentiality and The Duty to Warn in The AIDS Context," *Dickinson Law Review* 94, no. 2 (Winter 1990): 435–87.
37. Marshall, S. E. "Doctors' Rights and Patients' Obligations," *Bioethics* 4, no. 4 (October 1990): 292–310.
38. Lappé, M. "Ethics and Public Health." In *Public Health and Preventive Medicine*, ed. J. M. Last. 12th ed. Norwalk, CT: Appleton-Century-Crofts, 1986: 1867–77.
39. Armenian, H. K. "In Wartime: Options for Epidemiology," *American Journal of Epidemiology* 124 (1989): 28–32.
40. Gordis, L. and Gold, E. "Privacy, Confidentiality, and the Use of Medical Records in Research," *Science* 207 (January 11, 1980): 153–56.
41. American Medical Association. Council on Scientific Affairs and Council on Ethical and Judicial Affairs. "Conflicts of Interest in Medical Center/Industry Research Relationships," *Journal of the American Medical Association* 23 (May 23/30, 1990): 2790–93.

42. Kenney, M. *Biotechnology: The University-Industrial Complex*. New Haven, CT: Yale University Press, 1986.
43. Healy, B. et al. "Conflict-of-Interest Guidelines for a Multicenter Clinical Trial of Treatment After Coronary-Artery Bypass-Graft Surgery," *New England Journal of Medicine* 320 (April 6, 1989): 949–51.
44. Rothman, K. J. and Poole, C. "Science and Policy Making," *American Journal of Public Health* 75 (1985): 340–41.
45. Weed, D. L. "Science, Ethics Guidelines, and Advocacy in Epidemiology," *Annals of Epidemiology* 4 (1994): 166–71.
46. Blumenthal, D. et al. "University-Industry Research Relationships in Biotechnology: Implications for the University," *Science* 232 (June 13, 1986): 1361–66.
47. Relman, A. S. "Economic Incentives in Clinical Investigation," [Editorial] *New England Journal of Medicine* 320 (April 6, 1989): 933–34.
48. Richardson, H. S. "Specifying Norms as a Way to Resolve Concrete Ethical Problems," *Philosophy and Public Affairs* 19 (Fall 1990): 279–310.
49. Mackie, J. L. *Ethics: Inventing Right and Wrong*. New York: Penguin Books, 1977.
50. Mayer, K. H. "The Epidemiological Investigation of AIDS," *Hastings Center Report* 15, no. 4 (August 1985): S12–S15.
51. Dickens, B. M. "Legal Rights and Duties in the AIDS Epidemic," *Science* 239, no. 4840 (February 1988): 580–86.
52. Faden, R. R., Geller, G., and Powers, M., eds. *AIDS, Women and the Next Generation*. New York: Oxford University Press, 1991.
53. Fox, D. M. "From TB to AIDS: Value Conflicts in Reporting Disease," *Hastings Center Report* 16, no. 6 (December 1986): S11–S16.
54. Walters, L. "Ethical Issues in the Prevention and Treatment of HIV Infection and AIDS," *Science* 239, no. 4840 (February 5, 1988): 597–603.
55. The National Commission for the Protection of Human Subjects of Biomedical and Behavioral Research. *Research Involving Children*. Washington, DC: U.S. Government Printing Office, DHEW Publication, 1977.
56. Christakis, N. A. "Ethics are Local: Engaging Cross-Cultural Variation in the Ethics for Clinical Research," *Social Science and Medicine* 35 (1992): 1079–91.
57. Christakis, N. A., Fox, R. C., Faden, R. R., IJsselmuiden, C. B. et al. "Informed Consent in Africa," [letters and replies] *New England Journal of Medicine* 327 (October 8, 1992): 1101–02.
58. Christakis, N. A. "The Ethical Design of an AIDS Vaccine Trial in Africa," *Hastings Center Report* 8 (June/July 1988): 31–37EM.
59. Angell, M. "Ethical Imperialism? Ethics in International Collaborative Clinical Research," [Editorial] *New England Journal of Medicine* 319 (1988): 1081–83.
60. Barry, M. "Ethical Considerations of Human Investigations in Developing Countries: The AIDS Dilemma," *New England Journal of Medicine* 319 (1988): 1083–86.
61. Levine, R. J. "Informed Consent: Some Challenges to the Universal Validity of the Western Model," *Law, Medicine and Health Care* 19 (Fall–Winter 1991): 207–13.
62. De Craemer, W. "A Cross-Cultural Perspective on Personhood," *Milbank Memorial Fund Quarterly* 61 (1983): 19–34.
63. Council for International Organizations of Medical Sciences (CIOMS). "International Guidelines for Ethical Review of Epidemiological Studies," *Law, Medicine and Health Care* 19 (1991): 247–58; and CIOMS, *International Ethical Guidelines for Biomedical Research*. Geneva: CIOMS, 1993.

64. IJsselmuiden, C. B. and Faden, R. R. "Research and Informed Consent in Africa—Another Look," *New England Journal of Medicine* 326 (March 19, 1992): 830–34.

65. Ekunwe, E. O. and Kessel, R. "Informed Consent in the Developing World," *Hastings Center Report* 14 (1984): 22–24.

66. Mill, J. S. *Utilitarianism.* In *Collected Works of John Stuart Mill*, vol. 10. Toronto: University of Toronto Press, 1969.

67. Scheffler, S., ed. *Consequentialism and its Critics.* Oxford: Clarendon Press, 1988.

68. Kant, I. *Foundations of the Metaphysics of Morals,* trans. Lewis White Beck. Indianapolis, IN: Bobbs-Merrill Company, 1959.

69. Korsgaard, C. "Kant's Formula of Universal Law," *Pacific Philosophical Quarterly* 66 (1985): 24–47.

70. Herman, B. *The Practice of Moral Judgment* (Cambridge, MA: Harvard University Press, 1993).

71. Korsgaard, C. "Kant's Formula of Humanity," *Kant-Studien* 77 (1986):183–202.

72. Aristotle. *Nicomachean Ethics,* trans. T. Irwin. Indianapolis: Hackett, 1985.

73. Nussbaum, M. "Non-relative Virtues: An Aristotelian Approach." In *Ethical Theory, Character, and Virtue*, ed. Peter French, et al. Notre Dame, IN: University of Notre Dame Press, 1988: 32–53.

74. Foot, P. *Virtues and Vices.* Oxford: Basil Blackwell, 1978.

75. Pence, G. *Ethical Options in Medicine.* Oradell, NJ: Medical Economics Co., 1980.

76. Jonsen, A. R. "Casuistry: An Alternative or Complement to Principles?" *Kennedy Institute of Ethics Journal* 5 (1995): 237–51.

77. Jonsen, A. R. and Toulmin, S. *Abuse of Casuistry.* Berkeley: University of California Press, 1988.

78. Jonsen, A. R. "Casuistry as Methodology in Clinical Ethics," *Theoretical Medicine* 12 (December 1991).

79. Arras, J. D. "Getting Down to Cases: The Revival of Casuistry in Bioethics," *Journal of Medicine and Philosophy* 16 (1991): 29–51.

80. Jonsen, A. R. "Casuistry and Clinical Ethics," *Theoretical Medicine* 7 (1986): 67, 71.

3

Toward a Philosophy of Epidemiology

DOUGLAS L. WEED

The two great engines of progress in society are a desire to understand the world and a desire to improve it.[1] This sentiment, penned over a half century ago by the British philosopher Bertrand Russell seems ready-made for today's epidemiologists. Scientists seek to understand the causes of diseases and we, the health professionals, struggle to decide when best to apply the knowledge gained, evaluating interventions and using those found effective and safe to improve the public's health. Put another way, epidemiologists contribute to social progress through the coupled engines of science and technology,[2] acquiring and using knowledge to prevent and control diseases, protecting and promoting health.

The overarching thesis of this book is that the acquisition and use of epidemiologic knowledge should be guided by the theories, principles, case studies, and methods of bioethics. In several chapters of this book, practical implications of this thesis are developed. In this chapter our attention will be focused in a different yet complementary direction, examining some philosophical implications of this same thesis. Simply put, to what extent can ethics, so obviously useful to the practice of epidemiology, also be considered part of a much broader philosophy of epidemiology? What else is needed to create a philosophical foundation for epidemiology?

From a philosophical perspective, the acquisition and use of scientific knowledge requires much more than ethics alone. In the philosophy of science, for example, there are many relevant concerns about the nature, discovery, and growth of knowledge—that is, epistemic concerns—ideally suited to play companion roles in a philosophy of epidemiology, if one existed.

A philosophy of epidemiology, however, has not received much attention. Several explanations for this oversight are possible: perhaps it is not apparent why such an effort should be undertaken; what purpose would a philosophy of epidemiology serve? perhaps we are unclear about how to go about developing a philosophical foundation for epidemiology, even if we deem it a worthwhile venture; maybe as practitioners of a growing and essential professional public health discipline, we are simply too busy plying our craft to spend the time and effort to unearth our philosophical roots, which are likely to be deep and convoluted.

My aim in this chapter is to explore the need for and nature of philosophy in epidemiology. It will require the collaboration of epidemiologists and philosophers who seek to uncover the foundations of this basic professional health discipline. I begin with some history, documenting the extent to which we (a few epidemiologists and even fewer philosophers) are already moving toward a philosophy of epidemiology.

Historical Background

Philosophical concepts and problems have intrigued epidemiologists for years. One need not look very far to see the close and longstanding connectivity of ethics and epidemiology; the publication of the second edition of this book is evidence enough. However, epistemic concerns involving the study of how epidemiologic knowledge is gained have attracted attention for an even longer time. In 1927, 50 years before epidemiologists began their first formal foray into ethics,[3,4] Wade Hampton Frost described epidemiology in philosophical terms, as an "inductive science, concerned not merely with describing the distribution of disease, but equally or more with fitting it into a consistent philosophy."[5] Pointing out that the interpretation of evidence is a much greater challenge than designing and carrying out studies, Frost wrote that weaknesses in conclusions from observational epidemiology are as likely due to faults in logic as inaccurate or insufficient data.

Sixty years later, Frost's belief in the need for clear logic in the interpretation of epidemiologic evidence was echoed by Mervyn Susser in a letter commenting on the parallels between philosophy in medicine and in epidemiology. He noted that without an understanding of the logic of causal inference, the interpretation of epidemiologic evidence is "likely to be misleading or fruitless."[6]

Susser's letter appeared at a time when a debate was raging in the epidemiologic literature about the appropriateness of different methods of scientific reasoning. The debate began in 1975, with the publication of a paper by Carol Buck on Popper's philosophy for epidemiology, the first in a long series of articles on the logic of causal inference.[7] Popper's somewhat radical view of the philosophy of science dispenses, for all practical purposes, with induction as a method for acquiring scientific knowledge, replacing it with a method of creative conjectures and refutations that relies heavily on a hypothetico-deductive logic.[8–10] Buck discussed the application of a few selected Popperian ideas, including the need for creativity in formulating hypotheses as well as finding ways to increase the opportunity for refuting hypotheses, especially those to which an investigator is personally attached. Soon after Buck's paper appeared, critics within epidemiology voiced their concerns, more about Popper's philosophy per se than with Buck's limited application of it. Some noted the impossibility of dispensing with induction, since statistical inference and the practice of causal inference in epidemiology were better described in inductive than deductive terms. Others argued that epidemiology lacks a coherent body of theory important to the successful application of Popper's approach.[11–15]

A discussion of the role of logic in causal inference and of the epistemic foundations of epidemiology continued during the 1980s. A handful of investigators, captivated by the clear arguments and prescriptive tone of Popper's writings, examined the implications of using conjecture and refutation as a methodological guide and of developing theories from which empirically testable conjectures about disease causation could be deduced.[16–23] At times, the debate was contentious, and it certainly deserves much more attention than can be given here, where its complexities and missteps (such as the unfortunate and easily disputed claim that a "cult" of Popperian epidemiologists had been created) are less important than its impact on practice.[24–26]

Current Practice and the Philosophy of Science

At least two trends have emerged from the focus on Popper's logic of scientific discovery: first, refutation now appears as part of the lexicon when scientific evidence is evaluated and interpreted, providing investigators with a reason to look for and to value "negative" evidence, that fails to confirm or even refutes a hypothesis, combating the tendency to put more weight on confirmatory or "positive" findings in a weight-of-the-evidence analysis;[27] second, an interest in theoretical development in epidemiology seems to be taking root. Discussions of causal definitions, causal mechanisms, and causal models from which relatively simple yet testable predictions could be derived have begun to appear.[28,29] There are, for example, at least five different yet overlapping definitions for a "cause" in our literature: production,[30,31] necessity,[32–34] the sufficient component causes model,[35] probabilistic causation,[36] and counterfactuals.[37–41]

Epidemiologists' explorations into the development of theory is a far cry from the traditional approach wherein hypotheses are treated as nothing more than potential statistical associations between exposures and diseases, disconnected from biological or social theories of disease. Today, epidemiologic inquiry more often proceeds with some attention paid to the theories within which factor-disease hypotheses fit. Nevertheless, we cannot, for example, predict from theory the expected magnitude of a relative risk. Such a capacity would make our hypotheses highly testable, because they would be subject to a rigorous form of empirical refutation. We remain limited to observing whether or not the relative risk (or any other outcome measure) differs from unity (or from some other empirically generated expected value) by more than what a probability distribution can explain. Efforts to improve both the predictability and testability of epidemiologic hypotheses by actually applying a method of theory-based conjectures subject to refutation[18] may emerge from the increased interest in linking biological and social mechanisms with epidemiological explanations of disease occurrence. This transition from the traditional approach nearly devoid of theory, which many epidemiologists refer to as "black box" or "risk factor" epidemiology, to a new approach involving a broad appreciation for the theoretical diversity of epidemiologic hypotheses can be considered a shift so fundamental as to be revolutionary. To put it another way, many say that the paradigms of epidemiology are shifting, from the paradigm of "risk factor epidemiology" to that of "eco-epidemiology." Such a shift brings up another important contemporary trend in the philosophy of science, what some call the "paradigm" or "postmodern" view of contemporary science.[42–44]

Paradigms are Thomas Kuhn's big idea,[45] described in his now-classic book *The Structure of Scientific Revolutions*,[46] which has produced a dramatic change in the way most scholars think about the role of science in a postmodern society and especially about the ways in which the community of scientists affects scientific progress. Building on the earlier work of Fleck,[47] Kuhn posited that the history of science is best characterized as paradigmatic periods of puzzle-solving (also called "normal science"), occasionally interrupted by dramatic shifts in thinking (the "revolutions"). Epidemiology's history has been characterized in Kuhnian terms as having moved through four different periods of "normal (paradigmatic) science." It began with the theory of miasma during the first half of the 19th century, followed by contagionism (germ theory) until the middle of the 20th, followed by a "black box" or "risk factor" paradigm, nearly devoid of theory, which recently has shifted to the most recent paradigm, called "Chinese box" epidemiology, or "eco-epidemiology" in which social and biological theoretical contexts join hands to explain disease occurrence.

A Kuhnian interpretation of scientific change and progress has implications that go well beyond a tidy historical framework or structure of paradigms and revolutions. A Kuhnian view of scientific progress seriously questions at best and rejects at worst what many scientists see as their ultimate aim—ever-improving approximations to some ultimate, final truth about the nature of the world.[45] When paradigms are about shift, Kuhn observed that many scientists resist these changes in ways that can only be interpreted as irrational and emotional. Paradigm shifts resemble value-laden religious conversion experiences much more than rational applications of any form of logical reasoning.

Epidemiologic history bears out Kuhn's claims. Early contagionists, such as John Snow, were challenged and even ridiculed by the miasmists who believed that bad air (not contaminated water) was responsible for the cholera epidemics in 19th Century London.[48] More recently, there are epidemiologists who would give up on risk factor (black box) epidemiology and those who most vigorously defend this paradigm.[49,50] Once a paradigm has shifted, nearly all traces of the older (now defunct) set of scientific problems and solutions are altered or even erased. Textbooks, Kuhn noted, are the best evidence of this reconstruction of scientific history. They are rewritten in the face of paradigmatic change in such a way that students lose touch with their past. Newly trained practitioners have not studied their discipline from the perspective of the old paradigm, now considered to be not only irrelevant but more importantly, no longer an approximation to the truth. Evidence of this effect can also be found in epidemiologic textbooks.[51] Finally, Kuhn argued that a new paradigm does not build on the old but is more or less incompatible with it. He called this lack of compatibility incommensurability. Scientific change is not necessarily progressive change, and a new paradigm may or may not represent cumulative progress toward the truth, if that were ever achievable.[52]

Contrast Kuhn's value-laden perspective on scientific progress with Popper's intensely rational if skeptical approach. Popper's philosophy of science has no room for values, emotions, and conversion experiences. Theories rise and fall as they are tested by experience through observations and experiments, with the most rigorously tested emerging as victors in the race to find the best approximation to the truth, which Popper's skeptical philosophy makes the aim of science. Cumulative scientific progress is not only possible but expected, as new theories explain better and explain more than their predecessors. In a Kuhnian world, on the other hand, theories change and we are hard-pressed to know if we are actually making progress. We have no real way of knowing if we are on the right track (to the best explanation) because our observations and our interpretations of those observations cannot be disentangled from our belief systems, values, interests, and norms. There is nothing like a mind-independent, objective way to assess the validity of our theories by refutations of hypotheses, as Popper's philosophy would have us accept. In Kuhn's contrasting world, the clash or concordance between hypothesis and experimental observation is always underdetermined and science simply cannot provide proof nor disproof. Therefore, confirmations and refutations of hypotheses are equally problematic as guides to acquiring scientific knowledge.

Moving Forward: The Value of Philosophy for Epidemiology

Who is right: Popper and his followers or Kuhn and his followers? More importantly, what shall it be: a Popperian philosophy for epidemiology or some other?

Unfortunately, no clear and convincing answers to these questions are available, providing us with one of the most potent reasons for not pursuing epidemiology's philosophical foundations: not only that philosophers lack agreement on this particular debate, but more importantly, that philosophers may be unable to come to agreement about *any* philosophical foundation for epidemiology, if they were even inclined to discuss it. As Schlesinger writes in his commentary on the applicability of the philosophy of science for epidemiology, most scientists refuse to accept the suggestion that philosophers have produced anything like a deep understanding of the ultimate foundations of science, because philosophy lacks any palpable body of knowledge due to a complete absence of any agreed-upon, unchallenged results. It is as if anything goes and perfect anarchy prevails. Whenever one thinker makes a claim, someone else adopts a diametrically opposite position, while the majority of their colleagues disagree with both of them.[53]

Perhaps Schlesinger's pessimism is unwarranted, but if he is even partially correct, what is a budding philosopher of epidemiology to do? There are, many additional choices beyond Popper and Kuhn. If philosophers can not easily decide who has the best view of the nature of science, what value does reflective philosophical thinking bring to epidemiology?

To answer this question, let us assume that we bear no a priori hostility toward philosophy—that is, we have no antiphilosophical bias—a phenomenon described by philosophers who have observed that scientists often seem to reject philosophy because they believe it to be not just impractical but wrong about the nature of science.[45] I suspect that an additional problem is one of mutual incomprehension, in which scientists do not understand the philosopher's concerns and modes of thinking, while philosophers do not understand the actual practice of science, especially within the discipline of epidemiology, to connect their inquiries to the practice that convinces anyone that these inquiries matter.

With these assumptions and considerations in place, it is perhaps easier to understand why many philosophers believe that the value of their discipline for the practicing scientist is primarily, or even exclusively, to satisfy his intellectual curiosity about the fundamentals or foundations of science. Unfortunately, scientists who are not already interested in these issues are unlikely to be swayed by this argument. To make matters worse, it is not uncommon for philosophers to state that their discipline has no intention of improving scientific practice. As Lipton writes, "Philosophy is unlikely to directly improve scientific practices,"[45] a sentiment echoed by Schlesinger, who writes, "It is not important for the scientist to take an interest in the philosophy of science, if he expects to improve his technique or problem-solving skills. The story of philosophy is unlikely to contribute much to a scientist's competence. The importance of philosophy lies in its ability to satisfy one's 'abstract intellectual gratification'."[53]

Most notably the philosophers of medicine, like Pellegrino, who is both practitioner and philosopher despite his self-effacing claims to the contrary, believe strongly that philosophy has much to offer the practice of a professional discipline beyond (yet still including) its capacity to satisfy one's curiosity. Pellegrino argues that few issues are more fundamental to human well-being than the acquisition and use of medical knowledge, but the validity of that effort does not lie within the realm of medicine. That inquiry belongs to philosophy.[54,55]

It seems reasonable and hardly overreaching to rephrase Pellegrino's assertions in epidemiologic terms: few issues are more fundamental to the public's health than the appropriate acquisition and use of scientific knowledge, including (but not limited to) epidemiology. But the validity of the ends of epidemiology—that is, what it aims to achieve in both the advancement of knowledge and its application—is a trans-epidemiologic matter, meaning that the assessment of the validity and value of the ends of epidemiology lies outside the realm of epidemiological methods and instead in a philosophy of epidemiology.

Not everyone will be convinced by this argument, still perched perilously high above the everyday practice of the discipline. Adding something closer to our everyday professional concerns, something practical and useful, would strengthen the argument—for example, a demonstration of the utility of philosophical inquiry. Earlier in this chapter, I proposed two practical (and useful) changes to epidemiological practice that have emerged from the debate on the logic of discovery in science—from the so-called Popperian debate—that grabbed the attention of epidemiologists for twenty years: first, the recognition that refutation is a vital outcome of hypothesis testing; second, the need for a robust search for theory in epidemiology that can be linked to testable predictions.

Other useful ideas have also emerged from the contrary philosophical view, namely, from Kuhn's sociohistorical view of progress in a postmodern scientific world. Kuhn's work spawned a growth industry in philosophical discussions about "values" in science,[56,57] which become especially important in those situations in which validated quantitative decision methods do not exist. The best example in epidemiology is causal inference. Values can play a decisive role in the interpretation of epidemiologic evidence.[58] The practical implications are several: epidemiologists now recognize that values—both scientific values and social or ethical values—play an influential role in causal decision making, in part because of the impact of the lack of proof and disproof, or "underdetermination," and also because carefully validated methods of inference do not yet exist. That puts any effort to improve the methods of causal inference at the top of anyone's list, if epidemiology is to make progress in science and in the application of science in public health.

In sum, it is fair to say that philosophical inquiry in epidemiology (and largely by epidemiologists) has brought a wealth of ideas, concepts, and concerns into practice beyond the requirement for a logic of inference recognized by Frost (early on) and by others much later. A partial list would include refutation, predictability, testability, realism, causation and the logic of causal inference, objectivity and subjectivity, paradigms, values, as well as underdetermination and incommensurability. These have certainly contributed to a deeper understanding of the philosophical foundations of epidemiologic science and have helped satisfy our intellectual curiosity. Most importantly, they have provided a rich source of guidance for our research and practice agenda, especially in the area of causal inference, the central scientific problem of the discipline.

Ethics and Causation

To what extent does ethics play a role in this search for philosophical insight and practical progress? Specifically, does ethics play a role in a fundamental scientific problem like causal inference, so well suited to philosophical reflection? Put more broadly, is ethics something separate and distinct from these philosophical concerns listed above? Are ethics and the philosophy of science interconnected roots of the same tree—two major contributors to an overarching and all-encompassing philosophy of epidemiology? I turn now to proposing answers to these questions.

It may seem peculiar at this point in this chapter to introduce ethics. After all, this entire book is intended to be about ethics and not about the philosophy of science or philosophy in general. This entire book examines how ethics matters deeply to epidemiological practice and to its aims: the acquisition and use of scientific knowledge. Ethics in epidemiology begins with a deep understanding of the moral foundations of our practice, the topic expertly discussed by Tom Beauchamp. But in the end, ethics provides us with a vast repertoire of theories, principles, rules, and methods that guide our practice. The method of casuistry, for example, provides us with a way to categorize and learn from the many case studies and the specific dilemmas that characterize and define the epidemiologist's everyday practice. Professional ethics guidelines and other standards of conduct also reflect the profession's recognition that ethics plays a key role in everyday practice. I have no less appreciation for the fundamental principles of bioethics, such as nonmaleficence, beneficence, justice, and respect for autonomy, than I had thirty years ago when they were introduced to epidemiology. All the authors of chapters in this book recognize and appreciate the fact that ethics matters deeply to the practice of epidemiology.

With so much ethics and epidemiology on hand, it may not make sense why ethics and causation should be connected. Causation appears to be exclusively a scientific matter with obvious connection to the philosophy of science. What is the role of ethics in the practice of making causal claims? Is ethics as important a source of guidance and reflection for epidemiology's central scientific problem as philosophy of science itself? We certainly recognize that ethics plays an important role in a wide variety of other professional matters, from informed consent, privacy, and confidentiality to community-based interventions, disclosure of results, and public health practice. Ethical issues are prominent in genetic epidemiology, infectious disease epidemiology, and in international research. Finally, epidemiologists recognize that Institutional Review Boards (IRBs) and scientific misconduct are topics best examined in terms of ethics. All these issues are carefully examined in this book.

However, what about ethics and causation? I believe there is a central role for ethics in the practice of causal inference. Ethics plays a critical role in the practice of causal inference well beyond the well-worn phrase that it is "unethical to do a randomized clinical trial exposing people to a purported causal factor." Both the ethics of virtue and principle-based ethics play a prominent role in the practice of causal inference in epidemiology.

Consider the role of virtue ethics in causal inference. When an epidemiologist opines about causation, typically as part of a systematic narrative review of a body of scientific evidence in which causal criteria may be employed, we presume or hope that this same epidemiologist is a person of good character, a professional whose scientific integrity is beyond reproach, who sees excellence in every part of her practice, and who is honest, open, and critical in her application of the complex method of causal inference. In that same capacity, we recognize that an epidemiologist uses judgment (along with the causal criteria, meta-analysis, and all the rest) which, in its broadest sense, is a mental capacity that employs scientific reasoning, ethical reasoning, values, and virtue, especially the virtue of practical wisdom.[59] Virtue, in other words, plays a critical and often recognized role in what might appear to be a practice exclusively scientific and directly connected to the philosophy of science.

But there is more to the ethics of causal inference than virtue. Consider one of the main reasons epidemiologists seek causes in the first place. Who can deny that we work so hard to identify the causes of diseases because we are committed to providing an assessment of the possible harms that some factors bring to the people we have promised to help? Is this not a reflection of our fundamental allegiance to the principle of beneficence achieved through prevention? Epidemiologists have made a promise to society to prevent disease; a promise that is a commitment not only to the public's health but also to the science of disease causation.[60] These professional commitments go hand in had with the public good. Our science is driven as much by the principle of beneficence as it is by the principle of testability or predictability or, for that matter, a principle of uncertainty. That does not mean that our causal claims are biased in favor of premature preventive action or that causation is a simple matter easily determined. Our causal claims, to best help the public and to reflect the best scientific practice, should be as transparent, open, honest, and critical as any other essential decision. They should not come to fruition without a careful, critical, and comprehensive assessment of the available evidence to which the methods of causal inference are applied.

There is more to the ethics of causal inference than virtue and beneficence. The care we take to inform study participants, to protect the privacy and confidentiality of our clients, and to disclose results in a fair and open way, is a reflection of our deep appreciation for the role ethics plays in achieving scientific results in individual studies, whose hypotheses and tests are always some part of a causal explanation. These actions, which we see as direct applications of ethics to our practice, are as much about our desire to understand causation as they are about our desire to improve it.

Ethics runs through causal inference like the river of uncertainty itself. But by no means am I suggesting that the scientific problem of causation cannot be examined solely in terms of logic and refutation and underdetermination (and any other concept from the philosophy of science), keeping ethical ideas at bay. Similarly, it is reasonable to focus primarily on ethical matters, say, the ethics of international clinical trials, keeping fundamental philosophical concepts (like testability) just below the surface. What is at stake here is not whether philosophical concepts (from the philosophy of science) and ethical concepts (from bioethics) are relevant or worthy in their own right, but how best to improve the practice of epidemiology using ideas from both disciplines. Philosophical and ethical concepts (and methods and arguments and all the rest) can and should be used together for the purpose of improving epidemiology.

I understand epidemiology to be a profession for which a philosophy and an ethic not only exist but support in an essential and fundamental way every aspect of our practice. The causation problem is a good example. Just as the list of philosophical concepts that began with refutation and ended with incommensurability affect our practice of making claims about causation, so too the theories, principles, rules, and cases of ethics affect and even improve that same practice. Ethics, therefore, has as much to do with the practice of causal inference as the philosophy of science itself.

I do not draw as sharp a distinction between philosophy and ethics as exists in academia. I do not put them much farther apart on my intellectual bookshelf than mathematics and statistics. That does not mean they are not separate and distinct in their own academic environments nor that one or the other cannot be applied without addressing the other. Instead, I see no compelling reason to keep them immaculately separate in their application to the problems we face as professional epidemiologists. I see no reason not to tuck them both up under the umbrella notion of a philosophy of epidemiology, the topic to which I now return.

Developing a Philosophy *of* Epidemiology

Two pillars of a philosophical foundation for epidemiology are the epistemological concerns of the philosophy of science and the theories, methods, and case studies of bioethics. With that claim in hand, I return to the premise of this chapter and its central probative questions: Is it reasonable or even important to uncover the philosophical foundations of epidemiology? Is it important to develop a philosophy of epidemiology? The answer is "Yes." These foundations are already in place and have been fruitfully linked to practice. This effort in no way diminishes their capacity to satisfy our curiosity about such matters, but makes practical implications as important as intellectual gratification.

Up to this point, I have not distinguished between searching for epidemiology's philosophical foundations and developing a philosophy of epidemiology. But the time has now come to make that careful distinction and to better characterize the relationship between philosophy within which I include the philosophy of science, ethics, and ontological concerns, such as the nature of "public health" and the meaning of "causation" and "epidemiology." Three levels of interaction are possible, building on a similar scheme applied to philosophy and medicine[55] as well as to the philosophy of public health:[61] Philosophy *and*, *in*, and *of* epidemiology.

Philosophy and *Epidemiology*. Here the two disciplines retain their separate identities. Philosophers use epidemiologically relevant examples in their discussions and epidemiologists use philosophical concepts in their analyses, interpretations, and commentaries. The depth of the analysis is meaningful but relatively superficial from both a philosophical and an epidemiological perspective. An epidemiologist's reference to "refutation" in discussing the interpretation of results is a good example. Within philosophy, it is uncommon to find many epidemiological examples, although disease causation (typically in individuals) surfaces occasionally.

Philosophy in *Epidemiology*. In this next level of interaction, philosophical tools such as critical reflection, dialectics, or the examination of values and aims, are applied to problems within epidemiology. These problems could include the forms of logical reasoning as reflected in the everyday practice of epidemiology, theories of causal inference, underdetermination and incommensurability in contemporary practice, the relationship of observation to experiment, the meanings of the concepts of health and disease, and the entire range of issues encompassed by this book at the intersection of ethics and epidemiology. Although it is tempting to concede these efforts to the professional philosophers, I would argue that such a constraint is not necessary nor even desired. What really matters is that the problems are carefully and artfully examined as philosophical problems whose solutions, however tentative and worthy of challenge, impact the theory and practice of the discipline.

Philosophy of *Epidemiology*. At this deepest level of interaction, philosophy turns to the discipline of epidemiology in a very different way, examining the meaning of epidemiology, its nature, concepts, purposes and its ultimate value to society. A philosophy *of* epidemiology could also be described as a general theory of epidemiology, within which the cluster of problems examined in the philosophy *in* epidemiology are synthesized. These are the problems now seen as uniquely ethical or uniquely scientific in nature. A philosophy *of* epidemiology is more than synthesis; it is creative, fundamental, and comprehensive.

What a philosophy *of* epidemiology should not be is also important. It should not be a diluted or derivative version of a philosophy of public health. No one seriously doubts the fact that epidemiology is a vital component of public health, but its important connections to the practice of medicine and law imply that it is much more than one of a number of public health disciplines. It is a unique discipline with its own unique problems and thus its own philosophy. A philosophy *of* epidemiology should also not be a search for a single view. We should not look for *the* philosophy *of* epidemiology. It remains reasonable to examine epidemiology's problems from particular points of view, for example, from a refutationist perspective, a postmodern viewpoint, or from any number of others, including pragmatism, principlism, casuistry, and virtue theory. But a philosophy *of* epidemiology is unlikely to be found solely in any one of these perspectives. It will be as unique as the discipline itself.

A philosophy *of* epidemiology should not have unreasonable expectations placed on it. Epidemiology's fundamental problems include responsibility, evidence to action, and causation, which are not only philosophical in nature. They have historical, political, social, economic, and scientific roots. They are ultimately problems for the practice of the profession. Our responsibility to actively participate in prevention activities, for example, is a matter of considerable debate. For those who take on that responsibility, the problem of "evidence to action" becomes a critical part of everyday practice, whose solution partially depends upon the solution to the problem of causation.

Finally, a philosophy *of* epidemiology should not be relegated solely to philosophers, who may not understand the complexities, nuances, and challenges of this essential yet often misunderstood discipline.

Where Things Stand and Where Things Could Go

How best to proceed on our continuing journey to a philosophy *of* epidemiology is an issue worthy of consideration. It is doubtful that many epidemiologists are prepared to undertake a serious and sustained effort to develop the philosophical foundations of their own discipline for two very good reasons—resources and training. Significant funding from the usual sources seems unlikely. Few epidemiologists are intellectually prepared to examine their discipline using philosophical tools, unless they have received formal training in philosophy or have focused their interests on the job and with the assistance of experts. On the other hand, perhaps only a few such individuals are needed to build the necessary bridges between the profession and the philosophers, who, in turn, may not be encouraged to focus their interests on epidemiology per se, perhaps because no support for such efforts exists, or because they are not conversant in the language and customs of this unique discipline situated at the intersection of science, public health, medicine, and the law.

Efforts to educate and train epidemiologists in philosophy and ethics along with parallel efforts for philosophers to learn epidemiology (and statistics, biology, and other relevant disciplines) would seem to be important, following a model already developed for the humanities in medicine. There has been some discussion of such a proposal for epidemiology, the humanities, and public health.[62] Perhaps such training efforts will bear fruit.

In any case, the philosophical inquiries of epidemiologists, in whatever form they continue, are better for society than no effort at all. Developing a philosophy of epidemiology should be encouraged, supported, and examined for its capacity to improve the practice of epidemiology. It will be interesting to see, after another decade or so, to what extent epidemiology's philosophical reflections have driven the engines of social progress closer to their destinations. What causes will we have discovered, what explanations accepted, however provisionally? What interventions will we have undertaken? How much will the health of the public have been improved? Even if all these milestones have been reached, assigning credit to philosophical inquiry will be a tough achievement. That fact or premonition does not make me any less interested or committed to moving toward a philosophy of epidemiology.

References

1. Russell, B. *Marriage and Morals*. New York: Horace Liveright, 1929: 301.
2. Healy, M. J. R. "Truth and Consequences in Medical Research," *Lancet* 2 (1978): 1300–01.
3. Coughlin, S. S., "Historical Foundations." In *Ethics and Epidemiology*, 2nd ed., ed. S. S. Coughlin, T. L. Beauchamp, and D. L. Weed. New York: Oxford University Press, 2009.
4. Susser, M., Stein, Z., and Kline, J. "Ethics in Epidemiology," *Annals of the American Academy of Political and Social Sciences* 437 (1978): 128–41.
5. Frost, W. H. "Epidemiology." In *Papers of Wade Hampton Frost, M.D. a Contribution to Epidemiological Method*, ed. K. F. Maxcy. New York: Arno Press, 1977: 493.
6. Susser, M. "Philosophy in Epidemiology," *Theoretical Medicine* 12 (1991): 271–73.
7. Buck, C. "Popper's Philosophy for Epidemiologists," *International Journal of Epidemiology* 4 (1975): 159–68.
8. Popper, K. R. *The Logic of Scientific Discovery*. New York: Harper and Row, 1968.
9. Popper, K. R. *Conjectures and Refutations: The Growth of Scientific Knowledge*. New York: Harper and Row, 1968.
10. Popper, K. R. *Objective Knowledge: An Evolutionary Approach*. Oxford: University Press, 1979.
11. Davies, A. M. "Comment on 'Popper's Philosophy for Epidemiologists'," *International Journal of Epidemiology* 4 (1975): 169–71.
12. Jacobsen, M. "Against Popperized Epidemiology," *International Journal of Epidemiology* 5 (1976): 9–11.

13. Smith, A. "Comment on Popper's Philosophy for Epidemiologists," *International Journal of Epidemiology* 4 (1975): 171–72.
14. Francis, H. "Epidemiology and Karl Popper," *International Journal of Epidemiology* 5 (1976): 307.
15. Creese, A. "Popper's Philosophy for Epidemiologists," *International Journal of Epidemiology* 4 (1975): 352–53.
16. Rothman, K. J. "Causation and Causal Inference." In *Cancer Epidemiology and Prevention*, ed. D. Schottenfeld and J. F. Fraumeni. Philadelphia: W. B. Saunders, 1982: 15–22.
17. Maclure, M. "Popperian Refutation in Epidemiology," *American Journal of Epidemiology* 121 (1985): 343–50.
18. Weed, D. L. "An Epidemiologic Application of Popper's Method," *Journal of Epidemiology and Community Health* 39 (1985): 277–85.
19. Weed, D. L. "On the Logic of Causal Inference," *American Journal of Epidemiology* 123 (1986): 965–79.
20. Weed, D. L. "Causal Criteria and Popperian Refutation." In *Causal Inference*, ed. K. J. Rothman. Chestnut Hill, MA: ERI, 1988: 15–32.
21. Lanes, S. F. "The Logic of Causal Inference in Medicine." In *Causal Inference*, ed. K. J. Rothman. Chestnut Hill, MA: ERI, 1988: 59–75.
22. Susser, M. "Falsification, Verification and Causal Inference in Epidemiology: Reconsiderations in the Light of Sir Karl Popper's Philosophy." In *Causal Inference*, ed. K. J. Rothman. Chestnut Hill, MA: ERI, 1988: 33–57.
23. Maclure, M. "Demonstration of Deductive Meta-Analysis: Ethanol Intake and Risk of Myocardial Infarction," *Epidemiologic Reviews* 15 (1993): 328–51.
24. Greenland, S. "Probability versus Popper: An Elaboration of the Insufficiency of Current Popperian Approaches for Epidemiologic Analyses." In *Causal Inference*, ed. K. J. Rothman. Chestnut Hill, MA: ERI, 1988: 95–104.
25. Pearce, N. and Crawford-Brown, D. "Critical Discussion in Epidemiology: Problems with the Popperian Approach," *Journal of Clinical Epidemiology* 42 (1989): 177–84.
26. Beaglehole, R. and Bonita, R. *Public Health at the Crossroads.* Cambridge: University Press, 1999: 101.
27. Weed, D. L. "Weight of Evidence: A Review of Concepts and Methods," *Risk Analysis* 25 (2005): 1545–57.
28. Parascandola, M. and Weed, D. L. "Causation in Epidemiology," *Journal of Epidemiology and Community Health* 55 (2001): 905–12.
29. Weed, D. L. "Theory and Practice in Epidemiology." In *Population Health and Aging: Strengthening the Dialogue between Epidemiology and Demography. Annals of the New York Academy of Sciences,* 954 (2001): 52–62.
30. MacMahon, B. and Pugh, T. *Epidemiology: Principles and Methods.* Boston: Little, Brown, 1970.
31. Susser, M. "What Is a Cause and How Do We Know One?" *American Journal of Epidemiology* 133 (1991): 635–48.
32. Gordis, L. *Epidemiology.* 2nd ed. Philadelphia: W. B. Saunders, 2000.
33. Elwood, M. *Causal Relationships in Medicine: A Practical System for Critical Appraisal.* Oxford: University Press, 1988.
34. Last, J. M. A. *Dictionary of Epidemiology.* 4th ed. New York: Oxford University Press, 2001.
35. Rothman, K. J. "Causes," *American Journal of Epidemiology* 104 (1976) 587–92.

36. Olsen, J. "Some Consequences of Adopting a Conditional Deterministic Causal Model in Epidemiology," *European Journal of Epidemiology* 3 (1993) 204–09.
37. Karhausen, L. R. "The Logic of Causation in Epidemiology," *Scandinavian Journal of Social Medicine* 24 (1996) 8–13.
38. Holland, P. W. "Statistics and Causal Inference," *Journal of the American Statistical Association* 81 (1986) 945–60.
39. Rubin, D. B. "Estimating Causal Effects of Treatments in Randomized and Nonrandomized Studies," *Journal of Educational Psychology* 66 (1974) 688–701.
40. Pearl, J. *Causality: Models, Reasoning, and Inference.* Cambridge: University Press, 2000.
41. Lilienfeld, D. E. and Stolley, P. D. *Foundations of Epidemiology.* 3rd ed. New York: Oxford University, 1994.
42. Susser, M. and Susser, E. "Choosing a Future for Epidemiology: Eras and Paradigms," *American Journal of Public Health* 86 (1996): 668–73.
43. Susser, M. and Susser, E. "Choosing a Future for Epidemiology: II. from Black Box to Chinese Boxes and Eco-Epidemiology," *American Journal of Public Health* 86 (1996): 674–77.
44. Winkelstein, W. Jr. "Editorial: Eras, Paradigms, and the Future of Epidemiology," *American Journal of Public Health* 86 (1996): 621–22.
45. Lipton, P. "The Medawar Lecture 2004: The Truth about Science," *Philosophical Transactions of the Royal Society B* 360 (2005): 1259–69.
46. Kuhn, T. S. *The Structure of Scientific Revolutions.* 3rd ed. Chicago: University Press, 1999.
47. Fleck, L. *Genesis and Development of a Scientific Fact.* Chicago: University Press, 1981.
48. Vinten-Johansen, P., Brody, H., Paneth, N., Rachman, S., and Rip, M. *Cholera, Chloroform, and the Science of Medicine.* New York: Oxford, 2003.
49. Weed, D. L. "Beyond Black Box Epidemiology," *American Journal of Public Health* 88 (1998): 12–14.
50. Greenland, S., Gago-Dominguez, M., and Castelao, J. E. "The Value of Risk-Factor ('Black-Box') Epidemiology," *Epidemiology* 15 (2004): 529–35.
51. Bhopal, R. "Paradigms in Epidemiology Textbooks: In the Footsteps of Thomas Kuhn," *American Journal of Public Health* 89 (1999): 1162–65.
52. Weed, D. L. "Truth, Epidemiology, and General Causation," *Brooklyn Law Review* 73 (2008): 651–65.
53. Schlesinger, G. N. "Scientists and Philosophy." In *Causal Inference,* ed. K. J. Rothman. Chestnut Hill, MA: ERI 1988: 77–91.
54. Pellegrino, E. D. "Philosophy of Medicine: Problematic and Potential," *Journal of Medicine and Philosophy* 1 (1976): 5–31.
55. Pellegrino, E. D. "Philosophy *of* Medicine: Towards a Definition," *Journal of Medicine and Philosophy* 11 (1986): 9–16.
56. Kitcher, P. *The Advancement of Science: Science without Legend; Objectivity without Illusion.* New York: Oxford University Press, 1993.
57. Longino, H. E. *Science as Social Knowledge.* Princeton: University Press, 1990.
58. Weed, D. L. "Underdetermination and Incommensurability in Contemporary Epidemiology," *Kennedy Institute of Ethics Journal* 7 (1997): 107–27.
59. Weed, D. L. "The Nature and Necessity of Scientific Judgment," *Journal of Law and Policy* 15 (2007): 135–64.

60. Weed, D. L. "Science, Ethics Guidelines, and Advocacy in Epidemiology," *Annals of Epidemiology* 4 (1994): 166–71.
61. Weed, D. L. "Towards a Philosophy of Public Health." *Journal of Epidemiology and Community Health* 53 (1999): 99–104.
62. Weed, D. L. "Epidemiology, the Humanities, and Public Health," *American Journal of Public Health* 85 (1995): 914–18.

II

INFORMED CONSENT, PRIVACY, AND CONFIDENTIALITY

4

Epidemiology and Informed Consent

JEFFREY P. KAHN AND ANNA C. MASTROIANNI

Informed consent is a central concept and practice in the protection of both patients receiving clinical care and individuals participating in research. What began as a commitment to ethical principles has found its way into legal cases concerning the physician-patient relationship, federal policy, and international standards for ethical research on human subjects. The concept and practice of informed consent is interesting in the context of this book because of the unique place occupied by epidemiology. At times epidemiology focuses on providing benefit to individuals affected by illness or disease, which gives it the marks of clinical practice. At other times, it is focused on obtaining information about groups and populations without regard to particular individuals, which makes it more like research. A concrete example is public health surveillance, one of the primary tools of epidemiology. Epidemiological surveillance can be very difficult, and sometimes impossible, to carry out with the informed consent of the individuals from and about whom information is collected.

Given that there is a tension between informed consent and much of epidemiology, this chapter analyzes three core questions: (1) Does epidemiology require informed consent? If so, (2) why and under what conditions? Finally, (3) what special issues, if any, does epidemiology raise for the concept and practice of informed consent?

Does Epidemiology Require Informed Consent?

A central question for this chapter is whether epidemiology requires the informed consent of subjects. Epidemiology occupies an unusual space because it is sometimes focused on public health research (the study of disease patterns among large groups), sometimes practice (infectious disease tracing), and sometimes something in between (surveillance). To the extent that its focus is on the study of disease in groups and populations, epidemiology is squarely within the practice of public health as a staple of local, state, and national public health departments. The requirements and practices of obtaining informed consent might be viewed as paralleling those used in clinical medicine, though with different implications. While informed consent in clinical medicine exists to foster autonomous decision making by patients seeking health care, its goal in public health practice is to assure understanding and protect the right of self-determination of individuals from whom samples and/or information is sought.

Epidemiological research also plays a central role in public health. Its goal is to shed light on incidence, prevalence, and trends of disease across a variety of populations, including workers, students, and geographical groups. When public health efforts involve research that uses group or population data on disease incidence and prevalence, requirements for informed consent of subjects seem to follow from the same justifications on which informed consent in research relies. Consent in population settings can be onerous and rarely succeeds in achieving consent from all members of a population group under study. This problem is recognized in federal policies, which exempt from informed consent requirements any research on records or data such that "the information is recorded by the investigator in such a manner that subjects cannot be identified, directly or through identifiers linked to the subjects."[1] This exemption makes research using population information possible without informed consent, but only if the information lacks personal identifiers. While such epidemiological and other research focused on groups is possible without informed consent, the power of this research and its potential benefits are sometimes undermined by requirements of unidentifiable data.

So how might we answer the question that opened this section, "Does epidemiology require informed consent?" Our answer is a qualified, "Yes." Informed consent is required of subjects in epidemiological research and should be required when the rights and interests of those who are asked to take part in epidemiological practice deserve the sorts of protections offered by informed consent. The bases for such protections are discussed subsequently to place in proper context any discussion of informed consent in epidemiology.

Informed Consent as Autonomous Authorization

Before addressing moral issues specific to epidemiology, we review the meaning and conceptual basis of "informed consent." There are several thorough and excellent accounts of the history and theory of informed consent.[2,3] This section treats these subjects only as needed to guide the discussion in the rest of the chapter.

The objective of the practice of informed consent is to allow individuals to decide for themselves whether to agree to particular diagnostic tests, courses of therapy, or participation in a research project.[2-5] Informed consent is rooted in the notion that the moral principle of respect for autonomy, sometimes termed "respect for persons," is the foundational principle for justifying the practice by which individuals are free to decide whether to pursue a particular treatment or to participate in research. Only individuals who are sufficiently informed and make a voluntary decision can give an *informed consent.*

Faden and Beauchamp's analysis of informed consent requires that one must make an autonomous choice to give a truly informed consent. (Perfunctory signings of consent forms might constitute a legally valid consent without being a truly *informed* consent.) To be autonomous, actions must satisfy three criteria: (1) intentionality, (2) understanding, and (3) non-control.[2] *Intentionality* is the term used to refer to the purpose or plan of one's actions. It refers to a person's intention to act, or being purposeful. This point can be important when groups or communities have a cultural background that may have a strong impact on decision making. For example, some Southeast Asian cultures, such as the Hmong, defer to clan elders rather than engage in individual decision making.[6] In such cases individual intentionality is called into question, and so standard notions of consent are not easily applied. Second, a person must have sufficient *understanding* of what he or she intends. The "informed" part of informed consent presumes that sufficient information is shared with the individual through disclosure and that he or she has sufficient understanding of the information to make a decision that reflects his or her true intentions. This can be a challenge, for instance, in research involving individuals of limited literacy or limited English-speaking proficiency.[6] An individual can have different levels of understanding and an informed consent usually does not entail a full understanding. There need be only a *substantial* understanding of the nature of the proposed action and the positive and negative consequences of a decision.[2] Finally, *non-control* or voluntariness is also fundamental to autonomous actions. Its importance in informed consent is clear and unconditional as a key principle of both the Nuremberg Code and within *The Belmont Report's* articulation of the principle of respect for persons.[7,8] The amount of control over an individual's actions (his or her voluntariness) can be understood as residing on a continuum,[2] with three general types of influence that may undermine voluntariness. Ranked from least to most influence over voluntariness, they are (1) persuasion, (2) manipulation, and (3) coercion.

Persuasion is influence through appeal to reason. When a person is successfully persuaded, he or she acts because the information and reasons presented appeal as arguments. Such influence is free from control and therefore compatible with autonomous actions.[9] At the other end of the continuum is *coercion*, in which a person is caused to act in ways that are against his or her wishes under threat of harm.[10] A coerced action can never reflect autonomous choice because it relies on a response to a credible threat of harm, an example being, "Give me your money or I'll shoot!" On the continuum between persuasion and coercion is *manipulation*, by which influence is exerted over another by taking advantage of weaknesses or by devious behavior. Manipulation carries a sense of falsification or trickery because the manipulator usually has a goal of personal gain. Given the sense of dishonesty connoted by manipulation, it has little place as part of acceptable influence over autonomous decision making.

Informed Consent in Practice and Policy

The discussion thus far has laid out the conceptual and normative underpinnings of informed consent as autonomous decision making. What are the reasons for informed consent in practice and what does the answer to this question hold for our actions in policy? The short answer is that informed consent is a means to preserve the autonomy of individuals and to minimize harm to patients and research subjects. The policies that have evolved over time and the practices that have emanated from them aim to serve these stated goals. Epidemiologists might wonder what sort of harms might befall people as a result of their work and how informed consent is relevant. The epidemiologist's job would be much easier if demographic and other personal information about individuals were linked to disease registries, vital statistics, and other public records. As Capron has put it, a place where meticulously kept, fully linked data is available to epidemiologists would deserve to be called "epidemiologists' heaven." [11] However, such a place would not be free of ethical concerns.

The practice of and laws governing informed consent initially developed out of concerns that patients and research subjects need to be protected from harm at the hands of physicians and medical institutions. This idea dates to the early part of the 20th century, when paternalism on the part of physicians toward patients was the norm rather than the exception. In a groundbreaking 1914 New York State Court of Appeals opinion, *Schloendorff v. Society of New York Hospital*, Justice Benjamin Cardozo wrote that "Every human being of adult years and sound mind has a right to determine what shall be done with his own body; and a surgeon who performs an operation without his patient's consent commits an assault, for which he is liable in damages." [12] This statement came in response to a case brought by a woman who agreed to undergo exploratory surgery, but awoke from surgery to find that she had had a tumor removed by surgeons who deemed it necessary, but who did not ask her permission to do so.

This new legal recognition of the patient's right to give consent to treatment was based in law on respect for self-determination—or, in moral philosophy, on the principle of respect for autonomy. Only in the late 1950s and into the next decade was the notion of "informed" added to consent in the context of medical decision making. This early requirement for information centered on disclosure of relevant information to patients, focusing on the risks and potential benefits of particular courses of action.[13] The standard for what constituted adequate disclosure evolved from a standard focused on professional practice to a standard focused on what patients would need and want to know about risks and possible benefits. This legal evolution occurred in the context of cases addressing voluntary decision making by patients in clinical care.

A similar policy evolution in informed consent occurred in the context of research on human subjects. Starting in the late 1960s and into the mid-1970s, information about unethical research on human subjects was made public. Examples included the infamous Tuskegee Syphilis Study and other well-chronicled studies, such as those conducted at the Willowbrook State School and the New York Jewish Chronic Disease Hospital.[2] These research scandals led to the appointment of influential Congressional commissions, including the Tuskegee Syphilis Study Ad Hoc Advisory Panel[14] and the National Commission for the Protection of Human Subjects of Biomedical and Behavioral Research.

The various scandals pointed to several common problems in studies, including absent or inadequate consent. Also highlighted were the use of subjects from "vulnerable groups" and exposure of the subjects to risk without potential for benefit to them as individuals.[15] Federal officials in the mid and late 1970s focused the government's first federal policies relating to research participation on protecting subjects from harm, using the now-standard Federal nomenclature of "policies for the protection of human subjects."[1] Such protections, which exist in similar form today, included requirements for signed informed consent from all subjects, prospective review and approval of research by Institutional Review Boards (IRBs), assessment of risk-benefit balancing, and limitations on acceptable risk for subjects from groups deemed to deserve additional protections, such as children, prisoners, and pregnant women and fetuses.

Consent as Promotion of Self-determination

The history of informed consent indicates that consent has functioned as a means of promoting and protecting self-determination of individuals. Starting with the legal decision in *Schloendorff*, the concept of self-determination has provided justification for informed consent as a means to protect an individual's right to determine what will happen to his or her body. This idea was articulated later as the principle of respect for persons in *The Belmont Report*, drafted by the National Commission for the Protection of Human Subjects of Biomedical and Behavioral Research to address concerns with exploitation of human subjects in the aftermath of the disclosure of research scandals in the United States.[8] The application of this principle performs at least two functions in contexts in which informed consent is important:

A means to prevent violations of rights to self-determination and a mechanism for allowing informed decision making by individuals asked to participate in research or offered medical care. The second mechanism provides the impetus for important information to be shared and for appropriate risk-benefit balancing to be sought, since research subjects or patients must decide based on the realities of their situation and the information disclosed to them. In these ways, informed consent can help protect both patients and research subjects from the physical or psychological injuries that might occur in research or medical care. While both functions are important, they do not have equally obvious application in all cases in which informed consent may be practiced or required. For epidemiological practice and research, informed consent plays a lesser role in protection from harm, but has more obvious importance in protection from rights violations, as discussed subsequently.

Consent as Functioning to Minimize Research Harms

Since the balancing of the risks and potential benefits of research are best weighed by individuals, informed consent gives prospective research subjects the opportunity to decide (1) whether the risks posed in research constitute harms from their individual perspectives and (2) whether the risks are sufficiently outweighed by potential benefits to be acceptable to them.

The history of informed consent in biomedical research suggests that the perception of research risks has been focused primarily on the physical risks posed by research participation. This practice makes sense in the context of clinical trials, but quickly begins to feel out of place when applied to public health and behavioral research. In behavioral research, subjects may not experience physical risks, but they may be exposed to risks of psychological harm. Public health efforts, such as surveillance or epidemiological research, are less likely to carry psychological risk, except in limited cases in which individual disease status may be stigmatizing and is disclosed to the individual or others, and such efforts have little chance of carrying physical risk. For example, infectious disease testing programs can be critically important for assessing incidence and prevalence of infection. Disclosure of test results for a disease such as influenza might have little psychological impact, whereas disclosure of HIV status to individuals or others can have serious psychological or stigmatizing effects.

In public health contexts, individuals participating in research or those whose information is collected in surveillance efforts may require protection not only from physical or psychological harm but also from some violation of their rights (termed "wrongs"), such as rights to privacy and confidentiality. Because the conceptualization of consent that underpins laws and policies governing informed consent is based largely on reactions to the history of mistreatment of patients or research subjects, the emphasis in policy and practice for protecting individuals from harms or wrongs is both appropriate and understandable.

In addition to concerns about harms and wrongs to individuals, epidemiological studies on populations and groups raise additional issues. Findings related to particular groups can have implications for its members, even when no individual can be linked to his or her own result. For example, in epidemiological research on the prevalence of the BRCA1 genetic mutation (an indicator of an increased lifetime chance of developing breast or other cancers) among women of Ashkenazi ancestry, concerns were expressed about how findings might lead to the stigmatization of the group and even potential insurance or other forms of discrimination toward women identified with that group.[16] The notion that communities and their members can have interests separate from and in addition to those of individuals has led to recommendations for community consultation and even "community consent."[17] The idea of community consent is controversial, raising questions about what characteristics define a group or community, who the relevant stakeholders are, and who from the community or group is authorized to consent on the group's behalf.[18] Nonetheless, there is consensus that the interests of communities and groups ought to be taken into account when planning for, carrying out, and overseeing research involving definable communities (see Chapter 6).[18-20] This can entail public meetings and other forms of consultation with the groups and communities from whom subjects will be recruited, as well as publicity and information in places accessible to those who will be recruited into or affected by the research. These activities can be accomplished in ways that are consistent with research goals and individual consent while respecting the features of groups and communities involved in research.

Finally, policies and practices of informed consent play a useful function in creating an environment of accountability between professionals, patients or subjects, and the institutions in which clinical care, public health practice, and biomedical research are carried out. This environment leads to important expectations for practice on the part of those involved throughout both patient care and the research enterprise and is a crucial aspect of the environment that leads to trust.[15,21] History has proven that lapses in informed consent and inattention to sociocultural experiences in research and within the health-care system can undermine public health efforts and public trust overall.[22-25] Without trust on the part of patients, research participants, and society at large, neither the health-care system nor the research enterprise will function as it should.

Should There Be Special Rules of Informed Consent for Epidemiology?

Given the relevance of informed consent in epidemiology, should there be special rules for informed consent in this context? Should explicit informed consent be required less often than in other kinds of research, given the central role of epidemiology in public health?

Alexander Capron has described the tension in epidemiology as situated between deontological and utilitarian commitments.[11] A deontological or duty-based view holds that research can only proceed when those exposed to its risks knowingly agree to participate, based on ethical duties of truthfulness and respect for individual decision making. This is one type of justification for informed consent. By contrast, a utilitarian might hold that researchers have a moral duty to advance knowledge in ways that improve the good of the whole, based on ethical duties to engage in policies and actions that produce the greatest good for the greatest number of people. The fact that this objective can come at the expense of a few individuals harmed or wronged in research is an acceptable moral cost of serving the greater good. Capron proposes that there need not be a complete resolution of this tension, but that society must "weigh the value of knowledge (both for its own sake and as a means for improving life) against many other values, prime among them autonomy, beneficence [doing good for others] and justice."[11] We live with this tension in epidemiology, negotiating practices and policies that do their utmost to respect these values while collecting the knowledge critical to protecting society.

The challenge for surveillance and other epidemiological methods is how to achieve the laudable goals of public health that underpin efforts to understand illness and disease at the population level while respecting the concepts and principles underlying informed consent. The primary public health authorities in the United States have indicated that there is some flexibility in the need to obtain informed consent if an activity is classified as public health practice.[26,27] This can include (1) activities in which collected data are "directly relevant to disease control needs," and (2) public health surveillance activities in which collected data are "directly relevant to disease monitoring and control needs."[26] The justification appears to be that the expediency required by urgent public health needs outweighs the value of informed consent. Put another way, the potential risks of harms or wrongs to individuals from failing to seek their informed consent is outweighed by the benefit to society from obtaining important public health information. Although this factor is important, the same authorities stress that it is imperative to obtain informed consent whenever feasible.[26-28] For example, the Centers for Disease Control and Prevention (CDC) Epidemiology Program Office has directed that even when an activity is not classified as research ("nonresearch" or "public health practice"), "informed consent should be considered whenever possible for any data collection project involving living persons."[26] International ethical guidelines for epidemiological studies formulated by the Council for International Organizations of Medical Sciences (CIOMS) are more strongly worded, but they still allow for circumstances in which individual consent may not be feasible:

For all epidemiological research involving humans the investigator must obtain the voluntary informed consent of the prospective subject....Waiver of individual informed consent is to be regarded as exceptional, and must in all cases be approved by an ethical review committee unless otherwise permitted under national legislation that conforms to the ethical principles in these Guidelines.[20]

Even in exigent circumstances, such as disease outbreaks, investigators are expected at minimum to disclose information about the investigation and its purpose to the participants.[27] One professional organization states that decisions to "loosen or bypass" informed consent requirements should not be made by individual investigators, but should instead be subject to an appropriate review process.[29] One commentator has suggested that the reliance on exigency to justify waiving the need for informed consent could be overcome by "submit[ting] model protocols and survey methods developed to cover the more predictable investigation types for prior approval."[28] Presumably, this could include a standardized approach to informed consent. Underlying any decision about waiving or loosening informed consent requirements should be assurances that adequate confidentiality protections are in place to minimize the risks associated with the collection and subsequent use of the data.[26,27,29] (See Chapter 5 for a discussion of confidentiality.) For example, public concern about the confidentiality of data collected in a proposed comprehensive diabetes surveillance program in New York prompted the development of an "opt out" procedure for consent, arguably driven by strongly held views on privacy of medical information in the United States.[30]

Some different contexts and approaches in epidemiology make informed consent difficult, if not impossible, to achieve. From tracking individuals as part of disease surveillance, to assessing the prevalence of disease in at-risk populations, to attempting to understand the rates of injury in occupational settings, to assessing the effectiveness of school-based public health education, seeking the informed consent of individuals may easily raise practical and methodological challenges. For example, epidemiologists interested in understanding the course of HIV-related disease in HIV-infected members of the military would need to review medical records to identify appropriate individuals to study, raising questions about consent for records review. Because of the sheer quantity of records involved in such a review, it would be impossible to seek consent from all members of the military before accessing medical records to ascertain HIV infection. In another example, epidemiologists studying workplace injury could be hampered by the need for consent, as workers may be reluctant to participate out of fear of discovery and disclosure of injury-related information that might result in job termination. In addition, public health officials interested in assessing the effects of school-based drug and alcohol education or smoking-cessation may lose important data if consent from students or their parents is required before distributing even anonymous surveys about drug or tobacco use, since some students or their parents will refuse. In addition, the consent process may bias results if students know the purpose of the survey.

In these three examples, the quality of epidemiological information is undermined by the constraints created by attempts to meet the demands of the prospective informed consent of individuals. As we will now see, however, some adaptations may be available to achieve the aforementioned goals of informed consent while allowing important epidemiological work to go forward.

Additional Issues of Informed Consent

As described earlier, federal regulations permit research without informed consent if the research involves existing samples or records in which individuals cannot be identified, provided the research is IRB approved.[1] Capron has argued that while this waiver may be justified by the fact that anonymity adequately protects research subjects from the harms of research, it does not serve the goals of promoting the self-determination of those in research or engendering trust on the part of the public.[11] One suggestion for approximating the goals of informed consent is to seek out members of the community on whom the research will be carried out. Such representatives could participate in the planning and improvement of research. Such a process, whether termed "peer consultation"[31] or "community consultation"[17] can be seen as an adjunct to self-determination of individuals. In working with members of the group of interest, there is also transparency and the public reassurance that comes with it.

One approach to the use of existing records is to obtain permission from those who maintain them and are charged with their safekeeping. While not a substitute for, or even an approximation of informed consent, the permission of and cooperation from these custodians can perform an important function. Since the custodians of records (institutions, employers) have an important relationship with those whose information is sought, their permission could serve as evidence that there is some formal process for seeking use of such records. Examples include records that are held in large repositories that control access to them and provide necessary protections, including all assurances of confidentiality.[32]

In the past, when biomedical research was carried out in settings in which consent was impossible to obtain, such as in emergency settings and intensive care units, proposals had been made for what has been termed "deferred consent." In deferred consent, subjects are informed and debriefed after the research has been conducted.[33] Such processes are more accurately termed deferred *notification* because the research has already been performed and consent is achieved only after the fact, if at all. In the United States, deferred consent in these settings has been superseded by National Institutes of Health and Food and Drug Administration rules on research in emergency settings. These rules rely on community consultation and notification. Epidemiology might take a page from these approaches and give subjects or groups information after studies have been conducted in the form of an effective debriefing, with or without the option to have their information removed on request, and use processes of community consultation and notification where appropriate.

Conclusion

A challenge in epidemiology is how to achieve vital goals of public health while respecting the goals of informed consent. To gain information through the tools of epidemiology, the public health community ought to work with policy makers to seek flexible approaches to informed consent requirements where they can be justified, including adjuncts to individual consent in some cases.

References

1. U.S. Department of Health and Human Services. *Basic HHS Policy for Protection of Human Research Subjects.* 45 C.F.R. § 46 (2005).
2. Faden, R. R. and Beauchamp, T. L. *A History and Theory of Informed Consent.* New York: Oxford University Press, 1986.
3. Katz, J. *The Silent World of Doctor and Patient.* New York: Free Press, 1984.
4. National Bioethics Advisory Commission. *Research Involving Human Biological Materials: Ethical Issues and Policy Guidance.* 1999. Available at http://www.bioethics.gov/reports/past_commissions/nbac_biological1.pdf, accessed April 18, 2008.
5. President's Commission for the Study of Ethical Problems in Medicine and Biomedical and Behavioral Research. *Protecting Human Subjects: The Adequacy and Uniformity of Federal Rules and Their Implementation.* Washington, DC: U.S. Government Printing Office, 1981. Available at http://www.bioethics.gov/reports/past_commissions/Protecting_Human_Subjects.pdf, accessed April 18, 2008.
6. Andrulis, D. P., and Brach, C., "Integrating Literacy, Culture, and Language to Improve Health Care Quality for Diverse Populations," *American Journal of Health Behavior* 31 (2007); S122–S133.
7. "Nuremberg Code." In *Trials of War Criminals before the Nuremberg Military Tribunals under Control Council Law No. 10.* Vol. 2. Washington, DC: U.S. Government Printing Office, 1949: 181–82.
8. National Commission for the Protection of Human Subjects of Biomedical and Behavioral Research. *The Belmont Report.* Washington, DC: U.S. Government Printing Office, 1979.
9. Benn, S. "Freedom and Persuasion," *Australasian Journal of Philosophy* 45 (1967): 259–75.
10. Nozick, R. "Coercion." In *Philosophy, Science, and Method: Essays in Honor of Ernest Nagel*, ed. S. Morgenbesser, P. Suppes, and M. White. New York: St. Martin's Press, 1969: 440–72.
11. Capron A. M. "Protection of Research Subjects: Do Special Rules Apply in Epidemiology?" *Law, Medicine and Health Care* 19 (1991): 184–90.
12. *Schloendorff v. Society of New York Hospital*, 211 N.Y. 125, 105 N.E. 92 (1914).

13. *Salgo v. Leland Stanford Jr. University Board of Trustees*, 154 Cal. App. 2d 560, 317 P.2d 170 (1957); *Natanson v. Kline*, 186 Kan. 393, 350 P. 2d 1093 (1960); *Canterbury v. Spence*, 464 F.2d 772 (D.C. Cir. 1972).
14. Tuskegee Syphilis Study Ad Hoc Advisory Panel. *Final Report of the Tuskegee Syphilis Study Ad Hoc Advisory Panel*. Washington, DC: U.S. Government Printing Office, 1973. Available at http://www.research.usf.edu/cs/library/docs/finalreport-tuskegeestudyadvisorypanel.pdf, accessed April 18, 2008.
15. Mastroianni, A. and Kahn, J. "Swinging on the Pendulum: Shifting Views of Justice in Human Subject Research," *Hastings Center Report* 31 (2001): 21–28.
16. Modan, B. "The Genetic Passport," *American Journal of Epidemiology* 147 (1998): 513–15.
17. Weijer, C. and Emanuel, E. J. "Protecting Communities in Biomedical Research," *Science* 289 (2000): 1142–44.
18. Dickert, N. and Sugarman, J. "Ethical Goals of Community Consultation in Research," *American Journal of Public Health* 95 (2005): 1123–27.
19. "Policy for the Responsible Collection, Storage, and Research Use of Samples from Named Populations for the NIGMS Human Genetic Cell Repository," August 25, 2004. Available at: http://ccr.coriell.org/Sections/Support/NIGMS/CollPolicy.aspx?PgId=220, accessed April 18, 2008.
20. Council for International Organizations of Medical Sciences. *International Guidelines for Ethical Review of Epidemiological Studies* (provisional text pending printed version). Geneva: CIOMS, 2008. Available at http://www.cioms.ch/080221feb_2008.pdf, accessed April 18, 2008.
21. Mastroianni, A. "Sustaining Public Trust: Falling Short in the Protection of Human Research Participants," *Hastings Center Report* 38 (2008): 8–9.
22. Gamble, V. N. "A Legacy of Distrust: African Americans and Medical Research," *American Journal of Preventive Medicine* 9 (1993): 35–38.
23. Gamble, V. N. "Under the Shadow of Tuskegee: African Americans and Health Care," *American Journal of Public Health* 11 (1997): 1773–78.
24. Corbie-Smith, G. "The Continuing Legacy of the Tuskegee Syphilis Study: Considerations for Clinical Investigation," *American Journal of the Medical Sciences* 317 (1999): 5–8.
25. Smith Y. R., Johnson A. M., Newman L. A., et al. "Perceptions of Clinical Research Participation Among African American Women," *Journal of Women's Health* 16 (2007): 423–28.
26. U.S. Centers for Disease Control and Prevention, Epidemiology Program Office. Overview of Scientific Procedures, Section II.A., Research vs. Non Research, 2002. Available at http://www.cdc.gov/epo/ads/section-iia.htm, accessed April 18, 2008.
27. American College of Epidemiology, "Ethics Guidelines," January 2000. Available at http://www.acepidemiology.org/policystmts/EthicsGuide.htm, accessed December 12, 2007.
28. Cone, J. "Ethical Issues in Occupational Disease Outbreak Investigations," *Occupational Medicine* 17 (2002): 657–63.
29. International Society for Environmental Epidemiology. "Ethics Guidelines for Environmental Epidemiologists." 1999. Available at http://www.iseepi.org/about/ethics.html#Ethics_Guidelines, accessed April 18, 2008.
30. Fairchild, A. "Diabetes and Disease Surveillance," *Science* 313 (2006): 175–76.
31. Baumrind, D. "Nature and Definition of Informed Consent in Research Involving Deception." In *The Belmont Report: Ethical Principles and Guidelines for the*

Protection of Human Subjects of Research, Appendix Vol. II. Washington, DC: U.S. Government Printing Office, 1978: 23.1–23.71.

32. Citro, C. F., Iglen, D. R., and Marrett, C. B., eds. *Protecting Participants and Facilitating Social and Behavioral Sciences Research.* Washington DC: National Academy Press, 2003.

33. Levine, R. "Research in Emergency Situations: The Role of Deferred Consent," *JAMA* 273 (1995): 1300–02.

5

Privacy and Confidentiality in Epidemiology: Special Challenges of Using Information Obtained without Informed Consent

ELLEN WRIGHT CLAYTON

The ability to obtain information about individuals is expanding as a result of new technologies that permit the collection and manipulation of massive amounts of electronic data. The discipline of epidemiology uses such data about individuals to enhance our understanding of diseases and their causes. Some of these investigations lead in some cases to scholarly publications. In other cases, governmental agencies use the results of epidemiologic research to inform their policies. Public health agencies actively use certain types of personal health information to protect individuals. Sometimes, this can require revealing information about one person to another. The prototypical example is contact tracing, in which public health officials having learned that a particular person has a contagious disease track down others who have been exposed to provide treatment, or if appropriate, prophylaxis. Society values and increasingly requires research and public health activities because of their benefits for individuals and society.

These advances in science and in protecting public health come with a cost. The process of gathering, analyzing, and applying this information in many cases invades privacy and accesses data that some people believe should not be shared. Many people in the United States, Canada, and the United Kingdom are reluctant to permit their clinical records and stored tissues to be used for research.[1-7] They are even more reticent when these data and samples were collected in the course of clinical care without specific consent for other uses. This chapter addresses the particular challenges posed by epidemiology and public health activities conducted without informed consent since these are the most vexing. It should be noted, however, that informed consent, even when obtained, may not address all the harms and wrongs that may accompany invasion of privacy and breach of confidentiality. The goals of this chapter are to address the following questions:

- What values underlie privacy and confidentiality and what consequences follow from their breach?
- What values justify intrusion upon privacy and confidentiality without consent? Under what circumstances and by whom? How are these decisions to be made?
- What personal information can be disclosed? When? To whom?

The values of individual privacy, confidentiality, and public goods cannot always be reconciled, so trade-offs are often required. We then turn to the laws and regulations that address these issues, identifying some of the ways in which they conflict with or fail to address these ethical issues.

Privacy, Confidentiality, and Common Goods

People care about controlling personal information, even though they at times choose to sell it quite cheaply, for example, to obtain discounts at a grocery store. They may feel, for example, that their sense of identity depends in part on the ability to exclude others from some aspects of their lives. Control of information does not matter solely to individuals, however, for society also benefits from it. Social interactions are shaped in many ways by the individual's ability to control information about him- or herself. The U.S. Constitution, by reserving to the people those powers not expressly given to the government, embodies the notion that the government should not have unlimited access to the lives of its people.

Individuals also fear harms that may result from disclosure of information about them, harms that may occur in many aspects of a person's life. The case of HIV, particularly in the earlier years of the epidemic, illustrates these harms. Infected children were excluded from school and shunned by their peers. Workers were fired. People found themselves unable to obtain health and life insurance. The fact that HIV was more prevalent among certain populations, such as IV drug users, males with hemophilia, and homosexuals, meant that members of these groups were stigmatized even when they were not infected. Indeed, the problem of group harm has become an increasingly important issue in epidemiologic research and public health intervention.

On closer analysis, people assert two related, but separate interests regarding the control of personal information. The first interest is privacy, which means that people are entitled to keep private certain information. Whether this interest extends to information that cannot readily be linked with the individual, a question of particular import to much of epidemiology, is contested. Some argue that people may nonetheless be concerned, reasoning that people feel as if they have been wronged if a person comes into their house and examines their belongings, even if the intruder takes nothing and does not know whose house he entered.[8] Others, however, assert that no privacy interests worthy of protection remain if the investigator does not know to whom the information applies.[9]

The second interest is confidentiality, which means that under certain circumstances, a person can disclose his or her private information to another with the expectation that it will not be disseminated more broadly. For instance, the patient who discloses private information to her physician can expect that the physician will not reveal it to others.[10] The duty of many professionals both inside and outside of health care to honor confidentiality is based in part on respect for the person to whom the information applies. This duty has an important utilitarian purpose as well. People are more likely to reveal personal information if they believe that it will be protected by the individuals to whom they reveal it. The clinician, lawyer, or clergy may need such data to give appropriate advice. It may be very important for a physician to know, for example, that her patient engages in risky health behaviors, such as using illegal drugs or having unprotected sex with multiple partners.

As important as privacy and confidentiality are, these interests at times must give way to other goods. Several distinctions are critical here. One is that there are several different potentially desirable goals: first, the benefit of greater scientific understanding (research by epidemiologists and other investigators can increase the efficiency of health care and prevention activities and help eliminate health disparities); second, the assessment of the health status of the public for purposes of planning; and finally, intervention to protect specific individuals including those who are currently ill as well as those at risk, benefits that run both to the persons at risk as well as society at large.

It also matters who is pursuing these goals and under what auspices. Research is conducted by many people and organizations that can have a variety of interests and obligations. Investigators working for industry, for instance, have different pressures on them than do those in the academic environment, which differ in turn from those experienced by those who work for the government. All of these actors are accountable for their actions in different ways, and with varying degrees of public transparency. Surveillance and specific intervention can be performed by state actors who typically act with specific statutory or regulatory authority. Public health agencies, for example, are required by statute and regulation to collect a variety of information and to engage in contact tracing. They, however, are not the only actors who monitor and intervene. Employers, for example, can perform surveillance of the workplace, and health-care providers may decide to warn at risk relatives. The legal and ethical justifications for these actions by employers and clinicians may be less clear.

The variety of goods, actions, and actors makes it impossible to identify a single balance between privacy and confidentiality and other goods, both public and private, that applies in all circumstances. Some advocate that public goods and notions of solidarity have been underemphasized in many Western societies and that we must alter the balance to give less weight to individual autonomy.[11] Some commentators also urge that public health surveillance and intervention are central to the inherent functions of government, and so justify greater levels of intrusion on the individual in exchange for the benefits of living in society.[12,13] Others frame this point differently, arguing that the existence of legal authority resulting from the political process, from the votes of the people, provides greater legitimacy to the actions of public health agencies.[14]

The research enterprise and public health activities involve complex choices about which actions to pursue at what costs, including the impact on the privacy interests of individuals. The process by which these decisions are made is important. Research and public health practice depend on the public's trust, and transparency in decision making is particularly important to earn society's confidence in the face of great complexity. Mechanisms are needed, therefore, to make clear the trade-offs that are being made in epidemiologic activities and to ensure that the privacy protections agreed upon are implemented effectively. These include publicly accountable oversight with community participation.

Characteristics of Data Sets

A basic premise of contemporary professional ethics is that privacy and confidentiality should be compromised, if at all, only to the extent necessary to achieve the desired public goal. Several corollaries follow from this premise, some of which have implications for how data is obtained and stored. Investigators should use data sets that contain as few pieces of identifying information—for example, name, address, social security number, date of birth—as possible. In the past, even if researchers ultimately removed identifiers from data sets, they had to extract information from individual medical records initially by hand. This step necessarily invaded privacy. In this regard, the electronic medical record (EMR) is a two-edged sword. While permitting much greater access and hence potentially a much greater threat to privacy, the EMR now makes it possible to create data sets that contain no identifiers without ever looking at individual records. Indeed, much effort is now being devoted at Vanderbilt and other institutions to create de-identified data sets that combine information from medical records and genetic testing, which can then be updated as new clinical data becomes available.[15,16] The extent to which these efforts will be successful either in creating usable data for research or in truly protecting identity is currently the topic of research.

Even if new methods of creating de-identified but interactive data sets are effective, there will be situations in which identified information is required. The clearest example is contact tracing in public health interventions, which is justified by the need to prevent harm to specific individuals. Deciding when the cost of removing identifiers, in terms of both money and the loss of data that necessarily accompanies de-identification, is too great can be a more difficult problem.[17]

Epidemiologists should use the least amount of information necessary to achieve the desired result. In the past, the burden of extracting data could make it tempting to gather as much as possible to avoid the need to go back. Current information technologies can decrease the risk to privacy by making it easy to search a limited number of data categories without first extracting the data from other sources.

Data Security

All researchers have an obligation to protect the data they use. Epidemiologists and public health officials typically do an excellent job of this, but lapses and intentional breaches do occur from time to time.[18] One of the most notorious is the release to the press a decade ago of the names of almost 4000 people infected with HIV in the Tampa, Florida area.[19] In 2005, a Palm Beach County, Florida statistician accidentally emailed a confidential list of names of 6500 people with HIV/AIDS to almost 1000 other health department employees.[20] Events like these demonstrate the need for ensuring data security. Yet studies have revealed more pervasive gaps in the security practices of state public health agencies.[21] The importance of providing security cannot be understated, as patients have stated that they would be more comfortable with epidemiologic research if they were convinced that access would be limited to authorized personnel and that the information was actually secure.[22] Both mechanical approaches to protect data from hackers, such as encryption and firewalls, and policies of accountability and transparency are required.

The Challenge of Open Access to Research Data

Pressure is growing to make data used for research more broadly available. One reason for this pressure is the desire to combine datasets to increase statistical power of studies.[23] Greater availability of data also enables other investigators to conduct further analyses on other problems or to reanalyze the data to reaffirm or challenge the original conclusions. The forces behind open access are many. One is the basic, albeit embattled, ethos of science that resources should be shared to advance knowledge, particularly when the data was acquired in the course of publicly funded research.[24] Another is the desire of commercial entities to challenge the science on which regulatory decisions and the outcomes of litigation are based. The concerns of business led to the enactment of the U.S. Data Quality Act in late 2000, which allows individuals and companies to access and reanalyze data on which regulations are based. This statute has already been invoked on numerous occasions.[25] If sharing data is to be permitted, one major question is to what extent identifiers can and should be removed before data are shared with others.

Some Special Challenges for Research Design

Respect for privacy and confidentiality can affect the ability to recruit research participants. For example, when investigators ask clinicians to recruit their patients to be participants, some institutional review boards (IRBs) worry that this practice both creates the possibility of undue influence and invades the privacy of patients because their provider could know what they decided. As a result, it is becoming more common to use strategies that do not allow practitioners to know which of their patients are taking part in a research protocol and which are not. Some have argued, however, that these less direct approaches can make recruitment prohibitive because patients are often less receptive to requests from investigators they do not know.[26]

Other challenges abound as well. Epidemiologists trying to understand the myriad genetic and social factors that contribute to disease increasingly seek information about the relatives of research participants and the environments in which they live. In 2000, however, a man complained that his privacy was violated when his daughter received a questionnaire that included questions about family history as part of a twin study conducted by Virginia Commonwealth University. The Office for Protection from Research Risks (the predecessor to the Office of Human Research Protections) concurred, causing many investigators to wonder whether it would be possible to conduct research without the individual consent of each person about whom information was obtained.[27] One lesson learned from this event is that IRBs must consider the privacy interests of others in reviewing protocols. In light of this experience, Jeffrey Botkin proposed guidelines to help IRBs determine when informed consent from everyone about whom information is obtained is not required. In some cases, the family members are not human subjects because they are not readily identifiable or because the information sought is not private. In other cases, conditions exist that justify waiver.[28]

Using Research Results

THE PROBLEM OF GROUP HARM The purpose of conducting epidemiologic investigations is to use the knowledge gained to inform policy making or directed intervention. Individuals and groups, however, may be adversely affected as a result of such investigations. Even analyses of aggregated data without identifiers have the potential to harm groups and their members. One need only recall the stigmatization of homosexuals and males with hemophilia in the early days of the HIV epidemic. Although these consequences do not result from direct invasions of privacy or breaches of confidentiality, several efforts to increase transparency have emerged. Many projects now involve an aspect of community engagement,[29] which can range from setting up mechanisms for reporting general research results to the group or its representatives to full participation in the planning, execution, and publication of the research. The extent of the community's involvement depends on a variety of factors, including the severity of the foreseeable risk and the extent to which the group affected can be readily defined and has an identifiable form of self-governance.[30,31] In addition, investigators must take care in how they describe their findings and the groups to which they apply to avoid mischaracterization or overgeneralization.[32,33] One of the areas in which concern about the precision of reporting research results has been debated is the appropriateness of correlating social categories such as race with patterns of genetic variation.[34,35] Questions of group harm arise in almost every project that addresses stigmatizing conditions or socially disadvantaged groups.

DISCLOSING RESULTS TO RESEARCH PARTICIPANTS A common ethical question raised by the use of identified information is whether to disclose individual results to research participants. Consistent with many earlier commentators, the National Bioethics Advisory Commission suggested that

IRBs should develop general guidelines for the disclosure of the results of research to subjects and require investigators to address these issues explicitly in their research plans. In general, these guidelines should reflect the presumption that the disclosure of research results to subjects represents an exceptional circumstance. Such disclosure should occur only when all of the following apply:

a) the findings are scientifically valid and confirmed,
b) the findings have significant implications for the subject's health concerns, and
c) a course of action to ameliorate or treat these concerns is readily available.[36]

In projects that seek specific consent, IRBs might require the investigator to explain the concept of clinical utility and ask participants if they want to be recontacted, for what types of conditions (how serious, how treatable), and if so, how they want to be told (by their primary provider or directly). The IOM's Committee on Assessing Genetic Risks in an earlier report set out similar criteria and suggested further that an investigator who wishes to disclose personal results for which the participant had not previously consented needs to justify this desire to an oversight body.[37] This process ensures that the evidence of value meets these standards.

Not all agree with these recommendations. Many participants expect to receive results. Some commentators now urge that these desires should be fulfilled out of respect for individuals, even in the absence of demonstrated clinical utility.[38–41]

Disclosure, however, raises a number of difficulties. When research was conducted without consent at the outset, disclosing results reveals to an individual that information about them was being used in research. The person may be upset by this revelation since most people in the United States, when asked, believe their permission should be sought before data about them, especially data acquired in the course of clinical care, is used in research. The person may also feel trapped into getting information that he or she otherwise might not have chosen to receive. It is difficult to say no when someone says, "I know something about you that you do not know. Do you want to know it?" Yet when people are given a choice before testing, they often elect not to proceed.[42–44] Revealing results also promotes the therapeutic misconception, which is the frequently misplaced belief that the goal of research is to provide immediate clinical benefit to a particular research participant. Investigators themselves may overestimate the utility of a research result, perhaps reflecting their enthusiasm for their work. And finally, in the United States, it is usually illegal to disclose research results that were obtained in a laboratory that was not certified under the Clinical Laboratory Improvement Act (CLIA).[45] That law was enacted in part to ensure that patients receive their own, accurate test results by requiring optimal tracking and performance of tests. There is more opportunity for error in research laboratories, which typically do not follow the procedures mandated in the clinical setting.

DISCLOSING RESEARCH RESULTS TO RELATIVES AND CLOSE CONTACTS One common question in both clinical and research ethics is whether and when it is permissible or required to disclose information about a patient to another person at risk, thereby breaching the patient's confidentiality.[45] Historically, this issue has arisen primarily in two settings, the patient who has a contagious disease and the mentally ill patient who has threatened to kill another person. In both cases, disclosure is generally thought to be warranted to prevent serious risk of harm, although the procedures for warning differ dramatically in the two cases. States require that clinicians report specific infectious diseases to public health officials who then are responsible for contact tracing. As a result, there is little reason for the clinician directly to warn individuals put at risk by exposure to one of their patients whose illness is contagious. By contrast, a number of courts have held that a mental health professional can be subject to damages when a patient reveals a credible plan to harm a particular individual and then carries out the threat. More recently, commentators have considered whether it is ever appropriate to warn relatives about genetic risks.[46–49] Most have concluded that these disclosures are permissible, if at all,

only if several conditions are satisfied: (1) reasonable efforts to elicit voluntary consent to disclosure have failed; (2) there is a high probability both that harm will occur if the information is withheld and that the disclosed information will actually be used to avert harm; (3) the harm that identifiable individuals would suffer would be serious; and

(4) appropriate precautions are taken to ensure that only the genetic information needed for diagnosis and/or treatment of the disease in question is disclosed.[50]

Thus, even in the clinical setting, the burden that must be met to justify disclosure of information about one person without consent to others is quite high. Moreover, patients usually believe that they are personally obliged to warn individuals at risk and would prefer to make disclosures themselves.[22,51] Clinicians should work with patients who are reluctant to share information, seeking to understand the reasons for their reticence and offering to provide assistance. Overriding patients' refusals should be a course of last resort even in the clinic.

The bar should be even higher in the research setting. The finding must be sufficiently important to warrant disclosure to the research participant him- or herself, meeting the substantive and procedural criteria set forth in the preceding section. That hurdle alone would mean disclosure of research results to third parties is permissible only in very rare circumstances.

REGULATORY CHALLENGES In the United States, some of the most important bodies of applicable law are the Common Rule for the protection of human subjects in federally funded research[52] and the Privacy Rule promulgated under the Health Insurance Portability and Accountability Act (HIPAA) to govern disclosures of information collected in the course of health care.[53] Many states have privacy laws as well, but their provisions vary widely, which has led one group of analysts to propose a new model state public health privacy law.[54] (The widely differing provisions of international rules governing epidemiologic research and public health activities are beyond the scope of this discussion, but they create additional complexity in our increasingly globalized world.[55])

Further complicating the analysis is the fact that the federal laws apply differently to different activities within the broad spectrum encompassed within epidemiology. The Common Rule for the protection of research participants, for example, applies to federally funded research. The lines between research and public health activities such as surveillance, however, can be blurry, potentially creating uncertainty for public health actors.[56,57] Some argue, however, that public health agencies are and should be completely exempt from the Common Rule even when conducting research.[56] At the same time, health care providers and their institutions are often reluctant to provide patient information for public health purposes even though the HIPAA Privacy Rule permits them to do so.[58] When both rules apply, their provisions at times conflict.[59]

One strategy that can avoid some conflicts between the Common Rule and the Privacy Rule is using de-identified information. Unfortunately, the two rules have different approaches to deciding what is de-identified. The Common Rule says that it does not apply to research using information the investigator has recorded "in such a manner that subjects cannot be identified, directly or through identifiers linked to the subjects."[60] It then goes on to say that "[p]rivate information must be individually identifiable (i.e., the identity of the subject is or may readily be ascertained by the investigator or associated with the information) in order for obtaining the information to constitute research involving human subjects," hence subject to the Common Rule.[52] Concepts such as "readily ascertainable" are nowhere defined. The Office of Human Research Protection (OHRP) in a recent interpretation made clear its view that most research using coded information or specimens falls outside the coverage of the Common Rule.[61]

The Privacy Rule, which applies only to information, sets forth much more strict standards for information to be deemed de-identified and hence exempt from its coverage. Either a "person with appropriate knowledge of and experience with generally accepted statistical and scientific principles and methods for rendering information not individually identifiable, ... [a]pplying such principles and methods, determines that the risk is very small that the information could be used, alone or in combination with other reasonably available information, by an anticipated recipient to identify an individual who is a subject of the information," or 18 specific types of information must be removed (see Box 5.1).[62] Coded information can also be considered de-identified and hence exempt so long as the code itself is not derived from individual health information. Research using so-called "limited data sets" from which 16 of the 18 types of information have been removed is also exempt so long as the researcher has executed a data use agreement. As a result, epidemiology research conducted in an academic institution using minimally coded samples and information could be exempt from the Common Rule but still subject to the Privacy Rule and so require authorization under HIPAA before research can proceed.

Box 5–1. Eighteen HIPAA identifiers

1. Names
2. All geographical subdivisions smaller than a State, including street address, city, county, precinct, zip code, and their equivalent geocodes, except for the initial three digits of a zip code, if according to the current publicly available data from the Bureau of the Census: (1) The geographic unit formed by combining all zip codes with the same three initial digits contains more than 20,000 people; and (2) The initial three digits of a zip code for all such geographic units containing 20,000 or fewer people is changed to 000
3. All elements of dates (except year) for dates directly related to an individual, including birth date, admission date, discharge date, date of death; and all ages over 89 and all elements of dates (including year) indicative of such age, except that such ages and elements may be aggregated into a single category of age 90 or older

Continued

Box 5–1. Continued

---

4. Phone numbers
5. Fax numbers
6. Electronic mail addresses
7. Social Security numbers
8. Medical record numbers
9. Health plan beneficiary numbers
10. Account numbers
11. Certificate/license numbers
12. Vehicle identifiers and serial numbers, including license plate numbers
13. Device identifiers and serial numbers
14. Web Universal Resource Locators (URLs)
15. Internet Protocol (IP) address numbers
16. Biometric identifiers, including finger and voice prints
17. Full face photographic images and any comparable images
18. Any other unique identifying number, characteristic, or code (note this does not mean the unique code assigned by the investigator to code the data)

These rules leave major gaps in oversight. The Common Rule has never applied to institutions that do not receive federal funds, but the areas in which informed consent and IRB review are not required have gotten larger. While all agencies of the Department of Health and Human Services, including the Centers for Disease Control and Prevention, adhere to the Common Rule, its application to state public health agencies is less clear. Even for academic institutions that receive federal research funds, the Office of Human Research Protection (OHRP) acknowledged that, under its interpretation, most research involving coded samples and information is not legally required to undergo review by IRBs. The OHRP could only suggest that institutions conducting research identify some body or entity to provide supervision for these projects. For most academic institutions, this represented a major shift in policy, and many IRBs have continued to require some sort of review. The oversight required under the HIPAA privacy rule is less well specified than that of IRBs, and in any event, the Privacy Rule applies only to covered entities and exempts public health activities. The activities of public health agencies are subject to political supervision, which varies from state to state. In sum, different standards and procedures apply to the oversight of epidemiologic activities, and for a growing number of these endeavors, federal and state laws require no review at all. This legal patchwork is hardly conducive to the transparency in decision making that is needed to ensure that intrusions on privacy interests are identified, justified, and limited to the extent possible.

Conclusion

Epidemiologic investigators and public health agencies seek information about people for a host of reasons, which must be weighed against individuals' interests in their own privacy. Some basic principles should guide this process, despite the huge gaps in oversight that currently exist in U.S. law. Although privacy interests should always be invaded as little as necessary to achieve the desired goal, more urgent public goods may warrant greater intrusion on individual interests. The process by which these trade-offs are made must be transparent, and those who would intrude on personal privacy must be able to document their decisions and their actions if epidemiologists are to retain and build upon the public's trust.

ACKNOWLEDGMENT

I would like to thank Mark Rothstein for his helpful comments on an earlier version of this chapter.

References

1. Wang, S. S., Fridinger, F., Sheedy, K. M., and Khoury, M. J. "Public Attitudes Regarding the Donation and Storage of Blood Specimens for Genetic Research," *Community Genetics* 4 (2001): 18–26.
2. Baker, R., Shiels, C., Stevenson, K., Fraser, R., and Stone, M. "What Proportion of Patients Refuse Consent to Data Collection from Their Records for Research Purposes?" *British Journal of General Practice* 50 (2000): 655–56.
3. Goodson, M. L. and Vernon, B. G. "A Study of Public Opinion on the Use of Tissue Samples from Living Subjects for Clinical Research," *Journal of Clinical Pathology* 57 (2004): 135–38.
4. Willison, D. "Privacy and The Secondary Use of Data for Health Research: Experience in Canada and Suggested Directions Forward," *Journal of Health Services Research and Policy* 8, Suppl 1 (2003): S1:17–23.
5. Robling, M. R., Hood, K., Houston, H., Pill, R., Fay, J., and Evans, H. M. "Public Attitudes towards the Use of Primary Care Patient Record Data in Medical Research without Consent: A Qualitative Study," *Journal of Medical Ethics* 30 (2004): 104–09.
6. Schwartz, M. D., Rothenberg, K., Joseph, L., Benkendorf, J., and Lerman, C. "Consent to the Use of Stored DNA for Genetics Research: A Survey of Attitudes in the Jewish Population," *American Journal of Medical Genetics* 98 (2001): 336–42.
7. Wendler, D. and Emanuel, E. "The Debate Over Research on Stored Biological Samples: What Do Sources Think?" *Archives of Internal Medicine* 162 (2002): 1457–62.
8. Capron, A. M. "Protection of Research Subjects: Do Special Rules Apply in Epidemiology?" *Journal of Clinical Epidemiology* 44, Suppl. 1 (1991): 81S–89S.
9. Gostin, L. O. "Health Information: Reconciling Personal Privacy with the Public Good of Human Health," *Health Care Analysis* 9 (2001): 321–35.

10. Beauchamp, T. L. and Childress, J. F. *Principles of Biomedical Ethics*. 6th ed. New York: Oxford University Press, 2009.
11. Knoppers, B. M. "Of Genomics and Public Health: Building Public 'Goods'?" *Canadian Medical Association Journal* 173 (2005): 1185–86.
12. Gostin, L. O., Hodge, J. G., and Valdiserri, R. O. "Informational Privacy and the Public's Health: The Model State Public Health Privacy Act," *American Journal of Public Health* 91 (2001): 1388–92.
13. Hodge, J. G., Gostin, L. O., with the Council for State and Territorial Epidemiologists Advisory Committee. *Public Health Practice vs. Research: A Report for Public Health Practitioners Including Cases and Guidance for Making Distinctions*, 2004. Available at http://www.cste.org/pdffiles/newpdffiles/CSTEPHResRptHodgeFinal.5.24.04.pdf, accessed May 21, 2006.
14. Rothstein, M. A. "Rethinking the Meaning of Public Health," *American Journal of Law, Medicine, and Ethics* 30 (2002): 144–49.
15. Marshfield Clinic Research Foundation. *Personalized Medicine Research Project*, 2007. Available at http://marshfieldclinic.org/chg/pages/default.aspx?page=chg_pers_med_res_prj., accessed August 7, 2007.
16. Roden, D.M., Pulley, J.M., Basford, M.A., et al. "Development of a Large-scale De-identified DNA Biobank to Enable Personalized Medicine," *Clinical Pharmacology and Therapeutics* 80 (2008): 362–9.
17. Fefferman, N. H., O'Neil, E. A., and Naumova, E. "Confidentiality and Confidence: Is Data Aggregation a Means to Achieve Both?" *Journal of Public Health Policy* 26 (2005): 430–49.
18. Wynia, M. K., Coughlin, S. S., Alpert, S., Cummins, D. S., and Emanuel, L. L. "Shared Expectations for Protection of Identifiable Health Care Information: Report of a National Consensus Process," *Journal of General Internal Medicine* 16 (2001): 100–11.
19. Palosky, C. S. "AIDS Leak Sparks Privacy Concerns," *Tampa Tribune* October 7, 1996, 1. Available at http://www.lexisnexis.com/us/lnacademic/search/omesubmitForm.do, accessed October 20, 2008.
20. Henry J. Kaiser Family Foundation. *Palm Beach County, Fla., Official Accidentally E-Mails Confidential List of HIV-Positive People to Health Dept. Employees*. Available at http://www.thebody.com/content/art9263.html., accessed August 5, 2007.
21. O'Brien, D. G. and Yasnoff, W. A. "Privacy, Confidentiality, and Security in Information Systems of State Health Agencies," *American Journal of Preventive Medicine* 16 (1999): 351–58.
22. Plantinga, L., Natowicz, M. R., Kass, N. E., Hull, S. C., Gostin, L. O., and Faden, R. R. "Disclosure, Confidentiality, and Families: Experiences and Attitudes of Those with Genetic versus Nongenetic Medical Conditions," *American Journal of Medical Genetics Part C* 119C (2003): 51–59.
23. Office of Extramural Research, NIH. *Genome-Wide Association Studies (GWAS)*, 2007. Available at http://grants.nih.gov/grants/gwas/index.htm., accessed August 6, 2007.
24. Neutra, R. R., Cohen, A., Fletcher, T., Michaels, D., Richter, E. D., and Soskolne, C. L. "Toward Guidelines for the Ethical Reanalysis and Reinterpretation of Another's Research," *Epidemiology* 17 (2006): 335–38.
25. Rosenstock, L. "Protecting Special Interests in the Name of 'Good Science'," *Journal of the American Medical Association* 295 (2006): 2407–10.

26. Ward, H. J., Cousens, S. N., Smith-Bathgate, B., Leitch, M., Everington, D., Will, R. G., and Smith, P. G. "Obstacles to Conducting Epidemiological Research in the UK General Population," *British Medical Journal* 329 (2004): 277–79.

27. Amber, D. "Case at VCU Brings Ethics to Forefront," *The Scientist* 14 (2000): 1, available at http://www.the-scientist.com/article/display/11831/, accessed on October 20, 2008.

28. Botkin, J. R. "Protecting the Privacy and Confidentiality of Family Members in Survey and Pedigree Research," *Journal of the American Medical Association* 285 (2001): 207–11.

29. American College of Epidemiology. "Ethics Guidelines," *Annals of Epidemiology* 10 (2000): 487–97.

30. Kaufman, C. E. and Ramarao, S. "Community Confidentiality, Consent, and the Individual Research Process: Implications for Demographic Research," *Population Research and Policy Review* 24 (2005): 149–73.

31. Foster, M. W., Sharp, R. R., Freeman, W. L., Chino, M., Bernsten, D., and Carter, T. H. "The Role of Community Review in Evaluating the Risks of Human Genetic Variation Research," *American Journal of Human Genetics* 64 (1999): 1719–27.

32. International HapMap Consortium. "Integrating Ethics and Science in the International HapMap Project," *Nature Reviews Genetics* 5 (2004): 467–75.

33. Foster, M. W. and Freeman, W. L. "Naming Names in Human Genetic Variation Research," *Genome Research* 8, no. 8 (1998): 755–57.

34. Lee, S. S. "Race, Distributive Justice and The Promise of Pharmacogenomics: Ethical Considerations," *American Journal of Pharmacogenomics* 3 (2003): 385–92.

35. Foster, M. W. and Sharp, R. R. "Race, Ethnicity, and Genomics: Social Classifications as Proxies of Biological Heterogeneity," *Genome Research* 12 (2002): 844–50.

36. National Bioethics Advisory Commission. *Research Involving Human Biological Materials: Ethical Issues and Policy Guidance.* 2 vols. Vol. 1. Rockville, MD: National Bioethics Advisory Commission, 1999.

37. Committee on Assessing Genetic Risks, Division of Health Sciences Policy, and Institute of Medicine. *Assessing Genetic Risks: Implications for Health and Social Policy*, ed. J. E. Fullarton, L. B. Andrews, N. A. Holtzman, and A. G. Motulsky. Washington, DC: National Academy Press, 1994.

38. Kohane, I. S., Mandl, K. D., Taylor, P. L., Holm, I. A., Nigrin, D. J., and Kunkel, L. M. "Medicine. Reestablishing the Researcher–Patient Compact," *Science* 316 (2007): 836–37.

39. Bookman, E. B., Langehorne, A. A., Eckfeldt, J. H., Glass, K. C., Jarvik, G. P., Klag, M., Koski, G., Motulsky, A., Wilfond, B., Manolio, T. A., Fabsitz, R. R., and Luepker, R. V. "Reporting Genetic Results in Research Studies: Summary and Recommendations of an NHLBI Working Group," *American Journal of Medical Genetics A* 140 (2006): 1033–40.

40. Council for International Organizations of Medical Sciences. *International Ethical Guidelines for Biomedical Research Involving Human Subjects.* Geneva: Council for International Organizations of Medical Sciences, 2002.

41. Shalowitz, D. I. and Miller, F. G. "Disclosing Individual Results of Clinical Research: Implications of Respect for Participants," *Journal of the American Medical Association* 294 (2005): 737–40.

42. Barnoy, S. "Genetic Testing for Late-Onset Diseases: Effect of Disease Controllability, Test Predictivity, and Gender on The Decision to Take the Test," *Genetic Testing* 11 (2007): 187–92.

43. Geller, G., Doksum, T., Bernhardt, B. A., and Metz, S. A. "Participation in Breast Cancer Susceptibility Testing Protocols: Influence of Recruitment Source, Altruism, and Family Involvement on Women's Decisions," *Cancer Epidemiology Biomarkers and Prevention* 8 Pt 2 (1999): 377–83.

44. Cappelli, M., Surh, L., Humphreys, L., Verma, S., Logan, D., Hunter, A., and Allanson, J. "Psychological and Social Determinants of Women's Decisions to Undergo Genetic Counseling and Testing for Breast Cancer," *Clinical Genetics* 55 (1999): 419–30.

45. Clayton, E. W. "Informed Consent and Biobanks," *Journal of Law, Medicine, and Ethics* 33 (2005): 15–21.

46. Falk, M. J., Dugan, R. B., O'Riordan, M. A., Matthews, A. L., and Robin, N. H. "Medical Geneticists' Duty to Warn At-Risk Relatives For Genetic Disease," *American Journal of Medical Genetics* 120 (2003): 374–80.

47. Dugan, R. B., Wiesner, G. L., Juengst, E. T., O'Riordan, M., Matthews, A. L., and Robin, N. H. "Duty to Warn At-Risk Relatives for Genetic Disease: Genetic Counselors' Clinical Experience," *American Journal of Medical Genetics C Seminars in Medical Genetics* 119 (2003): 27–34.

48. Offit, K., Groeger, E., Turner, S., Wadsworth, E. A., and Weiser, M. A. "The 'Duty To Warn' a Patient's Family Members about Hereditary Disease Risks," *Journal of the American Medical Association* 292 (2004): 1469–73.

49. Lehmann, L. S., Weeks, J. C., Klar, N., Biener, L., and Garber, J. E. "Disclosure of Familial Genetic Information: Perceptions of the Duty to Inform," *The American Journal of Medicine* 109 (2000): 705–11.

50. United States. Congress. House. Committee on Government Operations. Human Resources and Intergovernmental Relations Subcommittee. *Genetic Testing: Predicting Disease or Diagnosis for Disaster?* Hearing before the Human Resources and Intergovernmental Relations Subcommittee of the Committee on Government Operations, House of Representatives, One Hundred Second Congress, second session, July 23, 1992. Washington: U.S. G.P.O. : For sale by the U.S. G.P.O. Supt. of Docs. Congressional Sales Office, 1993.

51. McGivern, B., Everett, J., Yager, G. G., Baumiller, R. C., Hafertepen, A., and Saal, H. M. "Family Communication about Positive BRCA1 and BRCA2 Genetic Test Results," *Genetics in Medicine* 6 (2004): 503–09.

52. Federal Policy for the Protection of Human Subjects. *45 CFR Part 46* Available from http://www.hhs.gov/ohrp/humansubjects/guidance/45cfr46.htm. Accessed October 20, 2008.

53. Health Insurance Portability and Accountability Act. "42 USC § 1301 et seq."

54. Burris, S., Gable, L., Stone, L., and Lazzarini, Z. "The Role of State Law in Protecting Human Subjects of Public Health Research and Practice," *Journal of Law, Medicine, and Ethics* 31 (2003): 654–62.

55. Lawlor, D. A. and Stone, T. "Public Health and Data Protection: An Inevitable Collision or Potential for a Meeting of Minds?" *International Journal of Epidemiology* 30 (2001): 1221–25.

56. Burris, S., Buehler, J., and Lazzarini, Z. "Applying the Common Rule to Public Health Agencies: Questions and Tentative Answers about a Separate Regulatory Regime," *Journal of Law, Medicine, and Ethics* 31 (2003): 638–53.

57. Amoroso, P. J. and Middaugh, J. P. "Research vs. Public Health Practice: When Does a Study Require IRB Review?" *Preventive Medicine* 36 (2003): 250–53.

58. Hiatt, R. A. "HIPAA: The End of Epidemiology, or a New Social Contract?" *Epidemiology* 14 (2003): 637–39.

59. Meslin, E. M. "Shifting Paradigms in Health Services Research Ethics," *Journal of General Internal Medicine* 21 (2006): 279–80.

60. 45 CFR § 46.101(4)(2007).

61. Office of Human Research Protections, and Department of Health and Human Services. *Guidance on Research Involving Coded Private Information or Biological Specimens*, 2004. Available at http://www.hhs.gov/ohrp/humansubjects/guidance/cdebiol.pdf., accessed July 2, 2005.

62. HIPAA identifiers. 45 CFR § 164.514 (2007).

III

BALANCING RISKS AND BENEFITS

6

Ethical Issues in the Design and Conduct of Community-Based Intervention Studies

KAREN GLANZ, MICHELLE C. KEGLER, AND
BARBARA K. RIMER

Community-based health intervention research includes studies with a variety of labels: community health research, public health intervention research, behavioral research, health education research, health promotion research, and community-based participatory research. Our definition of community-based intervention research and our use of this term are intentionally broad, and encompass community as the setting, target, and agent for change.[1] For purposes of this chapter, community-based intervention research investigates strategies designed to improve the health of individuals and populations through wider adoption of healthful behaviors, early detection and therapeutic practices, changes in public policies and institutional services to support healthier behaviors and community environments, mobilization of community resources to address priorities related to quality of life and community well-being, and combinations of these approaches. Community-based health intervention research includes research on, or with, defined populations in a wide variety of settings, including geographically defined communities, institutions such as worksites and schools, health-care delivery systems and other organizational networks, and the general public, such as the consumer marketplace. Community-based research covers the continuum from disease prevention and health promotion to treatment, rehabilitation, long-term care, and end-of-life care. Excluded from this broad category of intervention research are clinical trials in which the sole purpose is to test the efficacy of medical techniques to improve health status (even if the study is conducted partly in a community setting) and laboratory studies of human cognitions and behaviors.

Health research in community settings has increased and diversified dramatically over the past 30 years.[2,3] Initially, heightened interest in community-based health interventions was stimulated by the epidemiologic transition from infectious diseases to chronic diseases as the leading causes of death, rapidly escalating health-care costs, and data linking individual behaviors to increased risks of morbidity and mortality.[4,5] More recently, increased recognition of social ecologic models that acknowledge the power of social and environmental factors in shaping individual behavior has also fueled interest in community-based research.[6-9] Advances in medicine and genetics research have drawn attention to the need for compliance with evidence-based therapeutic regimens, participation in screening programs for disease susceptibility and early detection, and appropriate use of health services.[10] With these advances, new dilemmas have arisen, dilemmas involving ethics, law, and the study of human behavior.[11] The AIDS epidemic also has been a catalyst for health research in community settings as part of changing group and individual norms and behaviors that predispose people to AIDS.

Much community health research has been stimulated by the relatively high prevalence of chronic diseases such as heart disease, cancer, diabetes, and stroke. Two areas of chronic disease control have dominated: the first concerns individual lifestyle behaviors, such as smoking, diet, and physical activity, to prevent disease onset; the second is aimed at screening, early detection, and management of risk factors for chronic illness. The latter include, as major areas of research interest, hypertension, diabetes, and cancer. Injury prevention, HIV/AIDS prevention, immunization, and substance abuse prevention are also targets of community health research. These research areas have broad social, ethical, and economic implications for communities.

Recently, public and professional concern about ethical issues in research has grown. New ethical issues have arisen out of new health-related problems addressed by research, such as obesity prevention and the built environment,[12,13] and the expanded repertoire of methods used by community health researchers, including community-based participatory research.[14,15] The challenge of balancing scientific rigor and dynamic community research environments with ethical concerns has become increasingly complex. Historically, most attention on research ethics focused on clinical research involving individuals; the emergence of ethical examinations of preventive, educational, and health promotion research in communities is a newer development.[16,17]

In this chapter, we will examine the scientific, methodological, and practical foundations of community-based intervention research that bear on ethical concerns. The chapter begins with a discussion of the role of partnerships in community research, including partnership models and related ethical challenges, special considerations in working with vulnerable or disadvantaged communities, and suggestions for reconciling multiple agendas. We then discuss ethics related to methodologic issues in community-based intervention research, including intervention strategies, data collection, and study design. We also discuss ethical issues related to research participants, interdisciplinary and professional relationships, and relationships of science to society. The chapter concludes with a brief overview of ethical issues in conducting research with Internet communities or collecting data using the Internet and in community-based research in international settings.

Ethical Issues in Researcher–Community Partnerships

Effective community health interventions and intervention research call for scientists to collaborate with organizations that serve as gatekeepers for both successful implementation of interventions, as well as data collection. Community-based organizations can provide valuable resources for research such as endorsement and promotion of a research project, access to study participants and data collection settings, and local understanding of health problems and possible solutions. Partnerships between scientists and these organizations present challenging and often neglected problems regarding researchers' responsibilities to the participants and to the intermediary organizations or communities.[18] These problems include the extent of collaboration and shared decision making, whose research agenda is addressed, the risk of raising false hopes when preparing grant proposals, the sharing of data and research findings, and the responsibility to establish a long-term relationship with the community, or at a minimum, to leave the community with increased capacity or services. Addressing these issues early in a relationship increases the likelihood that damaging conflicts will be avoided, that both community members and researchers will benefit from the research, and that the community will be receptive to future research. The primary emphasis in community-based intervention research should not be on the advancement of researchers' careers or advances in scientific knowledge alone, but also on the individuals and communities whose health is at stake.

Continuum of Partnership Models

Almost all community-based research requires researchers to build a relationship with the community, or at a minimum, with a gatekeeper organization within the community. The rare exception is when researchers recruit participants through mass media and collect data through telephone interviews or mailed surveys, and never interact with community organizations or with community residents, except as research participants. A more common approach to designing and implementing community-based research is to establish a partnership with one or multiple organizations within the community. These partnerships fall along a continuum of possible degrees of involvement and interaction with communities. At one end, the community is simply the setting for research. A researcher may obtain the cooperation of an organization such as a local health department, hospital, school, or employer to provide demographic data and information about how to contact potential participants. In this model, the researcher typically approaches a gate-keeper organization with a research question in mind, and is seeking access to information about potential research participants and permission to recruit participants from specific institutions.

In the middle of the continuum are models where community input is actively sought, but researchers still drive the research process. A common approach for soliciting community participation is to establish a community advisory board (CAB) to provide input to investigators. CABs typically include members of the community and representatives from organizations that serve the community (who may or may not live in the community). CABs can be structured simply to allow members to provide input into a research effort so that members can participate as equal partners in the research endeavor. CABs and similar structures for community participation can provide concrete benefits to researchers such as gaining access to local leaders, resources, and technical skills, garnering citizen support and volunteer time, incorporating local values and symbols into intervention activities, developing local skills and competencies for future community problem-solving efforts, and enhancing local ownership and long-term maintenance of changes in the community.[19] CABs have been used as a means for obtaining input from community members in several of the large community trials of the past two decades. Typically, the intervention protocols were established by academic researchers, but community members were able to provide input into how the interventions were adapted and implemented in their own communities.

In addition to benefiting the researcher, community participation through CABs can provide benefits to community members and strengthen a community's capacity to address other issues of concern.[20,21] Community advisory boards can build planning, evaluation, and research skills among participants, strengthen ties across personal and organizational networks, and provide access to resources within the community and external resources such as specialized expertise or new funding opportunities.

Community-based participatory research (CBPR) is at the end of the continuum on which community members do more than provide input into the research. Instead, they share control over the research process. CBPR is an alternative to traditional research models in which outsiders control the questions, methods, interventions, indicators of success, and interpretation of results.[14] In CBPR, research questions often originate from community members. Community members are equal partners in designing the research and data collection methods, often collect the data themselves, aid in analysis and interpretation, and are coauthors on resulting presentations and publications. Research is geared toward action that benefits the community.

CBPR is a rapidly growing paradigm that acknowledges and values the unique strengths that all partners, both researchers and community members, bring to the research process.[22,23] According to Minkler and Wallerstein,[14] a variety of forces have fueled "increased attention on alternative orientations to inquiry that stress community partnership and action for social change and reductions in health inequities as integral parts of the research enterprise." These include an emphasis on health disparities, increased recognition of the need for community and social change, and disappointment in results from researcher-driven community interventions.[14]

Israel and colleagues[15] identify nine key "principles" or conditions of CBPR:

1. Recognizes community as a unit of identity;
2. Builds on strengths and resources within the community;
3. Facilitates collaborative, equitable partnership in all phases of the research;
4. Promotes colearning and capacity building among all partners;
5. Integrates and achieves a balance between research and action for the mutual benefit of all partners;
6. Emphasizes local relevance of public health problems and ecological perspectives that recognize and attend to the multiple determinants of health and disease;
7. Involves system development through a cyclical and iterative process;
8. Disseminates findings and knowledge gained to all partners and involves all partners in the dissemination process; and
9. Involves a long-term process and commitment.

Similar to partnership models in the middle of the continuum, CBPR partnerships often employ advisory boards or steering committees to obtain meaningful participation from communities. These collaborative structures provide a practical means through which researchers and community residents can jointly frame the research questions, design data collection instruments, establish data collection procedures, design and ensure the cultural appropriateness of intervention materials, gain access to intervention sites, implement interventions, interpret results, and disseminate the findings and institutionalize intervention activities.[24]

Ethical Issues in Establishing Researcher and Community Partnerships

Early issues to be faced in establishing a research partnership are how to define a community, and who legitimately represents the community's interests. "Community" is usually defined by a shared identity. This identity can be based on geography, such as county or city, or on ethnicity, culture, faith, or institutional affiliation.[25] Accordingly, an early step in building a research partnership is understanding how a community defines itself and its boundaries. According to Wallerstein and colleagues,[25] "it is shared identity and the institutions and associations that grow up within shared identity that allow the development of partnerships, and outside research partners must begin by getting to know how 'the community' is in fact defined by those with whom they hope to partner."

Ideally, community-based research projects build on existing positive relationships, either with the lead investigators, a colleague, or existing institutional connections. In CBPR, the community may initiate contact with a researcher. Quite often, though, a researcher initiates the relationship without any prior connections to the community.[26] In these situations, conducting a community assessment is a logical place to start, with one purpose being to identify and engage formal and informal leaders and organizations with strong ties to the community of interest.[27] Selecting the wrong partner—for example, one with a negative history with the community—can create unnecessary difficulties for the research project.

Other ethical problems concern who—researchers or community members—should control the research agenda and determine the research questions of interest, especially when the researchers are from outside the community. In CBPR, one of the basic tenets is that the research addresses an issue of concern to the community. Ideally, then, the research questions originate from the community or at least are generated in collaboration with the community. Fadem and colleagues identify "three ethical principles that lie at the heart of CBPR—respect for self-determination, liberty, and action for social change"[28] These principles are grounded in the belief that people can assess their own needs and have the right to address them.[28,29] In much community-based research, however, the researcher defines research topics and seeks community partners with shared interests. This behavior is a result of the fact that researchers' expertise tends to be focused on a limited number of content areas such as heart disease prevention or cancer screening, or that researchers are responding to an RFA that stipulates the problem. Given the heterogeneity of community types, it is usually possible to find a community partner with a shared interest, such as for example a local unit of the American Heart Association or American Cancer Society.

More obvious ethical issues can emerge when working with a disadvantaged community on an issue peripheral to their needs, and diverting resources, including the attention of community leaders and respected organizations to a lower priority concern.[30] A low-income African American community, for example, may be in dire need of economic development or community-oriented policing to reduce drug-related violence, but a financially strapped community-based organization may agree to divert its energies from advocacy efforts to participate in a teen pregnancy prevention project due to the lure of funding.

One practical approach to navigating these sometimes challenging, and always complex relationships between investigators and community partners is to develop guidelines for collaboration. At a minimum, these should address roles and responsibilities of various categories of partners (e.g., staff, investigators, and CAB members), rules for decision making, (including how decisions will be made and what types of decisions will be made jointly), human subjects protection and institutional review board (IRB) review (including who will be listed on IRB protocols and who needs to be formally trained in human subjects protection), stewardship of data, and rules for coauthorship on publications and presentations. There are often ways to reach compromises that permit both communities and researchers to meet their needs. An example related to coauthorship of peer-reviewed publications is to follow established international guidelines for authorship, but to also structure the research and paper writing process so that a substantive role in the design, conduct, and writing of results exists for nonacademic partners.

High-Risk and Vulnerable Communities

Due to the disproportionate burden of disease, disability, and premature death, there is likely to be increased intervention research directed to minority and low-income communities.[31,32] Despite the structures and policies of organized science that are designed to protect study populations, many members of minority and disadvantaged communities have a fundamental distrust of scientific research directed at them due to past injustices. This distrust is particularly evident in African American communities, where the abuses of the Tuskegee Syphilis Study, which sought to document the natural history of syphilis among poor black men in Alabama, have led to distrust of health researchers.[33]

Formal safeguards and reforms in research may be insufficient to change fears of harm and exploitation in vulnerable communities. The needs of communities to protect the welfare of their members and ensure long-term social benefit make community partnerships in which community members can help ensure sensitivity in design, conduct, and interpretation of findings especially important.[34] In order to produce high-quality, ethical research in minority and disadvantaged communities, both researchers and funding institutions need to overcome objections that community partnerships introduce unacceptable scientific biases and compromise methodological rigor. They also should address the current situation in which formal research consent procedure requirements often result in documents that are too difficult for most communities, especially disadvantaged communities, to understand.[35]

Communities are becoming more sophisticated in their interactions with researchers. Most notably, tribal communities are demanding accountability from researchers through the establishment of tribal institutional review boards. These boards have the power to deny access to researchers and to control publication of research findings.[25] The American Indian Law Center[36] developed a checklist for

Indian Health Boards to use in their decisions about whether to support particular research proposals. Some of the key questions on the checklist are:

* What are the expected benefits of the research to the tribes and local community, to the individual research subjects, and to society as a whole?
* What are the assurances regarding the confidentiality of data? Will the tribe or community be identified in the research report?
* Will the researcher agree to satisfy tribal, Health Board, and community concerns in final drafts and the final report?
* Is the researcher willing to attempt to find means of using local people and resources rather than import all resources?
* Is the researcher willing to deposit raw data in a tribal or tribally designated repository or otherwise share the data with the tribe?

There are special challenges for other vulnerable populations, such as children and youth: The usual requirement for active parental consent in all research with minors (age 18 or younger) may introduce biases in relation to participation in studies about subjects of a sensitive nature (e.g., sexual behavior, use of alcohol, tobacco, and drugs), or, even worse, may put young people at risk if their parents can demand access to research data collected from their children. A variety of strategies may be used to enhance parental consent and youth assent in community-based intervention studies,[37] though they are not often described in the literature. Most of the IRBs responding to a recent survey stated that they never grant parental waivers to allow minors to provide full consent on their own behalf,[38] although the regulations have some flexibility to ensure strong participant protections.

Reconciling Multiple Scientific and Community Agendas

Even when the value of collaboration between researchers and the communities they study is recognized, many complicated pragmatic issues remain. As Dressler[39] notes, "Negotiating such a collaborative relationship can demand skills, time, and patience perhaps notably lacking in some academic researchers. Similarly, the willingness of the community to enter into the long-term pact required for high-quality research can oftentimes necessitate a difficult shift in values." With their different agendas, researchers may have understandable reasons for conflicts with community leaders and residents. These may be science-based, such as believing randomization is the only way to ensure internal validity in an intervention research study, or more personal, such as feeling the need to publish study results in a timely manner without the delays inevitable in a collaborative writing process. However, the multiple needs of scientists and participating communities can all be accommodated with attention to five key areas: first, to increased sensitivity to ethnic and cultural habits and norms; second, to instilling trust through better communication; third, to considering communities as research partners not just sources of research subjects; fourth, to understanding and addressing important problems of communities, such as crime, poverty, racism, and violence; and fifth, to developing guidelines for collaboration or operating procedures that clarify how a relationship will function.[26,39] These matters are not intended simply to require researchers to compromise in order to satisfy community representatives. Openness to understanding each others' views should come from both residents and researchers. Sometimes the community partners need help dealing with political systems around issues such as crime or racial discrimination, which the researchers can help with before the research on the scientists' agenda can move ahead.

Methodological Issues and Ethics in Community-Based Intervention Research

A range of methodologies is used in community-based health intervention research. There is wide diversity in the choice of intervention strategies, data collection techniques, and study design. We will consider ethical issues in the context of these methodologies.

Intervention Strategies

Contemporary community interventions may address health problems at one or more levels of the social ecology: they may focus on intrapersonal factors (such as knowledge, attitudes, behavior), interpersonal processes (family relationships, social support, social networks), institutional factors (organizations and their norms or rules), community factors, and public policy.[7,40] Interventions generally labeled as health promotion include not only educational and motivational strategies but also organizational change, policy directives, laws, economic supports, and community activation.[41] For example, successful tobacco control programs have used a variety of strategies, such as mass media campaigns, community coalitions, increased prices through excise taxes, retailer education, reduced financial barriers for cessation therapies, provider reminder systems, telephone counseling, and smoking restrictions.[42] Programs to increase use of mammography screening and Papanicolaou tests among women have also used diverse approaches: printed and audiovisual materials, cost reduction through free screening, reduced copayments and expanded insurance coverage, outreach and advocacy using lay health advisors, telephone counseling, education of community physicians, one-on-one education through allied health professionals, and modification of delivery system factors such as hours of operation and availability of child care.[43] Other community-based health interventions range from environmental health interventions [17] to studies of remote intercessory prayer.[44–46] Some interventions that involve passive community recipients may seem paternalistic to the targeted audiences.

Methods of Data Collection

The unit of observation in community-based intervention research may be individuals, groups, organizations, or communities defined by geographic or political boundaries. In addition, data may be collected both directly (by asking questions or conducting observations) and indirectly (by reviewing records and archival sources). The most common methods for collecting data from individuals is survey research using self-administered written questionnaires, and telephone or face-to-face interviews. However, use of medical, educational, occupationally related, or public record sources may allow for unobtrusive measurement and verification of self-reported data. Linkages are increasingly being made to large databases, such as Medicare files. Access to these databases requires investigators to document specific data requests and the need for them, and involves close scrutiny of ethical issues. Biologic information such as blood pressure, serum cholesterol levels, body weight, saliva thiocyanate levels, and urinary cotinine may serve as proxy measures of behavior, indicators of risk level, or biomarkers of behavior change. Contemporary ethics board regulations (e.g., those based on federal Health Insurance Portability and Accountability Act (HIPAA) rules in the United States) may require extra consent procedures, depending on the sources and personal identification on health and personal data.[47]

At the organizational or community levels, information about social structure and the physical environment may be obtained through interviews with key informants or by direct observation. For example, neighborhood nutrition environments have been assessed by observing food availability in a sample of stores or restaurants in a neighborhood.[48] Indirect indicators of enforcement of tobacco control policies or of consumers' eating patterns might include measures such as environmental tobacco smoke using nicotine monitors or cafeteria plate waste. These data collection approaches do not require informed consent of individuals, and involve collection of data about and sometimes from an entity such as a neighborhood, school, or worksite. This raises the question of how and to what extent is it necessary to protect the privacy of social groups, organizations, and communities when individuals are not the focus of the research. The answer to this question depends, at least in part, on the extent to which the information is generally available to researchers and the public.

Community intervention researchers increasingly are using qualitative methods to obtain greater in-depth information and to learn about unique cultural groups or high-risk populations. Qualitative methods are especially useful in their ability to "capture and communicate" stories.[49]

Major qualitative data collection techniques include interviews, observations, focus groups, and document review.[49] Qualitative interviews ask open-ended questions that allow respondents to answer in their own words. Observations result in detailed descriptions of an event or experience, such as behaviors, interpersonal interactions, or organizational processes.[49] Focus groups allow for in-depth exploration of topics in a group setting. Documents include written and other material from program or organizational records and include progress reports, attendance records, meeting minutes, photographs, correspondence, and so forth.

Study Designs

Randomized, controlled experiments remain the most rigorous type of design in community-based intervention research. However, numerous variations on randomized controlled trials are also employed because of practical and political considerations such as the reluctance of organizations or participants to take part in a study where they may be randomized to a no-treatment control group. In some studies, randomization to different conditions is performed on a unit larger than the individual. This technique is both scientifically justified and necessary if the intervention involves organizational change and where social networks would create excessive contamination between groups (such as cross-talk within the organization), which happens in many worksite health intervention studies. However, when an "organization" is the unit of randomization, individuals may not have a personal choice about whether or not to participate, even though community-level interventions may be directed at these individuals.[50] This again raises the issue of community consent, in addition to the more traditional research participant consent.

Some have argued that "respect for communities" should be added as a principle to supplement the individualistic interpretation of protecting human subjects as represented in the Belmont Report.[24,51] Quinn[24] states that CABs are one way to achieve community consultation and to implement a community consent mechanism. She argues that "some form of consultation in the process of informed consent can help ensure that researchers gain an understanding of the social context in which community members assess the risks and benefits of research."

It can be difficult or ethically unacceptable to recruit groups or individuals to participate in research without their receiving the benefit of some type of intervention or service. Control groups, in particular, can also raise ethical issues in some situations where control group participants feel they are being denied the benefit of a potentially valuable intervention. Hence, additional design variations may include using modified control groups (such as usual care or "wait-list" control), before–after comparisons, and combinations of cohort and cross-sectional samples for evaluation. Wait-list and before–after comparisons enable all participants to receive the intervention over time. Usual care control groups ensure that control group participants are not denied standard care as a result of the research.

Interdisciplinary Health Research Traditions and Ethical Concerns

Community-based intervention research is, by its nature, eclectic and interdisciplinary. It draws on perspectives and tools from such diverse disciplines as psychology, sociology, anthropology, communications, statistics, biology, epidemiology, and marketing.[40] An important consequence of this interdisciplinary approach is that the codes and standards of conduct, as well as the identification and resolution of ethical dilemmas, may differ among the groups involved.[52-54] Psychology, with its emphasis on individual behavior, has been the basis for many of the research studies and methodologies used; sociological approaches are particularly important to the study of organizations and social structures within communities. Social science traditions may conflict with those of biomedical researchers,[53] and these differences may cause ongoing challenges for social and behavioral scientists due to the composition of ethics review boards, the guidelines used for health behavior research, and unevenness in IRB deliberations about social research investigations.[54]

There is substantial overlap between public health and medicine in health interventions carried out in clinical settings. However, the ethical issues most salient for community-based intervention research are derived primarily from the traditions of the social sciences and public health sciences, and only secondarily from biomedical ethics. A fundamental distinction has been made between public health ethics and traditional medical ethics references (e.g., see the work of Powers and Faden[55]). Medical ethics has its roots in the rights and respect due to individuals in their relationships with physicians and other health-care professionals, whereas many view the central concerns of public health ethics to be maximizing the welfare of the community or society as a whole and social justice.

Ethical conflicts arise in public health interventions when decisions must be made about distribution of health resources and priorities for programs, and when standards for health protection are at stake. They also occur in public health research due to concerns about privacy, autonomy, and the equitable treatment of individuals.[56] In both medicine and public health, conflicting obligations sometimes result from the dual roles of practitioner and scientist. From a public health viewpoint, decisions about community research design depend primarily on three factors: first, anticipated kind and extent of benefit to the public and to scientific knowledge; second, degree of restriction of individual rights needed to achieve the benefit; and third, balance between risks and benefits attendant to participation in the research. Although research seldom warrants entirely sacrificing individual rights and liberty for the public good, this perspective of public health as an independent value can influence decisions regarding the design and conduct of community health intervention research.[57,58]

Ethical Issues Related to Research Participants

Ethical considerations impose both restrictions and responsibilities on researchers. Ethical guidelines are vital to community intervention research to ensure that studies have worthwhile goals, and to protect the welfare of research participants. Several ethical principles in community-based intervention research relate to research participants, These principles include respect for autonomy, beneficence, justice, privacy, and avoidance of deception.[59–61]

Respect for Autonomy

Autonomy involves respect for the rights and ability of individuals and groups to make decisions for themselves.[61] In public health practice, it is accepted that there are some situations in which autonomy must be limited to protect the public's health, such as the requirement of immunization against communicable diseases. But in most cases, respect for autonomy becomes the central ethical principle and infringements of autonomy are not permitted.

In community-based intervention research, respect for autonomy is the reason for obtaining informed consent and the justification of rules of voluntary data provision and participation in interventions as well as the avoidance of excessive inducements to participate, or incentives for research participants, such as large cash payments to low-income participants. Elements of disclosure in informed consent include a statement of purpose, explanation of procedures, and a description of discomforts and risks that participants might experience as discussed by Robert Levine in Chapter 12. Although in the past the standards of disclosure could be community standards or "reasonable person" standards, they are often much more stringent today following the enactment of the HIPAA rules[62] in the United States.

One ethical question regarding informed consent concerns how specific a researcher must be about the study aims when the provision of complete information may lead to refusal to participate, behavior change in anticipation of the study, or biased responses to measures used for evaluation. For example, it is common for consent forms in randomized trials to state that participants will be assigned to one of two different educational programs, without reference to specific differences or the fact that one program is enhanced in some manner. Decisions regarding disclosure should be carefully weighed so that information is as complete as possible without severely compromising research methodology.

In some cases, consent for participation has been obtained for the group, organization, or community, and individuals become research subjects without their consent by virtue of belonging to a relevant group or community. An example of this is a cluster randomized trial (a study in which intact groups rather than individuals are the units of randomization) of a school-based tobacco prevention program, in which schools that agree to participate are assigned to receive one strategy or another, or serve as "controls." However, in this type of situation in which all individuals within the participating schools receive the intervention such as a tobacco use prevention curriculum or a smoke-free school environment, the individuals do have free choice about participating in terms of whether they answer questionnaires or interviews. When information from medical records or employment records on factors such as use of preventive services or absenteeism are used as measures, individual subjects may not be approached directly for their permission. Although these assessment methods raise ethical questions, they are sometimes justified—for example, when research questions are significant and the risk of harm to subjects is very low and precautions to protect privacy are taken.

Program or study attrition compromises internal and external validity of community-based intervention studies. A strategy to ameliorate the problem of attrition is the use of incentives such as small gifts, payment to participants, or reimbursement for inconvenience or travel expenses. Although this practice may be perceived as manipulative or restrictive of freedom to withdraw from participation, such compensation usually does not compromise ethics if incentives do not involve unreasonable enticements and if they do not have even the appearance of constituting coercion. It is even possible that, for some groups, small incentives covering extra expenses of time or effort involved in the research enable a broader base of participants to take part. Although this example should probably be regarded as a reimbursement, different IRBs take different stands on incentives:[63-65] some may view any compensation as potentially coercive or manipulative while others permit some incentives, but define a level that is unacceptable. It is true that a small incentive for a poor person could have a very different impact than the same incentive offered to a middle-income person.

Beneficence

The principle of beneficence requires that researchers minimize risk to participants and maximize the potential benefits both to subjects and to society.[61] Potential risks to participants include psychological distress resulting from participation in research, physical danger, respondent burden, and loss of self-esteem and anxiety. In chemoprevention studies, there may be a risk of toxicity associated with the drugs. The potential benefits of research should be judged in terms of the direct benefits to participants, as well as the prospects that the findings will improve the health of populations, often different from the research population. One group of people should not be expected to bear risks unduly, which is especially true for socioeconomically disadvantaged and underserved populations.

The concept of beneficence has unique implications for community-based intervention research in which screening or health examinations might result in the identification of at-risk individuals. In such situations, provisions should be made for referral and follow-up to protect the welfare of participants, even if it means violating the study plan. It is unethical to recruit people into screening programs without providing for treatment should abnormalities arise. Investigators are responsible for minimizing risks to participants by examining the potential risks, and ensuring that they are unlikely, minor, and reversible if they occur. Measures for the early detection of any physical or psychological harm should also be taken.[59,60]

Another aspect of beneficence in the conduct of health-related research is the obligation to act on important interim findings. For example, in interim analysis, a fear-arousing communication designed to motivate people to quit smoking could be found to generate significant anxiety but minimal behavior change. Under such circumstances, it would be unethical to continue the trial without substantive modification to the intervention. Alternatively, interim analysis could show a clear improvement in psychosocial or medical outcomes associated with an intervention. It would then be reasonable to offer the more effective strategy to all communities or participants. Accordingly, the research questions could focus on identifying subgroups that are most or least likely to benefit, based on individual or organizational factors.

Justice

Ethical principles of justice concern the fair distribution of benefits and burdens of research among potential subjects.[55,61] According to utilitarian principles of justice, the public benefit should be maximized, potentially justifying a relaxing of the requirement that *each research participant* receives an equal share of the benefits from the research.[66] Justice-based considerations are relevant to selection of research subjects and communities, and to randomization of subjects or organizations to receive different interventions. For example, investigators may need to make a choice between studying those most in need of an intervention and selecting a more accessible or practical population. Further, such decisions may be imposed by funding sources, such as government research set-asides that are available only for studying selected minority groups or women.

Meeting requirements of distributive justice is particularly challenging when individuals or communities are assigned to control or comparison groups that do not receive the intervention hypothesized to be most effective. The control subjects may be burdened disproportionately by data collection requirements without receiving the benefits of services. One such study where it was charged that withholding a full intervention was unethical was the recent Kennedy Krieger Institute's study of lead abatement in public housing.[56] Although this accusation was controversial, some critics felt that all efforts should be made to reduce lead exposure across those potentially exposed.[56] In some studies, the use of a minimal intervention such as an educational brochure may provide an acceptable level of benefit. Another common solution to this problem is the use of a delayed control group design, wherein the intervention is delivered during a later phase of the study, or the intervention materials or services found most effective are provided to all groups at the conclusion of the investigation. However, this solution may require special resources that are not always available as part of research funding. Investigators should take particular care not to make promises they cannot keep, for it is easy to offer delayed treatment and much harder to follow through.

Privacy

Conflicts can arise in research when individuals' rights to privacy are at odds with the goal of obtaining knowledge to improve public health. Dimensions of privacy include the sensitivity of information, the setting being observed, and plans for dissemination of information and its linkage to the subjects' names. Anonymity may not be possible in cohort studies or record linkages; however, privacy should be protected to the extent feasible. Names should be destroyed as soon as they are no longer needed, and the anonymity of individuals should always be protected in reporting results. In the United States, HIPAA regulations impose strict guidelines on the use of "protected health information," which can be defined very broadly by some IRBs. [35,67] Although HIPAA greatly limits access to participants' medical or health-care records, it is possible to obtain partial or complete waivers when a study could only be completed with direct access to such information (like insurance claims information). In such cases, researchers must demonstrate how they will protect subjects' privacy and only use the specific information needed to answer a research question so the public's health may be improved.

Early community health research often involved fictitious names for communities being studied, though the location of community research is not usually concealed today. Currently, the use of pseudonyms for research communities may not accomplish its intended purpose because of the difficulty of maintaining secrecy when descriptive information is provided and/or institutional affiliations are listed for authors and those acknowledged. An alternative is to use a general description of the study's locale (such as region or state). Community-based intervention studies that use indirect data collection methods and unobtrusive measures preserve privacy if they collect data at the level of the environment, community, or other aggregate unit of observation, and if individuals cannot be identified. These may be appropriate techniques for testing environmental interventions for health promotion.

Guarantees of confidentiality are essential when research is being conducted in settings where individuals work, receive services, and are educated. For example, high school students may be reluctant to respond to surveys in a smoking prevention study if they have reason to believe that their parents, teachers, or school administrators will have access to the information that they provide. Parent or teacher access to information about tobacco use could lead to disciplinary action or punishment. Although the provision of aggregate data to cooperating organizations is usually justified, it is critical that participants be protected from any possible repercussions of disclosure of information they provide in the course of research. In community studies, investigators should avoid situations in which workers are collecting personal data on people they know, which is a real issue since researchers are increasingly hiring indigenous community workers or long-time residents.

It is also ethically unjustified to study very private areas of life without subjects' prior permission. Research on AIDS risk reduction, as well as studies of other sexually transmitted diseases and unwanted pregnancy, which are potentially of great public health importance, often entail highly personal questions about sexual practices and drug use. Participants must be assured of strict confidentiality, and any exceptions should be disclosed. One way to address this problem is to study repeated cross-sectional samples of anonymous participants rather than identifiable cohorts. However, sampling error could lead to erroneous interpretations of behavior change. That is, a new sample of participants may be different in important ways from those included in the original sample.

Deception

Several types of deception are of particular concern in community-based intervention research; for example, deliberately lying about the research purpose and manipulation of information within an intervention involving persuasive communication.[59] Deception is common in laboratory-based psychological experiments, and in fact was used in some classic, albeit controversial, social psychological investigations such as Milgram's[68] studies of obedience to authority and Asch's experiments on the effects of social pressure.[59,60,69] In community-based studies of human behavior, deception has been used in studies of response to simulated emergencies, discrimination, and prejudice.

Deceptive research methods have revealed important problems in health care that would probably not have been acknowledged if deception was totally avoided. Rosenhan[70] used eight "pseudopatients" to study the treatment of patients confined to mental health facilities and to evaluate how normal behavior would be interpreted by hospital staff following a psychiatric diagnosis. He found that the treatment environment and diagnostic labels were more powerful determinants of staff treatment of patients than their actual behavior.

Reasons for deception in community research include methodological control, external validity, and pragmatic factors (time, money, access).[60] Alternatives such as forewarning participants, role-playing, or use of hypothetical scenarios are methodologically weaker because they are not the same as real-world situations. A review of studies using deception found that, while it is considered "morally wrong," research participants often say that they enjoy it, do not mind being deceived, and do not mind the invasion of their privacy.[69] As long as risks and potential harms are minimal and the protocol has been approved by an ethics review committee, short-term deception is sometimes a justifiable technique for answering important research questions that cannot otherwise be resolved. Studies involving deception may be ill advised in minority communities especially where there is a tendency to distrust medical and government researchers.

Informed Consent and Health Literacy

An increasing challenge in community-based intervention research involves the vocabulary used to communicate required elements of informed consent to potential study participants. It has been suggested that some of the groups most needing protection—vulnerable groups, low-income persons, and minorities—are not well served by the highly technical requirements of ethics committees.[47] The readability levels of consent forms are usually at the 10th grade level or above,[71] and are often beyond the 12th grade level for HIPAA notices.[35] This is most often the case even though many IRBs publish readability standards between the 5th and 10th grade levels.[71] The balance between compliance with regulations and the quality of communication with potential participants is a difficult one to achieve.

Ethical Issues Related to Professional Relations and Interactions

Researchers who conduct community-based intervention research interact not only with research participants and their communities, but also with other professionals both within and outside their primary disciplines, and with the public at large. Relationships with funding sources, professional colleagues, practitioners, and legislators and policy makers may present ethical dilemmas such as conflict of interest, as well as biased conduct and interpretation of research and the use of research findings in practice and policy arenas. Professional codes of ethics include attention to principles of research integrity in areas of funding, relationships, data use, and communication.[59]

In recent years, there has been an enormous increase in requirements that investigators complete continuing professional education on the responsible conduct of research—via courses, seminars, or online tutorials. It is less clear how many of these programs address professional conduct issues, as the greatest emphasis is typically on protection of human subjects. Other chapters in this volume provide more detailed up-to-date coverage of the issues of professional conduct that are of concern to community-based intervention researchers, such as funding and sponsorship, publications and reporting, and the use of research findings to influence public health practice and policy.[58]

Emerging Ethical Issues: Globalization, Internet Research, and Protection of Subjects

Health research in the 21st century is marked by increasing use of the Internet for research, and the growth of international intervention studies. Although there are universally acknowledged principles for protection of human subjects (named above), the actual rules and oversights are put in place within countries. Industrialized countries usually have their own guidelines and monitoring for ethical research,[72,73] which may not be identical to those in the United States.

Community health intervention research in countries that are less economically developed is needed, because of the burden of infectious and communicable diseases such as HIV/AIDS, diarrheal diseases and malaria, and the prevalence of cigarette smoking and environmental health concerns. Research ethics systems may not even be in place in some locations, where they are greatly needed. A recent study of 46 member states of the World Health Organization (WHO) African Region found that many countries do not have formal Research Ethics Committees, although some have ad hoc review mechanisms.[74] Anecdotal reports suggest that bribery or demands for payment from researchers are common practice in some countries. Further, the populations' vulnerability and low literacy levels raise questions about the applicability of voluntary informed consent in non-Western settings.[75] There may be a mismatch between U.S. consent regulations and the infrastructure, culture, and context of underdeveloped countries, so that the complex processes that work in the United States often seem not to fit in the developing world.

The Internet offers health researchers unique access to participants, and some research shows that Internet-based behavior-change interventions, can be both feasible and effective, for issues such as weight loss.[76] A review of many Internet-based health behavior change programs concluded that they are in an early stage of development and many consumers would not choose a web-program to improve health risk behaviors.[77] Clearly, though, these programs are increasing rapidly. Human research using the Internet raises ethical issues such as the assurance of confidentiality, the ability to protect participants from harm, and the viability of truly informed consent.[78] Varnhagen and others[79] studied participants' reading and recall of informed consent documents presented by paper or computer. They found little difference in the amount of time spent reading documents in the two different media, but there was somewhat greater recall when consent forms were presented in a paginated rather than a continuous format in both media.[79] There is at least initial evidence that informed consent can be achieved as successfully on the Internet as with paper-format methods. Nevertheless, there are many challenges in designing Internet-based consent methods that fully disclose appropriate information yet do not serve as an untenable barrier to participation. These include assuring full understanding of the information and that the actual participant is the person providing consent.

Summary and Conclusions

Ethical principles are vital to community-based intervention research, to ensure that the research addresses worthwhile goals, to protect the welfare of individuals and communities participating in the research, and to help establish and maintain effective community partnerships and professional relations. Technical proficiency must be accompanied by sensitivity to values and ethics, and a sense of social responsibility. There are few ready-made formulas for making difficult decisions. In this chapter we have tried to present some familiar issues and to analyze new problems of growing concern to community researchers.

As health investigators strive to conduct innovative, high-quality research, they should take precautions to safeguard participants' privacy and autonomy, and optimize their receipt of benefits from the research. Special care should be exercised to protect the rights and interests of vulnerable populations, including children, older adults, minorities, and high-risk populations. Communities and individuals should be consulted and their wishes respected in the conduct of research. At the conclusion of a study, efforts should be made to offer the most effective treatment or program to all participants. Bias in reporting results should be avoided, and scientists should fulfill their obligations for responsible use of research knowledge for public health, medical practice, and social policy. Moreover, public health investigators should form partnerships with ethicists or members of IRBs to identify proactively the ethical implications of research and to ensure that basic ethical principles are not violated. Finally, there should be a continuing search to improve the nature of information provided to participants in studies and to preserve informed consent as an ethical foundation of community-based research.

ACKNOWLEDGMENTS

The preparation of this paper was supported in part by a Georgia Cancer Coalition Distinguished Research Scholar award to Karen Glanz. The authors thank Else Henry for her assistance with preparation and editing of this chapter.

References

1. McLeroy, K., Norton, B., Kegler, M., Burdine, J., and Sumaya, C., "Community-Based Interventions," *American Journal of Public Health* 93 (2003): 529–33.
2. Merzel, C. and D'Afflitti, J. "Reconsidering Community-Based Health Promotion: Promise, Performance, and Potential," *American Journal of Public Health* 93 (2003): 557–74.
3. Mittelmark, M. (1999). "Health Promotion at the Communitywide Level: Lessons from Diverse Perspectives." In *Health Promotion at the Community Level,* ed. N. Bracht. 2nd ed. Thousand Oaks: Sage Publications,1999.
4. McGinnis, J. M. and Foege, W. "Actual Causes of Death in the United States," *Journal of the American Medical Association* 270 (1993): 2207–12.
5. Mokdad, A. H., Marks, J. S., Stroup, D. F., and Gerberding, J. L. "Actual Causes of Death in the United States, 2000," *Journal of the American Medical Association* 291 (2004): 1238–45.
6. Institute of Medicine. *The Future of the Public's Health in the 21st Century.* Washington, DC: National Academies Press, 2003.
7. McLeroy, K., Bibeau, D., Steckler, A., and Glanz, K. "An Ecological Perspective on Health Promotion Programs," *Health Education Quarterly* 15 (1988): 351–77.
8. Stokols, D., Grzywacz, J., McMahan, S., and Phillips, K. "Increasing the Health Promotive Capacity of Human Environments," *American Journal of Health Promotion* 18 (2003): 4–13.
9. Stokols, D. "Establishing and Maintaining Healthy Environments: Toward a Social Ecology of Health Promotion," *American Psychologist* 47 (1992): 6–22.
10. Institute of Medicine. *Implications of Genomics for Public Health. Workshop Summary.* Washington, DC: National Academies Press, 2005.
11. Wilkinson, J. and Targonski, P. "Health Promotion in a Changing World: Preparing for the Genomics Revolution," *American Journal of Health Promotion* 18 (2003): 157–61.
12. Sallis, J. and Glanz, K. "The Role of Built Environments in Physical Activity, Eating, and Obesity in Childhood," *Future of Children* 16 (2006): 89–108.
13. Gordon-Larsen, P., Nelson, M. C., Page, P., and Popkin, B. M. "Inequality in the Built Environment Underlies Key Health Disparities in Physical Activity and Obesity," *Pediatrics* 117 (2006): 417–24.
14. Minkler, M. and Wallerstein, N., eds. *Community-Based Participatory Research for Health.* San Francisco, CA: Jossey-Bass, 2003.
15. Israel, B., Schulz, A., Parker, E., Becker, A., Allen, A., and Guzman, J. "Critical Issues in Developing and Following Community-Based Participatory Research Principles." In *Community-Based Participatory Research for Health*, ed. M. Minkler and N. Wallerstein. San Francisco, CA: Jossey-Bass, 2003: 53–76.
16. Buchanan, D. "A New Ethic for Health Promotion: Reflections on a Philosophy of Health Education for the 21st Century," *Health Education and Behavior* 33 (2006): 290–304.
17. Resnik, D. B., Zeldin, D. C., and Sharp, R. "Research on Environmental Health Interventions: Ethical Problems and Solutions," *Accountability in Research* 12 (2005): 69–101.
18. Dickert, N. and Sugarman, J. "Ethical Goals of Community Consultation in Research," *American Journal of Public Health* 95 (2005): 1123–27.
19. Bracht, N., Kingsbury, L., and Rissel C. "A Five-Stage Community Organization Model for Health Promotion: Empowerment and Partnership Strategies."

In *Health Promotion at the Community Level: New Advances,* ed. N. Bracht. 2nd ed. Thousand Oaks, CA: Sage Publications, 1999: 83–104.

20. Norton, B., Burdine, J., McLeroy, K., Felix, M., and Dorsey, A. "Community Capacity: Theoretical Roots and Conceptual Challenges." In *Emerging Theories in Health Promotion Practice and Research: Strategies for Improving Public Health,* ed. R. J. DiClemente, R. A. Crosby, and M. C. Kegler. San Francisco, CA: Jossey-Bass, 2002: 194–227.

21. Goodman, R., Speers, M., McLeroy, K., Fawcett, S., Kegler, M., Parker, E. et al. "An Initial Attempt at Identifying and Defining the Dimensions of Community Capacity to Provide a Basis for Measurement," *Health Education and Behavior* 25 (1998): 258–78.

22. Green, L., George, M., Daniel, M., Frankish, C., Herbert, C., Bowie, W. et al. *Study of Participatory Research in Health Promotion: Review and Recommendations for the Development of Participatory Research in Health Promotion in Canada.* Vancouver, British Columbia: Royal Society of Canada, 1995.

23. O'Fallon, L. and Dearry, A. "Community-Based Participatory Research as a Tool to Advance Environmental Health Sciences," *Environmental Health Perspectives* 110 (2002): 155–59.

24. Quinn, S. "Ethics in Public Health Research," *American Journal of Public Health* 94 (2004): 918–22.

25. Wallerstein, N., Duran, B., Minkler, M., and Foley, K. "Developing and Maintaining Partnerships with Communities." In *Methods in Community-Based Participatory Research,* ed. B. Israel, E. Eng, A. Schulz., and E. Parker. San Francisco: Jossey-Bass, 2005: 31–51.

26. Suarez-Balcazar, Y., Harper, G., and Lewis, R. "An Interactive and Contextual Model of Community–University Collaborations for Research and Action," *Health Education and Behavior* 32 (2005): 84–101.

27. Eng, E., Moore, K., Rhodes, S., Griffin, D., Allison, L., Shirah, K. et al. "Insiders and Outsiders Assess Who is 'the Community': Participant Observation, Key Informant Interview, Focus Group Interview, and Community Forum." In *Methods in Community-Based Participatory Research,* ed. B. Israel, E. Eng, A. Schulz, and E. Parker. San Francisco, CA: Jossey-Bass, 2005: 77–100.

28. Fadem, P., Minkler, M., Perry, M., Blum, K., Moore, L., and Rogers J. "Ethical Challenges in Community-Based Participatory Research." In *Community-Based Participatory Research for Health,* ed. B. Israel, E. Eng, A. Schulz, and E. Parker. San Francisco, CA: Jossey-Bass/Wiley, 2003: 242–262.

29. Minkler, M. and Pies, C. "Ethical Issues in Community Organization and Community Participation." In *Community Organizing and Community Building for Health,* ed. M. Minkler. New Brunswick, NJ: Rutgers University Press, 1997: 120–138.

30. Khanlou, N. and Peter, E. "Participatory Action Research: Considerations for Ethical Review," *Social Science and Medicine* 60 (2005): 2333–40.

31. Institute of Medicine. *Unequal Treatment: Confronting Racial and Ethnic Disparities in Healthcare.* Washington, DC: National Academies Press, 2002.

32. Cooper, S. P., Heitman, E., Fox, E. E., Quill, B., Knudson, P., Zahm, S. H. et al. "Ethical Issues in Conducting Migrant Farmworker Studies," *Journal of Immigrant Health* 6 (2004): 29–39.

33. Shavers, V. L., Lynch, D. F., and Burmeister, L. F. "Racial Differences in Factors That Influence the Willingness to Participate in Medical Research Studies," *Annals of Epidemiology* 12 (2002): 248–56.

34. Murphy, F. G., Jackson, P. A., Johnson, P. S., Ofili, E., Quarshie, A., and Nwigwe, C. "Informing and Consenting Disadvantaged Populations for Clinical and Community-Based Research Studies," *American Journal of Health Studies* 19 (2004): 246–53.

35. Walfish, S. and Watkins K. "Readability Level of Health Insurance Portability and Accountability Act Notices of Privacy: Practices Utilized by Academic Medical Centers," *Evaluation and the Health Professions* 28 (2005): 479–86.

36. American Indian Law Center. *Model Tribal Research Code*. Albuquerque, NM: American Indian Law Center, 1999.

37. Leakey, T., Lunde, K. B., Koga, K., and Glanz, K. "Written Parental Consent and the Use of Incentives in a Youth Smoking Prevention Trial: A Case Study from Project SPLASH," *American Journal of Evaluation* 25 (2004): 509–23.

38. Wagener, D. K., Sporer, A. K., Simmerling, M., Flome, J. L., An, C., and Curry, S. J. "Human Participants Challenges in Youth-Focused Research: Perspectives and Practices of IRB Administrators," *Ethics and Behavior* 14 (2004): 335–49.

39. Dressler, W. W. "Commentary on Community Research: Partnership in Black Communities," *American Journal of Preventive Medicine* 9 (2003): 35–38.

40. Glanz, K., Rimer, B., and Lewis, F., eds. *Health Behavior and Health Education: Theory, Research and Practice*. 3rd ed. San Francisco, CA: Jossey-Bass, 2002.

41. Green, L. and Kreuter, M. *Health Promotion Planning: An Educational and Ecological Approach*. 3rd ed. Mountain View, CA: Mayfield Publishing Co., 1999.

42. Hopkins, D., Briss, P. A., Ricard, C. J., Husten, C., Carande-Krulis, V., Fielding, J. et al. "Reviews of Evidence Regarding Interventions to Reduce Tobacco Use and Exposure to Environmental Tobacco Smoke," *American Journal of Preventive Medicine* 20 (2001): 16–66.

43. Legler, J., Meissner, H. I., Coyne, C., Breen, N., Chollette ,V., and Rimer, B. K. "The Effectiveness of Interventions to Promote Mammography among Women with Historically Low Rates of Screening," *Cancer, Epidemiology, Biomarkers and Prevention* 11 (2002): 59–71.

44. Leibovici, L. "Effects of Remote, Retroactive, Intercessory Prayer on Outcomes of Patients With Bloodstream Infection: Randomized Controlled Trial," *British Medical Journal* 323 (2001): 1450–51.

45. Halperin, E. C. "Should Academic Medical Centers Conduct Clinical Trials of the Efficacy of Intercessory Prayer?" *Academic Medicine* 76 (2001): 791–97.

46. Hobbins, P. B. "Compromised Ethical Principles in Randomized Clinical Trials of Distant, Intercessory Prayer," *Journal of Bioethical Inquiry* 2 (2005): 142–52.

47. Green, L. A., Lowery, J. C., Kowalski, C. P., and Wyszewianski, L. "Impact of Institutional Review Board Practice Variation on Observational Health Services Research," *Health Services Research* 41 (2006): 214–30.

48. Glanz, K., Sallis, J. F., Saelens, B. E., and Frank, L. D. "Healthy Nutrition Environments: Concepts and Measures," *American Journal of Health Promotion* 19 (2005): 330–33.

49. Patton, M. Q. *Qualitative Research and Evaluation Methods*. 3rd ed. Thousand Oaks, CA: Sage Publications, 2001.

50. Eldridge, S. M., Ashby, D., and Feder, G. S. "Informed Patient Consent to Participate in Cluster Randomized Trials: An Empirical Exploration of Trials in Primary Care," *Clinical Trials* 2 (2005): 91–98.

51. Weijer, C. "Protecting Communities in Research: Philosophical and Pragmatic Challenges," *Cambridge Quarterly of Healthcare Ethics* 8 (1999): 501–13.

52. American Psychological Association. APA Ethics Code 2002. Available at https://www.apa.org/ethics/, accessed June 25, 2006.
53. Hoeyer, K., Dahlager, L., and Lynoe, N. "Conflicting Notions of Research Ethics: The Mutually Challenging Traditions of Social Scientists and Medical Researchers," *Social Science and Medicine* 61 (2005): 1741–49.
54. DeVries, R., DeBruin, D. A., and Goodgame, A. "Ethics Review of Social, Behavioral, and Economic Research: Where Should We Go From Here?" *Ethics and Behavior* 14 (2004): 351–58.
55. Powers, M. and Faden, R. R. *Social Justice: The Moral Foundations of Public Health and Health Policy.* New York: Oxford University Press, 2006.
56. Buchanan, D. R. and Miller, F. G. "Justice and Fairness in the Kennedy Krieger Institute Lead Paint Study: The Ethics of Public Health Research on Less Expensive, Less Effective Interventions," *American Journal of Public Health* 96 (2006): 781–87.
57. Wynia, M. K. "Judging Public Health Research: Epistemology, Public Health and the Law," *American Journal of Bioethics* 5 (2005): 4–7.
58. Glanz, K., Rimer, B. K., and Lerman, C. "Ethical Issues in the Design and Conduct of Community-Based Intervention Studies." In *Ethics and Epidemiology,* ed. S. S. Coughlin and T. L. Beauchamp. New York: Oxford University Press, 1996: 156–77.
59. Babbie, E. "The Ethics and Politics of Social Research." In *The Practice of Social Research, 6th edition,* ed. E. Babbie. Belmont, CA: Wadsworth Publishing Co., 1992: 462–82.
60. Diener, E. and Crandall, R. *Ethics in Social and Behavioral Research.* Chicago: University of Chicago Press, 1978.
61. Beauchamp, T. L. and Childress, J. F. *Principles of Biomedical Ethics, 6th edition.* New York: Oxford University Press, 2009.
62. Health Insurance Portability and Accountability Act of 1996. Available at http://www.hhs.gov/ocr/hipaa/, accessed on June 28, 2006.
63. Grant, R. W. and Sugarman, J. "Ethics in Human Subjects Research: Do Incentives Matter?" *Journal of Medicine and Philosophy* 29 (2004): 717–38.
64. Emanuel, E. J. "Undue Inducement: Nonsense on Stilts?" *American Journal of Bioethics* 5 (2005): 9–13.
65. Klitzman, R. "The Importance of Social, Cultural, and Economic Contexts, and Empirical Research in Examining 'Undue Inducement'," *American Journal of Bioethics* 5 (2005): 19–21.
66. Coughlin, S. S. and Beauchamp, T. L. "Ethics, Scientific Validity, and the Design of Epidemiologic Studies," *Epidemiology* 3 (1992): 343–47.
67. Breese, P., Burman, W., Rietmeijer, C., and Lezotte D. "The Health Insurance Portability and Accountability Act and the Informed Consent Process (Letter)," *Annals of Internal Medicine* 141 (2004): 897–98.
68. Milgram, S. "Behavioral Study of Obedience," *Journal of Abnormal and Social Psychology* 67 (1963): 371–78.
69. Christensen, L. "Deception in Psychological Research: When is its Use Justified?" *Personality and Social Psychology Bulletin* 14 (1988): 664–75.
70. Rosenhan, D. L. "On Being Sane in Insane Places," *Science* (January 1973): 250–58.
71. Paasche-Orlow, M. K., Taylor, H. A., and Brancati, F. L. "Readability Standards for Informed-Consent Forms as Compared with Actual Readability," *New England Journal of Medicine* 348 (2003): 721–26.

72. Anderson, W. P., Cordner, C. D., and Breen, K. J. "Strengthening Australia's Framework for Research Oversight," *Medical Journal of Australia* 184 (2006): 261–63.
73. Downie, J. and McDonald, F. "Revisioning the Oversight of Research Involving Humans in Canada," *Health Law Journal* 12 (2004): 159–81.
74. Kirigia, J. M., Wambebe, C., and Baba-Moussa, A. "Status of National Research Bioethics Committees in the WHO African Region," *BMC Medical Ethics* 6, no. 10 (7 pages), 2005.
75. Molyneux, C. S., Wassenaar, D. R., Peshu, N., and Marsh, K. " 'Even if They Ask You to Stand by a Tree All Day, You Will Have to Do It (Laughter)...!' Community Voices on the Notion and Practice of Informed Consent for Biomedical Research in Developing Countries," *Social Science and Medicine* 61 (2005): 443–54.
76. Tate, D. F., Jackvony, E. H., and Wing, R. R. "Effects of Internet Behavioral Counseling on Weight Loss in Adults at Risk for Type 2 Diabetes: A Randomized Trial," *Journal of the American Medical Association* 289 (2003): 1833–36.
77. Evers, K. E., Cummins, C. O., Prochaska, J. O., and Prochaska, J. M. "Online Health Behavior and Disease Management Programs: Are We Ready For Them? Are They Ready For Us?" *Journal of Medical Internet Research,* 7 (2005): e27.
78. Keller, H. E. and Lee, S. "Ethical Issues Surrounding Human Participants Using the Internet," *Ethics and Behavior* 13 (2003): 211–19.
79. Varnhagen, C. K., Gushta, M., Daniels, J., Peters, T. C., Parmar, N., Law, D. et al. "How Informed is Online Informed Consent?" *Ethics and Behavior* 15 (2005) 37–48.

7

Ethical Issues in the Interaction with Research Subjects and the Disclosure of Results

ANDREA SMITH AND PAUL A. SCHULTE

Notorious cases of violations of subjects' human rights and dignity, stemming largely from Nazi medical experimentation during the 1930s and 1940s, motivated the development of ethical codes for research involving human subjects, notably the Nuremburg Code[1] and the Helsinki Declaration.[2] Along with recognizing the need to protect research participants from harm came a conviction that research subjects and patients have the right to be informed about the risks and potential benefits of their participation in a study, as well as their right to refuse involvement at any point during the research. The practice of disclosure has been further reinforced by related developments such as the 1978 *Belmont Report* of the National Commission for the Protection of Human Subjects in research,[3] the right-to-know,[4] and workers notification[5] movements, as well as various efforts by professional organizations to formulate codes of ethics for health researchers.[6-8] More recently, cases of conflict of interest[9,10] point to the need for further guidelines in obligations of full disclosure.

Research subjects have the right to expect that epidemiologists will conduct their research in accordance with established ethical principles. Autonomy entails that potential research participants are viewed and treated as self-determining and able to freely choose to participate in research without coercion or manipulation.[11] Autonomy also implies that those who are not capable of self-determination (e.g., children) are to be protected from exploitation. The ethical principle of respect for persons, which is closely related to the principle of respect for autonomy, means that individuals themselves are in the best position to protect their lives and interests if they are informed about a known risk. Respect for persons is the ethical ground upon which full disclosure to the research subject is based.[12] Some object to an unlimited practice of disclosure, expressing concern that the disclosure of aggregate or individual test results may result in harms that outweigh the benefits of the disclosure. However, evidence suggests that most research participants want research results returned to them, and that the risk of harm is less than originally estimated.[13]

In order for the practice of full disclosure to become a routine part of epidemiologic research, there remains a need for an overview of the ethical and practical issues involved in implementing disclosure, particularly as it relates to each facet of study design and execution. Even those intent on implementing full disclosure often face difficulty putting it into practice. One reason is that the return of test and of study results requires planning and resources that are often not identified by funding agencies and investigators. For example, there are often extra costs due to the increased complexity in maintaining confidentiality, the disclosure strategy itself, and follow-up.[14] These costs are not merely financial. The practice of full disclosure requires time, with investigators needing to generate lay summaries and individualized results, to contact participants, and to coordinate appropriate follow-up, all of which may require extending the duration of the study.[15] If the return of results is to be effective and ethical, disclosure should be considered during the design and funding of studies,[8] and not be merely added as an afterthought.

Developments in epidemiologic methods such as large-scale cohort studies and the increased use of molecular and genomic samples have created new challenges in disclosure. Since epidemiology is focused on populations, disclosure should be motivated by population-level bioethics, public health ethics, and clinical bioethics. Here, we review various aspects of epidemiologic studies that affect the reporting of results: (1) subject recruitment and informed consent, (2) privacy and confidentiality, (3) interpretation of test and study results, (4) communication of individualized test results, and (5) communication of study results. Our review is not exhaustive of the issues pertaining to disclosure of results. Rather, our hope is that through engaging key issues we can provide support and motivation for more widespread adoption of good practices.

Before we proceed to these practices, we analyze a few basic terms.

Disclosure: What Is It?

Most epidemiologists freely use the concepts of *disclosure* and *results*, but there are facets of each notion that are rarely discussed. By *results*, we mean not only the epidemiologic findings of a study, but also each individual's psychological, medical, or biological test result. *Results* refers not only to group comparison values (such as incidence rates or risk ratios), but also to the interpretations of summary statistics in terms of the subsequent risk to members of the studied population. In other words, returning results is not merely providing aggregate findings, it also implies providing interpretation—that is, on the extent to which an individual is at risk of a disease. Provided appropriate individual-level risk factor information is available, such individual-specific results can be quantified as an individual risk-function through the use of statistical models.[16]

By *disclosure,* we mean the act of informing or notifying study subjects (either as a group or individually) of individualized test or study results, and the risks and potential benefits implied by those results. We also include the communication of all risks and potential harms attending the participation in a study, as well as communication of all conflicts of interests of investigators. The actual provision of information is but one dimension of disclosure. *Disclosure* also includes the broad dissemination of research results through relevant publications, policy forums, and news reports. Communicating results can be complex, because what one person says is not always what another hears, with personal beliefs, opinions, and experiences influencing one's understanding of risks and objectives. This can lead to a scenario in which disclosure was adequate, but the subject's comprehension is inadequate. Thus, when communicating results, it is critical to understand disclosure as part of a process of communication, anticipating how the communication will be received and tailoring one's activities accordingly.[17,18]

Subject Recruitment and Informed Consent

With few exceptions, returning individual test or study results is usually not the first communication between investigators and study participants. The initial contact often occurs when recruiting individuals to participate in research or when seeking permission to use their medical records. It is respect for the individual's autonomy that prescribes that researchers seek their informed consent. As discussed in Chapter 4, potential research subjects must be told the nature and the purpose of the study, its duration, who the investigators and the sponsors are, the methods and procedures to be used, and all potential risks and benefits of participating in the study.[2] Potential research subjects should be informed of all conflicts of interest, as they may bias the investigators and the findings and result in harm to participants through the manipulation or improper application of ethical and scientific principles. Further, conflicts of interest can undermine the public's trust in research.[19] The motivation here is the principle of autonomy, as all information relevant to an individual's decision to participate in a study must be provided to them.

Obtaining informed consent is a process that can be characterized as having three components: (1) disclosing information, (2) securing understanding, and

(3) receiving consent, all of which are frequently centered on the administration of a consent form. Before a participant is asked to sign the consent form, an oral explanation is generally provided and time is allocated to answer the participant's questions. The consent form describes the study and the tests to be administered, although a limited and readable description may suffice (e.g., "tests of kidney function or damage") as opposed to a detailed list.

During the informed consent process it should be made clear to participants which results will be disclosed and how they will be returned. Limitations of tests, and their potential meaning for individual participants and for research findings in general, should be explained.[20] Participants must also be informed of the potential risks and benefits of receiving the results. These include the immediate risks (e.g., risks of anxiety or psychological distress), as well as potential long-term risks (e.g., potential impact on insurance coverage).[14] Some commentators have expressed concern over the temporal lag between recruitment and return of results, and have suggested that it may be important to discuss the potential risks and benefits of receiving the results prior to their return.[21] Clearly, investigators are required to consider potential ethical consequences of their disclosure protocol prior to subject recruitment, so as to ensure that their strategy is both ethically justifiable and practically feasible with available resources. Moreover, with the use of diagnostic imaging techniques and other tests with the possibility of incidental findings (e.g., neuroimaging), it becomes important to develop a strategy to account for how findings will be treated.[22,23]

A key characteristic of autonomy is voluntary choice, which raises the need to consider how coercion and manipulation of subjects can occur during recruitment and consent. The consent process must be free of fraud, deceit, or duress, and persons must be told explicitly that they can refuse to participate at any time during the study and that there is no penalty for nonparticipation. Similarly, potential research subjects must understand that they have a right to refuse receiving their individual results or study results at any time without repercussions. One proposed option is to invite participants to request their individual test results during the consent process.[20]

Depending on the nature of the study, location of recruitment and interviews can raise concerns about coercion and autonomy.[24] Investigators can manipulate subjects by inadvertently overstating the scientific contribution of a particular study, or by exaggerating the personal benefits and minimizing the risks. This highlights the need for researchers to recognize their vested interest in encouraging full participation and to be vigilant in how it affects the process of disclosure.

Manipulation can also manifest in the form of undue inducements. Inducements normally considered reasonable (i.e., adequate compensation for participation) may sway individuals' decision to participate when they are in economically vulnerable or marginalized populations.[24,6] Any use of incentives greater than the costs incurred by research subjects can only be viewed as ethically acceptable in studies where their participation carries no more than minimal risk for participants.[25]

Another such undue incentive includes offers of medical care, or the perception that medical care will be received. Often there is a blurred line between research and medical practice for participants, and investigators, because the two occur simultaneously. The distinction between research and medical practice is clarified when one considers that research activities are tests and interventions undertaken with the aim of benefiting scientific knowledge, whereas medical treatment is done with the direct intent of benefiting individual patients.[3] However, even when it is made clear to participants that they are not going to be receiving medical benefit or direct treatment, it is possible that they may still expect that they will be informed of any clinically significant findings.[22] Thus, it is necessary that any medical care or treatment received by a patient that is directly related to the study must be made explicit to research participants.

When recruiting participants and informing them of the risks and benefits of their involvement, researchers should detail the study's purposes and the intended uses of the data. Yet, it is the nature of scientific investigation that there will remain analyses that, while at the time of recruitment were unspecified and unknown, are of central importance to the research program. Thus, the question may arise as to whether specimens collected for one particular purpose can be ethically used for a related, but different, research purpose. Consider, for example, during a study of premalignant effects of a carcinogen, a new assay is developed that allows for assessment of a different mutation than the one stipulated in the study's consent form. In this case, how should a researcher proceed? Does this closely related endeavor require new consent, or given that it is consistent with the study's original expressed purpose, does consent still apply?

How to place limits on conducting additional analyses unrelated to the original purpose of the study is unclear.[26,27] This question plagues research involving repositories of biological specimens (biobanks), in which specimens can be stored and, in the future, tested using as-of-yet unavailable assays for currently unformulated research questions. Proposed solutions have included enabling participants to specify the uses to which they consent.[28] Others have argued that the requirement for detailed and specific informed consent is unduly burdensome and that a blanket informed consent remains the most appropriate.[29] These proposals suggest that a professional consensus has yet to emerge. If the tests are conducted, one must consider what should be done with the results from additional assays. Whether an investigator is responsible for communicating these new, or additional, findings to participants should be guided by the general considerations of respect for persons. Finally, a question arises over the ownership of and access to biologic specimens. For example, are the researchers the only ones able to access banked materials, or are other investigators, even other nonscientific interests (such as insurance companies, commercial interests, or employers) able to access banked specimens? Ownership of specimens and specifics about access, storage, and disposal should be detailed during the consent process.

Similar concerns can arise during the use of administrative data that have been collected for one purpose, and then used for another. Administrative data may not require informed consent, provided that such data are fully nonidentifiable, publicly available, and that the study involves minimal risk for research subjects.[8,25] In these cases, research participants will need to be protected through other mechanisms, such as through encryption and formal ethics review.[7]

Privacy and Confidentiality

When a person agrees to participate in research, he or she expects that the information or biological specimens provided will be used only for the purposes communicated to them during the informed consent process. Participants' cooperation should be recognized by respecting their right to confidentiality and privacy, as discussed in Chapter 5. Specifically, information detailing their involvement in the study and the information collected should not be distributed in a way that identifies him or her individually to any other parties (e.g., other noninvolved investigators or staff, employers, insurers, or lawyers).

Disclosure of personal information to other parties violates both privacy and confidentiality. Privacy is a concept that denotes controlled access to a participant and his or her personal information, and respect for privacy means that any personal information disclosed should only be with the consent of the participant.[30] Confidentiality implies that private or sensitive information revealed by a research participant will be protected from being revealed to others.[30] In some exceptional circumstances, there may be limits to an investigator's ability to maintain confidentiality such as disclosure ordered by court of law or necessitated by a public health emergency. Research participants should be informed of the types of situations in which confidential information may be released. Although standard practices of privacy and confidentiality—such as removing personal identifiers, data encryption, and maintaining security of data through proper storage—have been widely adopted in principle, their implementation in practice is often defective. Unauthorized dissemination or reporting of personal results intrudes on subjects' privacy and violates their confidentiality. If inappropriately disclosed, personally identifiable data collected under the auspices of research can result in harm to participants. Disease labels and risk factor status carry powerful connotations, and with them comes the potential for stigmatization and marginalization.[31] Possible outcomes of unwarranted disclosure include discrimination, stigmatization, and denial of opportunity, all of which can affect research subject's ability to obtain or keep insurance, employment, or financial credit.

Breeches of confidentiality may occur inadvertently. During the data-collection period, such unwarranted disclosures can arise when inadequately trained researchers or staff link the identity of subjects to other personal identifiers. Even if safeguards are undertaken to maintain privacy and confidentiality during the collection, analysis, and storage of data, opportunities for violating privacy and confidentiality arise in the publication stage. The most common scenario is when data sets or analyses containing enough covariate information to allow for the identification of particular subjects are published. Although rarely the case, this scenario is a possibility in small or pilot studies, or studies in which subjects have particularly unique characteristics. Thus, it is generally the case that statistical stratification which results in cell sizes of five persons or less are not published.[8] In addition to adversely affecting individual research subjects, such instances of unwarranted disclosure threaten public trust that researchers will conduct the study in ways that protect research participants.[7] This can place epidemiologic research in a precarious position of waning public support for funding and diminished public participation in studies.

Genetics raises a number of issues about privacy. With the ability to investigate the whole genome, the ethical concerns that have arisen from single gene studies will be exacerbated as investigators move toward conducting Genome Wide Association Studies (GWAS) in large cohorts or in combinations of cohorts. The utility of the GWAS approach will be maximized as the genetic data may be posted in widely accessible databases.[32] Although such approaches may be powerful research tools and resources, they have the potential to allow an individual in the database to be identified. Consequently, the privacy of individuals in such large databases is in jeopardy. Underlying the privacy issues is the nature of the original informed consent, the safeguards in the database assembly procedures, and the limitations on the use of the database by other investigators.

Concerns about privacy and confidentiality are also applicable to groups and populations. Groups may have a right to confidentiality of unlinked data. Just as individuals can be stigmatized by the disclosure of personal information, so too can a group or community. Epidemiologists have a responsibility not to inadvertently disclose information about a group or community that could put a community at risk or otherwise cause harm without any overarching public good. As with confidentiality of an individual's information, a breach of group confidentiality may potentially be justifiable in the face of a public health emergency. In such cases, investigators have a responsibility to act to prevent the stigmatization or marginalization of the group or community and its members.[7]

Interpretation of Test and Study Results

Investigators are often confronted with the question of what to reveal to study participants during the course of each study. Since epidemiologic research has the potential for social, political, and economic implications, accurate interpretation of research findings is critical. Communicating the results of an epidemiologic study requires appropriate interpretation of findings from both a scientific and ethical perspective. Researchers have an obligation to maintain the fidelity and accuracy of results[2] and to conform to scientific principles. This responsibility suggests that epidemiologists ought to use the most reliable and valid measures for the purposes of interpretation of results. It is important to ensure that the epidemiologic interpretation, as opposed to clinical interpretation of a result is made clear.[33] Participants may anticipate the return of results with clinical significance, even where results are only interpretable at the population level.[34] Participants also may want action; they may seek recommendations to ban or promote a drug, restrict an environmental hazard, or attribute a particular risk factor as the cause of their disease. Frequently, individual studies alone do not provide enough conclusive data to support such calls for action. Without exaggerating or minimizing their findings, researchers must juggle the responsibility of providing the most definitive recommendations justifiable by their studies.[7]

There are several dimensions of interpreting results that bear on disclosure. These include: (1) the use of group data as the basis for identifying an individual's risk; (2) whether or not surviving or healthy subjects are at the same risk as the overall study population from which measures of risk were calculated; (3) the use of appropriate thresholds for statistical significance; and (4) the difficulties of interpreting novel biological markers. We will explore each of these in turn.

Epidemiologic protocols summarize the characteristics of one group compared with that of another group, and such data do not necessarily bear on the experience of any particular individual within the group.[35] It is imperative that researchers uphold their responsibility to provide accurate interpretation of results by explicitly acknowledging that the epidemiologic measures of risk are group-specific. Inferences drawn from one level of analysis and applied to another are susceptible to fallacious reasoning. In the case of individual-level inferences drawn from population-level data, the risk is that these inferences are subject to the ecological fallacy.[36,37] Whether measures of risk derived from the study population are applicable to individual members depends on probability.

Much of what falls under the umbrella of public health pertains to identifying the persons or members of a group who may be at higher risk. In the event of a positive association between exposure and disease, individuals with the outcome of interest may be more likely to be those with the highest exposures or those who are most susceptible. Surviving or healthy subjects may not be at the same risk as the high-risk persons. If researchers provide these healthy subjects with the results derived from high-risk individuals without clarifying that such findings are not likely to be applicable to them, they may be misinformed that they are at higher risk than they actually are.

Finally, with regards to statistical tests, correct interpretation means one should bear in mind the likelihood of Type I and II errors, as statistical certainty in test results is amongst the considerations that affect researchers' ability to interpret results. Thus, appropriate tailed test and p-values should be selected. When a study involves multiple comparisons it may be necessary for researchers to distinguish their findings based on a priori hypotheses from those based on a posteriori hypotheses. In the case of a posteriori hypotheses a stricter test of statistical significance might be warranted. Similarly, if relevant, uncertainty in results (e.g., from statistical imprecision), should be acknowledged during the interpreting of results. These issues emphasize the value of adhering to the highest scientific standards as it facilitates ethical disclosure.

Problems with interpretation can also arise when using data derived from biological specimens. Given the extensive variation in genetic and biological factors,[38] it is vital that investigators recognize the role of this variation in interpreting test results. Failing to do so may lead to inappropriate inferences that will influence the interpretation and communication of biomarker results.[39] Thus, it is crucial that the range of biomarker values in the general population is known. Depending on the biomarker, the range of normal values can be quite expansive.

It is frequently the case that epidemiologic studies involve biological markers for which the "normal" range has not been established. This scenario arises in the use of technologies such as in genomics and neuroscience, for which the link between test results and health outcomes remains highly uncertain. In these cases, researchers are in a difficult position with respect to the interpretation of results from tests that are not yet validated, yet are suspected indicators of risk or susceptibility. Some suggest that only the test results with clear clinical validity or other interpretation that enables action (whether preventative or remedial) should be disclosed.[40] While the concern with not causing harm in the form of unnecessary worry or anxiety is one of benevolence, it can run counter to the principles of respect for persons, and can be considered paternalistic. One can envision scenarios where such test results, once validated, could prove to be invaluable to the research participant. With regards to returning such ambiguous test results, the key issue is to provide each subject with some perspective on their results, even if their exact epidemiologic or clinical meaning is not known. For example, providing subjects with both their own results and the statistical mean and range of the study groups results, or further details on the biological mechanisms suspected to be important, facilitates understanding.

Furthermore, biomarkers have multiple meanings, and can indicate an exposure, effect, or susceptibility,[41] with each of these uses having their own particular disclosure requirements and challenges. For example, not all biomarkers will be disease-related, and many may only represent normal variation that may or may not go on to be pathologic. Markers of susceptibility may also only be relevant in the presence of a specific type of exposure. These distinctions must be explained when communicating test results to subjects. The use of genetic analysis poses unique challenges in the interpretation of results due to a lack of validation.

Moreover, it must be borne in mind that such results may have an interpretation both for the research subject and their family due to shared genetic variation.

Population-Based Research Involving Low-Penetrance Gene Variants

Until recently there was little available guidance for addressing the ethical, legal, and social issues involved in population-based studies of low-penetrance gene variants. The guidance that did exist generally pertained to single genes of high penetrance that are investigated in family studies. The risks and benefits of population-based research involving low-penetrance gene variants can differ from those associated with the family-based research that has been the cornerstone of genetic epidemiology. As Beskow et al. observed, "Recommendations developed for family-based research are not well suited for most population-based research because they generally fail to distinguish between studies expected to reveal clinically relevant information about participants and studies expected to have meaningful public health implications but involving few physical, psychological, or social risks for individual participants."[42]

Recently developed consent materials address the distinction between genetic research expected to reveal clinically relevant information about individual participants and genetic research that does not. Population-based research involving genetics will not be expected to identify clinically relevant information. Beskow et al. did not recommend informing participants of individual results in these types of studies. However, they did note that the line between low and high penetrance may be difficult to define; therefore, they recommended that, "When the risks identified are both valid and associated with proven intervention for risk reduction, disclosure may be appropriate."[42]

Communication of Individual Test Results

Although acknowledged by some researchers, the responsibility for communicating both individual test results and overall study results is not universally recognized.[43] A recent international survey of longitudinal studies on aging found that only 70% of studies reported that they returned individualized test results to participants.[44] By communicating and explaining individualized test results, participants receive tangible benefits from their involvement, which may be used to protect or to promote their health.

The information provided to study subjects must include the probability of the outcome under study, its extent or severity, and the uncertainty associated with each test result.[20] This communication is best performed by individuals with the appropriate scientific and communications training. Whether results are returned through written correspondence, oral communication, or face-to-face interaction depends on the investigators' relationship with the participants, the nature of the investigation,[14] and the resources available. Whichever strategy is chosen, it must be discussed and agreed on by participants during the informed consent process.

To take an example, reporting individual test results of those tested for their HIV seropositive status is mandatory under U.S. Public Health Service (PHS) policy. Originally implemented in 1988, this applies to all intramural and extramural PHS activities, including domestic and foreign research and health services activities.[45,46] It requires that for HIV testing conducted or supported by PHS, those individuals whose results are associated with personal identifiers and are seropositive must be informed of their test results, and provided with the opportunity to receive appropriate counseling. Exceptions are made under special circumstances, set forth in the policy. The ramifications of such a policy on disclosure should be discussed with participants during recruitment and consent.

As part of considering in advance the potential harms and benefits posed to research participants, investigators should anticipate the consequences of the participants learning their results. With some test results, it may be best to enlist the aid of the subjects' physician or other appropriately qualified medical personnel in the communication of test results. For example, as part of a participatory research project on cardiovascular disease in Inuit communities, participants' test results were returned by mail to both research subjects and physicians.[47] Such activities serve to facilitate referrals to appropriate medical care and to afford participants further opportunities for discussing and understanding their individual test results. Again, such disclosure to other health professionals must be consented to by research subjects during recruitment.

Despite the ethical basis for disclosure, there is the possibility that even the warranted returning of individual test results may have harmful effects for both investigator and participant. Clearly, disclosure places additional burdens, financial and otherwise, upon investigators. Although full disclosure of individualized results facilitates and encourages participant retention, making it a particularly beneficial strategy for longitudinal studies, disclosing results before the conclusion of the study may introduce bias and cause participants to change their behavior, thus altering the outcome of the study.[7] In such ongoing studies, it is may be permissible to wait until the completion of the study before releasing individual test results, as investigators are also ethically required to ensure the scientific validity of their research. The obvious exception would be results that provide information of an immediate risk to a participant should be promptly disclosed, regardless of impact on the study.

Regarding potential harms resulting from disclosing individual test results to participants, several issues have been raised. In an occupational setting, such concerns have included an increase in illness behaviors such as workplace absenteeism among notified individuals.[48] A more common concern is that disclosure of individualized test results, particularly those whose values have no clear clinical interpretation, will cause more harm in the form of undue anxiety than benefit.[49] Thus, the question is raised: who should decide if information that pertains to a person is too anxiety-inducing and that disclosure should be avoided? Institutional Review Boards, investigators, and community advisory boards have been suggested. Such paternalism, while likely stemming from the best of intentions and consideration of nonmalfeasance, comes into direct conflict with subjects' right to autonomy. Further, limited disclosure means reducing or eliminating potential benefits for participants. In short, there does not appear to be ethical grounds for the limiting of disclosure. Evidence is mounting that suggests people wish to have results returned to them.[13] For example, Gustafsson Stolt and colleagues[50] found that in their work on neonatal screening, mothers were predisposed to respond positively to information about a baby's increased risk, seeing it as an opportunity rather than a source of anxiety. Indeed, many saw it as their right-to-know. Furthermore, in the anticipated event of anxiety, investigators can provide or encourage participants to access supportive measures, such as counseling or peer support.

Communicating Study Results

To Study Participants

Prior to the early 1980s, epidemiologists did not routinely notify research participants of study results. Debate over the return of study findings on mortality rates to subjects in a retrospective cohort of workers was the ethical basis of the practice.[51] Today, several ethical guidelines encourage the timely return of study results to research subjects,[6-8,52] although certainly not all. Many of the issues that characterize the communication of individual test results are shared by the communication of study results—accurate interpretation, appropriate information, acknowledging uncertainty, and providing the necessary follow-up. In cases where unlinked data are used, the study results should be communicated to the widest possible population or communities for whom such information is relevant.[6-8]

To help guide epidemiologists during the process of communicating study results to participants, Sandman[53] articulated some responsibilities of epidemiologists:

1. Tell the people who are most affected what you have found—and tell them first.
2. Make sure people understand what you are telling them, and what you think the implications are.
3. Develop mechanisms to bolster the credibility of your study and your findings.

4. Acknowledge uncertainty promptly and thoroughly.
5. Show respect for public concerns even when they are not scientific.
6. Involve people in the design, implementation, and interpretation of the study.
7. Decide that communication is part of your job and learn the rudiments.

The ethical obligation to return study results suggests that more emphasis needs to be placed on developing communication skills in epidemiology training programs.

The issues surrounding epidemiologists' task of drawing appropriate inferences across levels of analysis also bears upon the return of study results. Epidemiologic measures of association between outcomes and exposures are group results, and thus the main challenge is to accurately convey their relevance to individual research participants. An investigator could either underestimate the risks posed to individual group members, by attributing any findings to a few highly exposed or susceptible individuals, or overestimate the risks by failing to acknowledge the particular characteristics of individuals and their exposures that are characteristic of greater risk.

Likewise affecting epidemiologists is the communication of relative, absolute, and attributable risks to research subjects. The failure to distinguish between these risks and the inferences supported by them affects the trustworthiness of the research findings being communicated.[54] Consider, for example, a finding of a high relative risk of a rare disease. This finding would trigger a different communication and follow-up strategy than a finding of a lower relative risk of a more common disease. Whether unintentional or not, the selection of the measure of risk can exaggerate or trivialize the risk posed by a particular exposure.

Anticipating the needs of research participants upon the return of the study results may involve the coordination of appropriate follow-up. For some participants, follow-up may include referrals for further information, counseling, or support. Depending on the study, all research subjects may be in need of medical follow-up, to assess whether they have developed signs of the disease for which they are at risk and to implement preventative measures. This responsibility may not fall exclusively on the investigators' shoulders, and it may, for example, be shared by the institution at which the research is undertaken.

Once notified of research findings, many participants' next concern is what it implies about their own personal risk, and what they can do about it. In some cases, participants, either individually or collectively, seek legal redress for real or perceived damages, including heightened anxiety due to their high-risk status.[18] Although disagreement remains as to whether epidemiologists have the duty to advocate for policy or other interventions based on their findings, researchers can act as advocates for public health policy or interventions when such actions are vital and supported by evidence.

To the Scientific Community and Society

In addition to returning study results to participants and communities, epidemiologists also have an ethical obligation to communicate findings to their peers and other stakeholders (e.g., policy makers, funding agencies) to whom the findings may be of interest.[55] Most often, such communication is done by publishing the findings in peer-review scientific journals, or in the grey literature such as government reports, research institution reports, graduate theses, and so forth. Ad hoc methods such as whistle blowing may also be used as socially responsible means of disclosure. When reporting studies, it is important that sufficient detail of study design, methods, data, and sources of biases are provided so as to permit others to draw conclusions from the study and to enable an independent evaluation of the findings.[7] Publication should be done in a prompt manner. The lack of timely publication of research findings is an ethical issue and impacts the quality and validity of scientific inference in a research area by inhibiting the availability of all relevant evidence.

Cases of bias where research results are not published because of negative or other unwanted findings are of particular concern. For example, lack of timely publication was claimed when the asbestos industry allegedly prevented publication of industry-sponsored animal experimental data that documented the carcinogenicity of asbestos.[56] This and other similar examples illustrate the potential ethical ramifications of conflicts of interest when a third party with vested interests in a particular result has financial or intellectual control over the study. Ethical guidelines for epidemiologists uphold the principle that publication is obligated, regardless of the results.[6–8] Furthermore, pressure to tone down or withdraw conclusions should be refused, as is consistent with the obligation to maintain the fidelity and accuracy of the results.[2]

Another reason for the failure to publish studies with statistically nonsignificant or negative results is because often they are never submitted for publication. Having lost interest is one reason commonly cited by investigators for not submitting results for publication.[57] At first glance, such decisions may seem to be lacking the ethical consequences of efforts to intentionally suppress or manipulate study findings, but such failure to publish still contributes to publication bias. Publication bias, regardless of its cause, may have an adverse effect on subsequent studies, notably meta-analyses or systematic reviews,[58] and ultimately may affect public health interventions and practice. Thus, in addition to being compensated according to the number of peer-review publications, we suggest that ethical considerations may also provide compelling reasons for investigators to submit all studies for publication. Publishing results is one of the benefits to society that stems from scientific research, and contributing to scientific knowledge should be one of the guiding motivations underlying epidemiologic research.

Lastly, as with the need to disclose all potential conflict of interests to potential research participants during the process of recruitment and informed consent, researchers are ethically obligated to disclose any material conflicts of interest to their collaborators, sponsors, research participants, journal editors, and their employer.[7] As with the need to disclose conflict of interests to research participants, investigators have an obligation to disclose all information relevant to the evaluation and interpretation of study results. This obligation is not to suggest that the existence of material conflicts means there is bias. Rather, with regards to conflict of interests, such disclosures enable scientific peers to evaluate whether any potential manipulation, intentional or otherwise, occurred. Full disclosure is also essential for public trust of epidemiologic research, as such transparency helps to garner the public's confidence that researchers are adhering to proper ethical and scientific standards.

Disclosure and Vulnerable Communities

While bioethics is often heavily focused on concern for autonomous choice and individual rights, public health is motivated to protect the public at large, and thus investigators are required to consider populations.[59,60] Because of epidemiologists' concern with public health issues of justice, they must also seek fairness in the distribution of benefits and harms associated with their research.[3] Hence, special attention should be given when returning study results to those populations vulnerable to coercion, exploitation, and discrimination due to social and economic marginalization.[24]

Conclusions

It is unlikely that this chapter alone will move epidemiologists toward the universal adoption of the practice of full disclosure, but we hope we have covered enough ground to persuade the reader that disclosure has ethical appeal. Funding agencies, educational institutions, and ethics review boards should all play a role in encouraging full disclosure to become a common practice.

The ethical principle of beneficence implies an obligation to act in the best interests of research participants. For epidemiologists, beneficence has the further connotation of an obligation to act in the best interests of society. Our discussion of disclosure and the consequence of communicating results highlights the importance of researchers' responsibilities. Disclosure obligations are largely contingent upon whether the study results are valid and reliable; hence research must incorporate a good rationale, study design, execution, and analysis. When an epidemiologic finding is disclosed, at the very least the research participants and the public should have confidence that all efforts were made to ensure that the findings were valid, given the current state of knowledge. Without the confidence that epidemiologists conduct their research in an ethically and scientifically rigorous fashion, many public health functions epidemiologists perform may become more difficult or even impossible.

ACKNOWLEDGMENTS

The authors would like to acknowledge Mitchell Singal, who contributed to this chapter in the first edition and upon which this version is based. We also thank the editors of this volume for their helpful comments.

NOTE

The findings and conclusions in this chapter are those of the authors and do not necessarily represent the views of the National Institute for Occupational Safety and Health.

References

1. *Nuremburg Code.* Trials of War Criminals before the Nuremberg Military Tribunals under Control Council Law No. 10. Vol. 2, pp. 181–82. Washington, DC: U.S. Government Printing Office, 1949.
2. World Medical Association. *Declaration of Helsinki: Ethical Principles for Medical Research Involving Human Subjects.* 52nd World Medical Association General Assembly, Edinburgh, Scotland, October 2000.
3. National Commission for the Protection of Human Subjects of Biomedical and Behavioral Research. The Belmont Report: Ethical Principles and Guidelines for the Protection of Human Subjects of Research. Washington, DC: U.S. Government Printing Office, 1978.
4. Baram, M. S. "The Right-To-Know and the Duty to Disclose Hazard Information," *American Journal of Public Health* 74 (1984): 385–90.
5. Sattler, B. "Rights and Realities: A Critical Review of the Accessibility of Information on Hazardous Chemicals," *Occupational Medicine* 7 (1992): 189–96.
6. Council for International Organizations of Medical Sciences. International Guidelines for Ethical Review of Epidemiological Studies. Geneva, Switzerland: World Health Organization, 1991.
7. American College of Epidemiology. "Ethics Guidelines," *Annals of Epidemiology* 10 (2000): 487–97.
8. International Society for Environmental Epidemiology. Ethics Guidelines for Environmental Epidemiologists. Soskolne, C. L. and Light, A. "Towards Ethics Guidelines for Environmental Epidemiologists," *The Science of the Total Environment* 184 (1996): 137–47.
9. Gilman, P. "A Conflict-of-Interest Policy for Epidemiology," *Epidemiology* 17 (2006): 250–51.
10. Hardell, L., Walker, M. J., Walhjalt, B., Friedman, L. S., and Richter, E. D. "Secret Ties to Industry and Conflicting Interests in Cancer Research," *American Journal of Industrial Medicine* (November 2006) [Published online].
11. Weed, D. L. and McKeown, R. E. "Ethics in Epidemiology and Public Heath I. Technical Terms," *Journal of Epidemiology and Community Health* 55 (2001): 855–57.

12. Fernandez, C. V., Kodish, E., and Weijer, C. "Informing Study Participants of Research Results: An Ethical Imperative," *Institutional Review Board* 25 (2003): 12–19.

13. Partridge A. H., Wong, J. S., Kundsen, K., Gelman, R., Sampson, E., Bishop, K. L., Harris, J. R., and Winer, E. P. "Offering Participants Results of a Clinical Trial: Sharing Results of a Negative Study," *Lancet* 365 (2005): 963–64.

14. Fernandez, C. V., Skedgel , C., and Weijer, C. "Considerations and Costs of Disclosing Study Findings to Research Participants," *Canadian Medical Association Journal* 170 (2004): 1417–19.

15. Fernandez, C. V., Kodish, E., and Weijer, C. "Importance of Informed Consent in Offering to Return Research Results to Research Participants," *Medical and Pediatric Oncology* 41 (2003): 592–93.

16. Schulte, P. A. "The Epidemiologic Basis for the Notification of Subjects of Cohort Studies," *American Journal of Epidemiology* 121 (1985): 351–61.

17. Hampel, J. "Different Concepts of Risk – A Challenge for Risk Communication," *International Journal of Medical Microbiology* 296 (2006): 5–10 Suppl.

18. Schulte, P. A. "Ethical Issues in the Communication of Results," *Journal of Clinical Epidemiology* 44 (1991): 57S–61S.

19. Resnik, D. B. "Disclosing Conflicts of Interest to Research Subjects: An Ethical and Legal Analysis," *Accountability in Research* 11 (2004): 141–59.

20. Shalowitz, D. I. and Miller, F. G. "Disclosing Individual Results of Clinical Research – Implications of Respect for Participants," *Journal of The American Medical Association* 294 (2005): 737–40.

21. Fernandez, C. V., Shurin, S., and Kodish, E. "Providing Research Participants with Findings from Completed Cancer-Related Clinical Trials – Not Quite as Simple as it Sounds," *Cancer* 107 (2006): 1419–20.

22. Illes, J., Kirschen, M. P., Karetsky, K., Kelly, M., Saha, A., Desmond, J. E., Raffin, T. A., Glover, G. H., and Atlas, S. W. "Discovery and Disclosure of Incidental Findings in Neuroimaging Research," *Journal of Magnetic Resonance Imaging* 20 (2004): 743–47.

23. Illes, J., Kirschen, M. P., Edwards, E., Stanford, L. R., Bandettini, P., Cho, M. K., Ford, P. J., Glover, G. H., Kulynych, J., Macklin, R., Michael, D. B., and Wolf, S. M. "Ethics – Incidental Findings in Brain Imaging Research," *Science* 311 (2006): 783–84.

24. Cooper, S. P., Heitman, E., Fox, E. E., Quill, B., Knudson, P., Zahm, S. H., MacNaugton, N., and Ryder, R. "Ethical Issues in Conducting Migrant Farmworker Studies," *Journal of Immigrant Health* 6 (2004): 29–39.

25. Bolumar, F., Barros, H., Florey, C., Olsen, J., Osler, M., Skjaerven, R., Diaz, M. J. T., and Zielhuis G. *Good Epidemiological Practice (GEP): Proper Conduct in Epidemiologic Research.* International Epidemiology Association, 2004. Available on-line at http://www.dundee.ac.uk/iea/GEP07.htm

26. Schulte, P. A. and Sweeny, M. H. "Ethical Considerations, Confidentiality Issues, Rights of Human Subjects and Uses of Monitoring Data in Research and Regulation." Proceedings of the Symposium on Human Tissue Monitoring and Specimen Banking: Opportunities for Exposure Assessment, Risk Assessment and Epidemiologic Research. *Environmental Health Perspectives* 103 (1995): S69–S74.

27. Maschke, K. "Alternative Consent Approaches for Biobank Research," *The Lancet Oncology* 7 (2006): 193–94.

28. Hansson, M. G., Dillner, J., Bartram, C. R., Carlson, J. A., and Helgesson, G. "Should Donors be Allowed to Give Broad Consent to Future Biobank Research?" *The Lancet Oncology* 7 (2006): 266–69.

29. Knoppers, B. M. "Biobanks: Simplifying Consent," *Nature Reviews Genetics* 7 (2004): 485.

30. McKeown, R. E. and Weed, D. L. "Ethics in Epidemiology and Public Health II. Applied Terms," *Journal of Epidemiology and Community Health* 56 (2002): 739–41.

31. Nelkin, D. and Tancredi, L. *Dangerous Diagnostics: The Social Power of Biological Information.* New York: Basic Books Inc., 1989.

32. Couzin, J. and Kaiser, J. "Closing the Net on Common Disease Genes," *Science* 317 (2007): 820–22.

33. Shields, P. G. "Understanding Population and Individual Risk Assessment: The Case of Polychlorinated Biphenyls," *Cancer Epidemiology, Biomarkers & Prevention* 15 (2006): 830–39.

34. Schulte, P. A. "Interpretation and Communication of Molecular Epidemiologic Data." In *Molecular Epidemiology: Principles and Practices*, ed. P. A. Schulte and F. P. Perera. San Diego: Academic Press, 1993: 233–50.

35. Schulte P. A. "Epidemiologic Basis for the Notification of Subjects of Cohort Studies," *American Journal of Epidemiology* 121 (1985): 351–61.

36. Rockhill, B. "Theorizing about Causes at the Individual Level while Estimating Effects at the Population Level: Implications for Prevention," *Epidemiology* 16 (2005): 124–29.

37. Diez-Roux, A. V. "Bringing Context Back into Epidemiology: Variables and Fallacies in Multilevel Analysis," *American Journal of Public Health* 88 (1998): 216–22.

38. Buchanan, A. V., Weiss, K. M., and Fullerton, S. M. "Dissecting Complex Disease: The Quest for the Philosopher's Stone?" *International Journal of Epidemiology* 35 (2006) 562–71.

39. Smith, A. and Robert, J. S. "Is the Cup Half-Full, or Half-Empty? Some Conceptual and Normative Dimensions of Toxicogenomics." In *Genomics and Environmental Regulation: Science, Ethics, and Law,* ed. R. Sharp, G. Marchant, and J. Grodsky. Baltimore, MD: John Hopkins University Press, 2008.

40. Deck, W. and Kosatsky, T. "Communicating Their Individual Results to Participants in an Environmental Exposure Study: Insights From Clinical Ethics," *Environmental Research* 80 (1999): 223S–29S.

41. Schulte, P. A. "The Use of Biomarkers in Surveillance, Medical Screening, and Intervention," *Mutation Research* 592 (2005): 155–63.

42. Beskow, L. M., Burke, W., Merz, J. F., Barr, P. A., Terry, S., Penchaszadeh, V. B., Gostin, L. O., Gwinn, M., Khoury, M. J. "Informed Consent for Population-Based Research Involving Genetics," *Journal of the American Medical Association* 286 (2001): 2315–21.

43. MacNeil, S. D. and Fernandez, C. V. "Informing Research Participants of Research Results: Analysis of Canadian University Based Research Ethics Board Policies," *Journal of Medical Ethics* 32 (2006): 49–54.

44. Dukeshire, S., Kits, O., Strople, G., Chipman, T., Kirkland, S., Raina, P., and Wolfson, C. "Return of Individualized Test Results to Participants in a Longitudinal Population-Based Study." Poster presented at the 34th Annual Scientific and Education Meeting of the Canadian Association on Gerontology, Halifax, NS, 2005.

45. OPRR Reports: Policy on Informing Those Tested About HIV Status, 1988.

46. OPRR Reports: Guidelines for Institutional Review Boards for AIDS Studies, December 26, 1984.

47. Ebbesson, S. O., Laston, S., Wenger, C. R., Dyke, B., Romenesko, T., Swenson, M., Fabsitz, R. R., MacCluer, J. W., Devereux, R., Roman, M., Robbins, D., and Howard, B. V. "Recruitment and Community Interactions in the GOCADAN Study," *International Journal of Circumpolar Health* 65 (2006): 55–64.

48. Sands, R. G., Newby, L. G., and Greenberg, R. A. "Labeling of Health Risks in Industrial Settings," *Journal of Applied Behavioral Sciences* 17 (1985): 359–74.

49. Markman, M. "Providing Research Participants with Findings from Completed Cancer-Related Clinical Trials," *Cancer* 106 (2006) 1421–24.

50. Gustafsson Stolt, U., Liss, P.-E., Svensson, T., and Ludvigsson, J. "Attitudes to Bioethical Issues: A Case Study of a Screening Project," *Social Science and Medicine* 54 (2002): 1333–44.

51. Bayer R. "Notifying Workers At Risk: The Politics of the Right-To-Know," *American Journal of Public Health* 76 (1986): 1352–56.

52. Canadian Institutes of Health Research, Natural Science and Engineering Research Council of Canada, Social Sciences and Humanities Research Council of Canada. *Tri-Council Policy Statement: Ethical Conduct for Research Involving Humans,* 1998 (with 2000, 2002, 2005 amendments).

53. Sandman, P. M. "Emerging Communication Responsibilities of Epidemiologists," *Journal of Clinical Epidemiology* 49 (1991): 541–50.

54. Rockhill, B., Newman, B., and Weinberg, C. "Use and Misuse of Population Attributable Fractions," *American Journal of Public Health* 88 (1998): 15–19.

55. Weed, D. L. and Mink, P. J. "Roles and Responsibilities of Epidemiologists," *Annals of Epidemiology* 12 (2002): 67–72.

56. Hardy, H. and Egilman, D. "Corruption of Occupational Medical Literature: The Asbestos Example," *American Journal of Industrial Medicine* 20 (1991): 127–29.

57. Dickersin, K., Min, Y. I., and Meinert, C. L. "Factors Influencing Publication of Results," *Journal of the American Medical Association* 267 (1992): 374–78.

58. Dickersin, K. "Systematic Review in Epidemiology: Why Are We So Far behind?" *International Journal of Epidemiology* 31 (2002): 6–12.

59. Bayer, R. and Fairchild, A. L. "The Genesis of Public Health Ethics," *Bioethics* 18 (2004): 473–92.

60. Callahan, D. "Individual Good and Common Good: A Communitarian Approach To Bioethics," *Perspectives in Biology and Medicine* 46 (2003): 496–507.

8

Ethics in Public Health Practice

ROBERT E. McKEOWN AND R. MAX LEARNER

Ethical challenges and controversy are occupational companions for public health practitioners. From emergency responses to outbreaks such as SARS and the devastation of Hurricane Katrina and preparedness for the predicted pandemic influenza to routine surveillance and implementation of public health policies and programs, public health practitioners are frequently confronted by ethical questions that require careful, principled, and rational analysis and response.

In this chapter we outline a perspective that can serve as a foundation for addressing ethical concerns in public health practice. Our perspective is informed by the approach of Alasdair MacIntyre,[1] whose definition of practice is the starting point for the foundation we propose below. This approach, which starts with the goal (*telos*) of public health and views practice as directed toward fulfillment of that goal and related goods, provides a common ground on which we can base further discussions.

Considerations of value are essentially related to the ends of public health, but are also critical in our assessment and implementation of the means by which we achieve those ends. The task of ethics then involves a continuing examination of means and ends in an iterative process that includes refining the definition of the end, evaluating appropriate means, and balancing the range of sometimes competing values, virtues, obligations, and principles that guide our practice. This approach is grounded in the view that we cannot disentangle questions of value from those of science from which the means are derived. Thus, in this perspective, ethics also comes into play in scientific considerations within public health practice. In an analogous approach, Madison Powers and Ruth Faden[2] have proposed a view of social justice in which the basis for evaluating the justice of a set of principles or policies is the ends or purposes the principles are intended to achieve and the adequacy of the principles for achieving those ends in concrete life situations. They propose that the overarching end toward which justice is directed is human well-being, which is composed of six essential, distinct, but interrelated dimensions: health, respect, self-determination, personal and social attachment, reasoning, and personal security. In their view, the emphasis on ends to be achieved implies that "empirical judgments of how various inequalities affect one another in concrete circumstances are ineliminable moral data," and that "achieving justice is an inherently remedial task, constantly shifting in its specific requirements as social circumstance themselves change (p. 5)."[2] This is consistent with our position that ethics in public health practice requires ongoing examination of means and ends with continuing adjustments relating ends and means to professional values, virtues, obligations, and principles.

This approach also has implications for our understanding of responsibility, which we see as an obligation to work toward ends to which we have committed, a position that has been developed elsewhere.[3,4] In professional public health practice, responsibility can be viewed as accountability, as reliability, and as commitment to or for someone or something. All of these enter into considerations of ethical practice of any profession, including acceptance of responsibility as a commitment to the fundamental ends of a profession itself, and all can be seen in the case studies later in this chapter.

We start with general comments about ethics as a prelude to a fuller discussion of the goal and mission of public health, followed by a case study on ethical issues raised by the public health response to the SARS epidemic. We then examine the nature of public health practice including the values embodied within it and their implications for practice, together with the role of values in the evaluation of science-based means to achieve public health ends. The latter issue leads to a more extended discussion of the research versus practice distinction, with a case study drawn from clinical practice, but with public health implications. Central to concerns surrounding the research–practice distinction is the ability to respond quickly to events, so the case study leads into a discussion of the concepts of preventive and procedural ethics, which is, in turn, followed by another case study on preparations for pandemic influenza. The nature of public health's mission and practice requires us to examine ethical problems in ways that may differ from clinical biomedical ethics, so we provide a discussion of some of those differences and make explicit certain characteristics of public health ethics, followed by a section on the role of a human rights perspective for public health. After a final case study on response to hurricane

Katrina, we discuss some ethical aspects of statistical analysis and error rates, before a summary and conclusion.

Foundations for Ethics in Public Health Practice

MacIntyre defines practice as a "coherent and complex form of socially established cooperative human activity through which goods internal to that form of activity are realized."[1] Public health practice spans policy and program development, implementation, evaluation, regulatory activities, health promotion and intervention, and, in some cases, provision of direct health services. Given this scope, it is unavoidable that public health professionals, institutions, and agencies will face, and sometimes generate, tension between competing values and obligations. Despite this breadth of scope and diversity, public health professionals share many core values and obligations, and also experience similar ethical dilemmas. Our view is that the mission of public health sets forth a common overarching goal that unifies the otherwise disparate disciplines of public health. This mission and closely related shared values, especially those related to justice, respect for persons, and the importance of health for personal and social well-being, constitute the foundation for addressing unavoidable tensions and trade-offs.

Public health professionals are often called upon to determine avenues of health investigation, protocols for research or surveillance, courses of action, and public policies that are intended to protect or promote health but that may also have uncertain scientific bases. These choices sometimes place constraints on fundamental rights, impose risks, or allocate resources or benefits unequally. Thus, it is inevitable that public health professionals will face trade-offs due to competing values and obligations. The task of ethics then becomes determining when such trade-offs are necessary, adjudicating among unavoidable trade-offs and conflicts in the context of the mission to protect and promote health, and justifying the chosen alternative.

As discussed by Tom Beauchamp in Chapter 2, ethics is a discipline concerned with the reasoned and critical judgment of human actions and decisions that have moral content, including an account of the ends, values, obligations, principles, and rules which guide that judgment.[5,6,7,8,9] Inevitably a principle of selectivity comes into play in any account of ethics or of a specific ethical decision. Each account is partial and provisional, shaped by core concerns, focusing on those features relevant for resolution of the issue at hand, and framed by the overarching end.

The relative importance or place of specific ethical values, principles, and obligations differs among professions, though it is characteristic of professions that each has common values and obligations, as well as a commitment to knowledge and excellence in the discipline.[6,10] Even within a profession, there may be relatively more or less emphasis on a particular ethical value or obligation according to professional roles or specialties. For example, maintaining confidentiality plays a different, and arguably more important, role for the public health professional involved in disease transmission contact tracing than for the food service inspector. In keeping with MacIntyre's definition of practice, shared ends, core values, and fundamental duties internal to the practice of a profession provide the basis for the ethics of the profession of public health. To lay a foundation for ethics in public health practice, we turn now to the nature and the mission of public health, for that defines the end toward which practice is directed.

The Institute of Medicine's (IOM) influential 1988 report, *The Future of Public Health*,[11] defined the mission of public health as, "The fulfillment of society's interest in assuring conditions in which people can be healthy." The substance of public health has been characterized, at least since the first quarter of the 20th century, as "organized community efforts aimed at the prevention of disease and promotion of health."[12] Public health practitioners are committed to work toward the desired end of assuring conditions that contribute to the public's health, which includes conducting the epidemiologic research needed to determine what those conditions are and how they contribute to well-being.

The IOM statement also makes explicit the claim that society has an interest in the health of people. It is not clear whether "society's interest" in the health of the population is because society holds the public's health to be a societal good in itself or because health is instrumental to attaining other goods or desired ends. Powers and Faden provide helpful insight into this issue in the context of their delineation of a broader concept of human well-being that includes health as one of six essential and distinct dimensions, described below. In their view, the value of each dimension is both in achieving a certain state, such as being healthy, and in the role each plays in the achievement of other dimensions of well-being or other goods.[2] To illustrate, historically, happiness and well-being have been accepted as legitimate ends for purposes of ethical analysis. It seems reasonable to consider health as a similar end as well as an essential contributor to happiness and well-being. In this sense, health is valued in its own right and for its own sake *and* as an instrumental good, desirable because it is necessary to achieve other desired ends.

A parallel question is whether the aim of public health is provision or attainment of health itself by and for people, or is the aim of public health to assure conditions and capabilities for people to pursue their own (or their community's health) if they so choose? The argument presented by Powers and Faden[2] is pertinent in making a distinction between the capabilities perspective[13] and their view of the dimensions of well-being, including health. They acknowledge that provision for or protection of capabilities is a critical component of achieving the dimensions of well-being, but hold that it is not only the capability, which after all may not be possible for some persons, such as children, but the achievement of the dimension itself that is desired. "Moreover," they write,

for most of the dimensions on our list, the focus on "capability of achieving it if one wishes" misunderstands the central aims of justice. While there is some truth in the notion that a part—but only a part—of what matters in being healthy is room to pursue our own health objectives if and to the extent that we wish, most of our dimensions are quite different. We want to be respected by ourselves and by others, not simply for us and others to have the capability to exercise respect if we, or they, so choose. We want to form attachments to others for our own sake and for reasons of sustaining just institutions and practices. What we want is the success of these attachments, not simply that some can form them if they so choose. Justice requires not just the capability for attachment if individuals wish to exercise it; rather it is essential for the capability to be developed and exercised for the success of other-regarding morality.... While to some degree both health and reason are matters for which the individual is largely the proper judge of how much achievement is worth pursuing, even here the emphasis on capabilities is misplaced. In some sufficient measure, the actual development and exercise of reason is essential to the functioning of society and the well-being of others, no less than respect. The same might be said of a certain level of good health.... The central concern of justice, then, is with achievement of well-being, not the freedom or capability to achieve well-being (p. 40).[2]

The mission of public health to create conditions in which people can be healthy may suggest a more limited view: that public officials and agencies can only design institutions, programs, and policies that enhance the ability of people and communities to achieve the level of health they choose, but cannot provide or create health. That is, public agents can develop policies and institutions that make it more likely people will gain, maintain, and exercise their capabilities for achieving health, thus creating conditions in which people can be healthy. However, the commitment of many public health professionals to "organized community efforts"[12] directed toward the prevention of disease and the promotion of health argue for some sense of obligation for promotion and achievement of health itself, and not only the conditions for health.

Finally, when considering the mission statement's claim that society has an interest in "assuring conditions in which people can be healthy," we see two important implications for public health ethics: (1) "Society's interests" may justify public health actions that infringe on individual autonomy; (2) As an expression of societal values, public health efforts must be evaluated both ethically and scientifically. Thus, the commitment of public health professionals to work toward the public's health is the basis for our responsibility, and society's interest in the public's health provides the justification for those actions and decisions that conflict with other responsibilities and values. Although the public's health is the essential, overarching end toward which practice is directed, ethical reflection also engages society's interests, more proximal ends, other dimensions of well-being, other values and obligations, and scientific judgments of means.

Case Study: Public Health Response to Severe
Acute Respiratory Syndrome (SARS)

It is in times of natural disaster or deadly epidemic that the ethical values guiding public health decisions are most starkly revealed. Emergency response to a major, life-threatening epidemic requires fast decisions and actions on the part of public health and medical leaders that may involve serious restrictions on individual liberties, such as quarantine; rationing of scarce vaccines, medicines, medical supplies, or medical transportation; reassessment of standards of medical care; and unequal treatment of individuals or groups.

In these situations, emergency managers must make decisions with consequences that affect the lives, welfare and rights of others.[14] Public health emergency managers have a fundamental moral responsibility to embrace the public welfare; protect the best interests of all, but especially the most vulnerable, and serve as responsible stewards of public resources. The following case study on the SARS outbreak illustrates the ethical tensions when public health actions to protect society from a deadly disease threat restrict individual freedoms.

In November 2002, a mysterious respiratory illness causing an atypical pneumonia emerged in Guangdong Province, China. Over the next eight months, 8098 cases of Severe Acute Respiratory Syndrome (SARS) and 774 deaths were reported by 29 countries in Asia, Europe, North America, Africa, and Australia. The greatest incidence of the disease occurred in China with 5327 reported cases; other significant outbreaks occurred in Hong Kong, 1755 cases; Taiwan, 346 cases; Toronto, 251 cases; and Singapore, 238 cases.[15] The emergence of this previously unknown contagious illness with a case fatality rate of 9.6% was an international public health emergency due to its rapid spread by travelers. The public health response provides examples of ethical issues in decision making, including decisions to use extraordinary public health powers involving isolation, quarantine, travel restrictions, and changes in standards of medical care.

The outbreak of SARS in Toronto, Canada led to extensive public health containment measures. The SARS outbreak began in February 2003, and was initiated by a traveler from Hong Kong. The World Health Organization issued an international travel advisory that recommended limiting travel to Toronto. Heightened surveillance measures were taken in many countries, including screening of airline passengers. Strict infection control practices and isolation of cases were implemented throughout Ontario province; even so, much of the disease transmission occurred in hospitals.[16] Surveillance, contact tracing, and quarantine of exposed persons were implemented. In the course of the outbreak, approximately 10,000 people were under quarantine in Ontario.[17] Hospitals were quarantined, visitors restricted, and admissions limited to probable SARS patients at some facilities, resulting in delay or denial of care for patients with other health conditions. Health care workers bore the brunt of the illness, representing nearly half of the cases in Toronto, as many jeopardized their own health to care for the sick. Risk communication to the public was very important, but difficult because little was known about the cause of the disease, its transmission, or its treatment.[18]

The public health response to control the SARS outbreak highlights the tension between individual interests and public health measures taken for the common good. Travel advisories recommended by the World Health Organization, the Centers for Disease Control and Prevention, and other national organizations served the important function of warning travelers of the potential risk of SARS. Although the travel advisories may have helped reduce the spread of SARS, there were severe economic impacts. The effectiveness of these advisories was demonstrated by sharp drops in the numbers of business and leisure travelers to Toronto, Singapore, and Hong Kong, and by losses in revenue for airlines, retail business, and tourism.[19]

Quarantine measures in Toronto relied heavily on voluntary compliance and were successful for the most part. Survey findings from a post-SARS study of public attitudes on quarantine and other public health measures in Hong Kong, Singapore, Taiwan, and the United States indicated that respondents prefer voluntary approaches to compliance and have unfavorable attitudes toward compulsory measures. In all countries, there was substantial approval for quarantine of people likely to have been exposed to an infectious disease: 95% of Taiwan respondents, 89% in Singapore, 81% in Hong Kong, and 76% in the United States approved. When asked if they still favored quarantine if people could be arrested for noncompliance, approval dropped markedly: 70% of Taiwan respondents, 68% in Singapore, 54% in Hong Kong, and 42% in the United States approved.[20] These attitudes provide some insight into public values regarding quarantine and other community outbreak control measures. Public health officials need to plan public awareness efforts in advance and communicate effectively about potential control measures, their practical consequences for individuals and families, the need for voluntary cooperation and the circumstances that might require compulsory measures.

The University of Toronto Joint Centre for Bioethics identified five major ethical concerns from the SARS outbreak and response: (1) individual freedom of movement versus quarantine restrictions to protect the public health; (2) privacy of health information versus revealing private medical information to prevent the spread of disease; (3) health care professionals' duty to care for the sick versus their personal risk and family obligations; (4) quarantine of hospitals to prevent the spread of SARS versus denial of medical care to patients who did not have SARS; and (5) a global health ethic of solidarity versus a "politics as usual" approach.[21]

For each of these ethical dilemmas, public health officials were called upon to place the common good and public health first, and to value equity and fairness for individuals; to communicate risks and response measures openly; to respect privacy and protect against stigmatization; and to use the least restrictive intervention in proportion to the threat. Health care providers have a professional duty to care for the sick, but also need to care for themselves. Caregivers must have the institutional supports, supplies, and equipment to protect their health and carry out their duties.

The Nature of Public Health Practice

Public health practice requires commitment to accountability, reliability, and ethical behavior. All of these enter into considerations of ethical practice of any profession, including acceptance of responsibility in terms of a commitment to the fundamental ends of a profession itself. These very general propositions constitute the basic framework for the ethical perspective developed in this chapter.

A Brief Historical Summary

The origins of public health practice may be traced to the Sanitary Movement of the 18th and early 19th centuries, with its focus on community characteristics, economic conditions, and environmental influences (see Chapter 1). Improvement of living conditions was seen as a means of improving health. The Sanitary Movement developed knowledge to influence public policy. This formative period of public health practice is still relevant because it reflects a multifactorial and contextual understanding of the determinants of health.

Scientific advances in bacteriology, chemistry, and medicine, as well as epidemiology, established the germ theory of disease in the late 19th century. These developments dramatically shaped public health practice. Public health laboratories were established, vaccines developed, and water treatment and dairy inspections initiated. Public education campaigns promoted disease control practices and sanitation. Tuberculosis and sexually transmitted diseases were brought under control by improved health practices and effective treatments. Malaria control efforts included draining of swamps and widespread pesticide use. Sharp reductions occurred in the incidence of communicable, food borne and vector borne diseases, and resulting mortality.[11,22]

By mid-20th century, public health attention shifted to chronic disease control and prevention, with emphasis on risk factor epidemiology and interventions directed toward individual behavior and lifestyle. Today the emphasis on genetic and cellular processes (a potential new "germ theory") and renewed interest in both psychosocial characteristics and broader contextual and environmental influences are seen as integral to personal and community health and well-being.[22,23,24,25] The threat of emerging infectious diseases continues to have global significance in an era of resurgent multidrug resistant tuberculosis, pandemic AIDS, and widespread distribution of vector borne diseases.

In each historical period, the dominant scientific approaches adopted to improve the public's health also raised ethical issues that were part and parcel of the method. Questions of value and scientific determinations cannot be disentangled in adopting public health measures to achieve agreed-upon ends.

The Contemporary Model of Public Health Practice

The modern ecological model of public health practice stresses the multiple dimensions that constitute our lives, relationships and environments, and, therefore, contribute to health and wellness or disease and disability. Public health practice inevitably encounters ethical dilemmas, tensions, conflicts, or trade-offs. Ethical analysis, therefore, is necessary for public health practice that is effective as well as ethically sound and responsible.

The 2003 IOM follow-up report[25] emphasized the "public" aspect of public health, that is, "healthy people in healthy communities." There has been a rich discussion in the public health literature on the definition and nature of public health and healthy communities.[26,27,28,29,30] Concepts of health and healthy communities entail different emphases in policy development, programmatic focus, evaluation, and allocation of resources, even different measures, all pertinent to ethical analysis of public health practice.[31,32,33] For example, viewing a healthy community primarily in terms of access to and provision of certain services has different implications for ethics than emphasizing characteristics such as social capital, general economic prosperity, and the level of income inequality, or more general human rights and social conditions. It is important to note that public health professionals increasingly recognize an organic notion of community, emphasizing that individual health is achieved or threatened by larger scale contextual factors, including social networks, environment, education, economic opportunity, and other characteristics of communities.

We believe most public health professionals would agree that a healthy community is not simply a collection of healthy individuals.[2,28] Defining what the common good is and determining how that shared value should be weighted versus individual goods or rights are among the most critical challenges facing public health ethics. For example, consider air pollution from an industrial plant. Clean air is a common good: when the air is polluted, some people in the community will suffer from respiratory problems and require medical care.

At the same time, economic opportunity is highly valued by communities: a factory offers employment and wages. Closing the factory to eliminate pollution may have severe economic consequences and ultimately result in poor health in the community. A balance must be struck between the amount of air pollution that the plant is allowed to release, the health consequences and their costs, and the rights of individuals to breathe clean air. Environmental protection programs regulate industrial pollution in an attempt to balance economic and health consequences, based on scientific knowledge, ethics, and societal values.

Public health and the determinants of health are multidimensional.[25,34] The meaning of *Public* can range from an aggregate of individuals to a community or corporate identity and even the global ecosystem. Understandings of *Health* range from the reductionist, biomedical model to broader, more encompassing views as reflected in the World Health Organization's (WHO) definition of health as "a state of complete physical, mental, and social well-being and not merely the absence of disease or infirmity."[35] The WHO definition can be taken to imply that health as absence of disease is secondary to health characterized by well-being and a number of other positive goods. This breadth creates difficulties at a number of levels, not least of which is the threat to a clear understanding of the domain of public health agencies and practitioners.

Typically, public health activities include health-related policy and regulation, health promotion, disease prevention and control, surveillance, and community-based program planning, implementation, and evaluation. Surely access to education and adequate housing are critical for healthy people and healthy communities, but public health professionals and agencies do not often see providing either of these services as part of their responsibility. If public health is responsible for everything that contributes to or threatens health, then it becomes too broad to have any meaningful focus.[9,26,27,34,36] Powers and Faden refer to this as the "boundary problem" in public health. Note that it results in a perception of public health as having "no real core, no institutional, disciplinary, or social boundaries" (p. 10).[2] In their view, situating health as an essential dimension for well-being allows for the better understanding of how harmful determinants, such as war, natural disasters, or environmental threats, can impact health as well as other dimensions of well-being. This points out, once again, that the definition and pursuit of an overarching end is not separable from reflection on the means, with regard to both scientific and ethical judgments.

The 2003 IOM report[25] also emphasized the importance of "intersectoral" collaborations, meaning public health agencies and professionals working with other institutions and entities in the community to achieve their common goals. Such coalitions, while pooling expertise and resources, also raise possibilities for conflicts that must be resolved for collaborative action to be successful.[29,33,36]

Resolution of these conflicts involves clarification of ends, evaluation of consistency of ends, assessment of means for achieving those ends, and respecting values that are shared. This process is the task of ethics.

There is a spectrum of targets of interventions undertaken by public health agencies, from individuals (as in vaccination) to environmental approaches such as monitoring and treatment of air and water, to broad social interventions to change individual behavior or community conditions.[37,38] Ethical analysis enters at each level: clarifying the goals of public health actions directed to the public and justifying the means employed, developing notions of corporate responsibility and accountability, and examining social norms and values that shape policy.

Values in Science and Practice

Values are embedded in research and practice, in both the pursuit and the application of knowledge. As discussed by Weed in Chapter 3, we rely on scientific principles and methods that shape our knowledge and understanding. Beyond that scientific and epistemological reliance, our pursuit of knowledge and application of it in practice exist within social, historical, cultural, professional, and disciplinary contexts. Public health practice is focused on a common good: the pursuit of health. In that regard MacIntyre writes: "goods...can only be discovered by entering into those relationships which constitute communities, whose central bond is a shared vision of and understanding of goods."[1]

MacIntyre's emphasis on communities and the social tradition is consistent with the IOM conclusion that, "The history of the public health system is a history of bringing knowledge and values together in the public arena to shape an approach to health problems."[11] The IOM has addressed some key issues directly in *On Being a Scientist: Responsible Conduct in Research,*[39] which speaks of the social role of science and the importance of values in science. The role of values is evident in funding decisions for research and prevention programs, implementation of screening recommendations, and the recent emphasis within public health on addressing health disparities. Our ability to act requires discussion of our shared vision and common values, the ultimate ends we seek, the means provided by science and resources, and the choices among competing intermediate ends. Because public health practice takes place in the social and political arena, there will be tensions among differing values and priorities. As Ruger has argued, we may agree on specific actions even when we disagree about the justifications for those actions.[36,40] The point is that decisions about public health practice involve weighing the evidence for the effectiveness of specific programs and the potential for differential benefits and harms. The process requires intentional reflection on the values that inform such decisions, including matters of justice and respect, especially for vulnerable populations.

The Distinction between Research and Practice

We have held that public health practice involves the application of knowledge gained through research toward the end of healthy people in healthy communities. It follows that science provides the means that we employ in our practice in order to achieve the end of health. This requires an iterative process of adjusting intermediate ends and means, which by its very nature invokes questions of value and obligation. We hold that we cannot disentangle questions of value from those of science in the process of applying what is gained from research to our pursuit of public health ends. This formulation also suggests that the transition from research to practice is characterized by reciprocal influences, as implementation in practice raises new questions for research, and research provides new options for practice.

The distinction between research and practice is, therefore, not an easy one. Nevertheless, the distinction is an important one. Consider, for example, the role of Institutional Review Boards. Their role is to oversee human subjects research, not to oversee practice. An oft-expressed concern is that such oversight can be and has been improperly used to impede public health practice, especially in responses to critical events, disasters, or outbreaks. Examples include surveillance activities, especially where there may be sensitive exposures or behaviors, such as sexually transmitted infections; rapid response teams collecting information in an outbreak or disaster in order to assess current health, to track patterns, and to prepare for future events; and oversight and monitoring to assure quality and evaluate program implementation and effectiveness. Specific examples include collecting information on airline passengers who may have been exposed to SARS when it is likely the results will not be known until the incubation period has passed, investigating possible adverse effects of a vaccine, and collecting data from survivors and relatives of victims of disasters to assess health status, access to services, and quality of response.

A characteristic frequently used to differentiate research and practice is whether the activity is designed to produce generalizable knowledge.[41,42] The Federal Policy for the Protection of Human Subjects (45 C.F.R., part 46, subpart A) defines research as "a systematic investigation, including research development, testing, and evaluation, designed to develop or contribute to generalizable knowledge." In contrast, according to the Centers for Disease Control and Prevention (CDC), practice is designed to "prevent or control disease or injury and improve health, or improve a public health program or service."[43] In practice, the intent of an investigation or study is to identify and control a health problem or improve a public health program or service. The data collected are needed to assess and improve the program or service, the health of the participants or the participants' community. Knowledge that is generated does not extend beyond the scope of the activity, and project activities are not experimental.

Obtaining and analyzing data are essential to the practice of public health. For many public health activities, however, the distinction between research and nonresearch is blurred. Because scientific principles and methodology are applied to both nonresearch and research activities in the practice of public health, knowledge is generated in both cases. Furthermore, at times the extent to which that knowledge is generalizable may not differ greatly in research and nonresearch. Thus, nonresearch and research activities cannot be easily defined by the methods they employ. Three public health activities—surveillance, emergency responses, and evaluation—are particularly susceptible to the quandary over whether the activity is research or nonresearch.

The distinction as described by CDC places considerable emphasis on the *intent* of the activity. Indeed, according to CDC, "a practice activity may produce generalizable knowledge provided this was not part of the primary intent from the outset. If the primary intent changes, what is initially deemed public health practice can become public health research."[43] This approach highlights the difficulty of determining clear lines of demarcation for research and practice when intent is central and can change for the same activity. It is a distinction that blurs upon examination. Consider, for example, public health surveillance activities, which are observational, typically involve no treatment, and are designed to monitor patterns of health, but which may also reveal important knowledge that applies to large populations. The initial intent of data collection may be purely for purposes of monitoring, but the intent may change as data accumulates and the research potential becomes more evident.

The Council of State and Territorial Epidemiologists (CSTE) explored this distinction in a report that considers definitions and distinguishing features of public health practice compared to public health research under several models.[41] The authors explore the legal foundation for the distinction and for the different ethical and procedural requirements of each. Ten case studies, nine of which were CDC-related, are presented in which a determination was required whether an activity constituted research or practice. After a summary of the facts of each case, the authors report the actual disposition of the case and then discuss what the case and the reasoning behind the determination can teach us about making these distinctions, especially with regard to criteria that are inadequate or factors that are discriminating in making a decision.

Based on their analysis, the report puts forward definitions and characteristics of public health research and practice that are influenced by the Federal Common Rule (45 CFR 46) that governs human subjects research and by the Privacy Act[44] in their emphasis placed on identifiable health information. The authors propose a set of guidelines reflecting multiple dimensions of the distinction between research and practice and reflecting the complexity of the question. No single one of the guidelines appears to be necessary or determinative, nor is it clear that there is some minimal threshold that constitutes a level of sufficient conditions that can be universally applied. We refer the reader to the report for a more extensive discussion of these guidelines and their application and for the case studies provided. For purposes of this chapter, we now outline the six guiding principles with brief comments.

1. *Legal authority.* Legal authorization to conduct an activity is typical for public health practice, whether the authorization is specific to an activity, such as establishing a disease registry with authority to collect information, or more general, as in the collection of data about a newly emerging threat under the broad mandate to protect the public's health.

2. *Primary intent.* In both the CDC statement and the CSTE report, the intent of the activity is central to determining whether it is research or practice, and the intent may change. CDC points out that practice activities may produce generalizable knowledge, but do not have that as the intent. If knowledge becomes the intent, then the activity, according to CDC, becomes research. The emphasis on generalizable knowledge plays a key role in definitions of research in both the Common Rule[42] and privacy regulations growing out of the Health Insurance Portability and Accountability Act of 1996 (HIPAA).[43] The primary difficulty here is that the same activity may be classified as research under one framing of the intent and classified as practice under a different framing, and the intent of the activity may change over time. For example, a surveillance project may produce generalizable knowledge without having been designed to do so. According to CDC, it would not be considered research. But if information collected, especially if identifiable, is used in further analysis that is intended to contribute to generalizable knowledge, then it becomes research and subject to review.

3. *Responsibility.* The report presumes that the investigator assumes responsibility to and for participants in research. By contrast, public health practitioners function in roles and under the authority of legal entities, while still maintaining their responsibility for actions that impact participants or recipients of the activity.

4. *Participant benefits.* Both the CSTE report and the CDC statement assert that public health practice is designed to benefit the persons or groups or communities that are the object of the activities. Though benefits sometimes also accrue to participants in research, the intent is for benefits to also extend to other persons or groups beyond the bounds of the particular project.

5. *Experimentation.* Both the CDC and CSTE documents include the experimental nature of the activity as a consideration in distinguishing research from practice. There is an implied distinction between "standard" or previously

"proven" approaches and novel or untested approaches. Hodge and Gostin characterize public health practice activities as relying on evidence-based or standard practices or "proven techniques" and conclude: "Thus, if any activity involves introduction of non-standard or experimental procedures, the activity is likely research rather than public health practice."[41]

6. *Subject selection.* The CDC and CSTE reports view selection of persons for research as intended to provide representative samples or reduce bias and thereby enhance generalizability. In public health practice, subject selection is based on program considerations, timing or stage of disease, or other factors related to prevention and control and not on considerations of bias or representativeness. The CSTE report argues that, in practice, project participants are "self-selected" due to some condition or risk or potential for health benefit, drawing a clinical parallel to those who need treatment. The report concludes:

Though drawing distinctions is critical, in many ways the objective of public health practice and public health research is the same: to perform public health activities that respect and protect the legal rights and ethical interests of individual participants while improving or promoting the public's health. . . . This objective should underlie all public health practice activities in the United States.[41]

The CDC Guidelines note that many of these characteristics, including statutory authority, methodological design, subject selection, and generation of new knowledge or hypotheses, may be found in both research and nonresearch practice activities. Their value as discriminating criteria, therefore, is limited, especially when viewed in isolation. General legal authority, for example, may exist for research activities when there is a legislative or regulatory mandate to conduct research on some condition or question. The issue of responsibility raises the need to explore who the responsible agent for public health activities is, what corporate responsibility means, and how it relates to the individual responsibility of practitioners representing the agency. When considering who benefits from research and from practice, it is clear that research participants frequently derive direct benefit, especially when they receive new treatments that prove effective. Similarly, even coercive public health actions, such as mandatory immunizations or quarantines, can benefit persons who are not quarantined or immunized by protecting them from exposure. This is the very basis for herd immunity, a fundamental concept in public health immunization policy. As for subject selection, the CSTE report seems to confuse self-selection with selection on the basis of specific disease conditions or other characteristics. Many research designs recruit participants specifically because they have some condition or characteristic or exposure of interest. Further, random selection does not guarantee generalizability, even under the optimal conditions of the randomized controlled trial, especially when there are stringent inclusion or exclusion criteria. Similarly, public health activities may target specific groups of people (e.g., the very young or very old) for some programs, without definitive evidence that such targeting actually reduces the occurrence of adverse events in the population. For example, influenza immunization campaigns are often targeted toward older adults and young children. Influenza vaccination of children may reduce the spread of influenza in the community, and thus benefit adults and the elderly as well. Conversely, under some conditions, public health practice may rely on randomization as a method of fair allocation of scarce resources. A lottery system, for example, may be used to choose recipients of influenza vaccine during a time of short supply, as in the autumn of 2004.

In spite of their limitations, the CSTE guidelines are likely to be influential because of their scope, the directness of the proposed approach, and the standing of CSTE among public health practitioners. The CDC guidelines constitute the official position of CDC for its activities. These criticisms of the guidelines are not intended to dismiss them. Rather they are meant to show the limitations of any one of them in isolation for making the determination of whether an activity is research or practice.

Case Study: Research or Practice?

At the time of this writing, these issues were at the center of a controversy surrounding a program implemented by Johns Hopkins University and intended to reduce catheter-related hospital infections in 67 cooperating hospitals in Michigan.[45,46,47] A complaint to the Office for Human Research Protections (OHRP) resulted in a finding by OHRP that the implementation of a checklist comprised of CDC-recommended procedures for catheter placement constituted human subjects research. As a result of OHRP determinations, the Johns Hopkins Institutional Review Board (IRB) suspended activity related to the project. Subsequent to considerable publicity, discussion, and further review, OHRP issued a revised statement indicating that the research/quality improvement project should be allowed to proceed.[48] Though OHRP continued to assert that the project as originally implemented constituted human subjects research and, thus, required at least expedited IRB review, the revised statement did acknowledge that the project would likely have been approved for waiver of consent and should not have been inhibited. The revised opinion gave approval for Michigan hospitals to continue implementation of the checklist program to reduce catheter-related infections without further OHRP scrutiny, and in fact "strongly" encouraged other hospitals to adopt it. In the initial ruling the determinative factors were not *what* was being done, or whether consent would be required for it to be done as part of hospital practice, but that it was called research. Analysis was conducted to determine if the checklist did indeed reduce infections significantly, and the results were published. As one commentator noted: "institutions can freely implement practices they think will improve care as long as they don't investigate whether improvement actually occurs. A hospital can introduce a checklist system without IRB review and informed consent, but if it decides to build in a systematic, data-based evaluation of the checklist's impact, it is subject to the full weight of the regulations for human subjects protection." [47]

From an ethical perspective a more fundamental question is: What difference should the distinction between research and practice make in our assessment of clinical or public health actions? There is no question that implementation of new practice guidelines or policy should be examined carefully for scientific evidence of effectiveness and for protection of patients. This is another instance when ethical values and principles cannot be disentangled from determination of scientific means. From the perspective of the patient, however, the determinative factors cited by OHRP in its original decision seem trivial and the requirements onerous to the point of interfering with care and threatening health and safety.[32,49] As MacQueen and Buehler write, "Regardless of whether public health projects are deemed to represent research or practice, it is essential that they be conducted ethically, emphasizing the need for public health ethics review mechanisms that are responsive to crises and sensitive to levels of risk, especially when projects involve vulnerable groups." [50] But these ethical considerations must be appropriate to the demands of the situation and the risks—to both health and autonomy—imposed by the threats and by the proposed response, and they should not be unduly burdensome either to practitioners or to those impacted by public health activities.

For the persons and communities affected, the issues are less likely to be whether something should be termed research or practice and more likely to reflect concerns about whether the activity provides benefits or imposes risks, whether participation or being subject to the action is voluntary or is coerced, whether the risks, if present, can be justified by potential benefit to the community, whether the program appears to be implemented fairly, whether the individual's rights and dignity have been respected, and similar questions. For purposes of answering these questions, it is less important whether the agents *intend* that the activity be one of research or practice, or whether the information gained is generalizable or not. What is critically important is that the activity be conducted responsibly. These are precisely the kinds of questions IRBs review, but they are fundamental to responsible conduct of research or practice quite apart from regulatory procedures. Practitioners should be sensitive to these issues even in the face of an emergency and formulate processes that incorporate such considerations efficiently and expeditiously.

Preventive Ethics and Procedural Ethics

In order to respond to critical situations expeditiously and ethically, public health agencies could develop an approach that combines preventive ethics and procedural ethics. Preventive ethics, as advocated for clinical practice by Lawrence McCullough, "adopts the strategy of anticipating, prospectively identifying, and addressing ethical challenges with the goal of preventing such challenges from becoming conflicts."[51] Consider, for example, surveillance programs. When these are designed and emergency responses are planned, there is intentional reflection on ethical concerns, whether inherent in the activities themselves, such as threats to privacy in surveillance or restrictions on individual autonomy in emergency situations, or as direct or indirect consequences of the actions. As programs are implemented, unanticipated problems are analyzed and corrections made when necessary for future implementation. This approach allows essential activities to proceed with greater confidence that ethical concerns have been addressed and, thereby, engenders trust by those affected by public health activities. For example, during the development of a new disease registry, planners examine and learn from ethical challenges encountered in other registries how to avoid similar problems or violations in the new program. Examples include training of staff in privacy issues and in technical aspects of protecting data, greater transparency, education of those included in the registry, and development of mechanisms for timely and compassionate response to concerns or objections.

Procedural ethics, which builds ethical considerations into the design of practice programs, is modeled after the concept of procedural justice as described by John Rawls in *A Theory of Justice*.[52] The concept, put simply, is that the focus is on designing processes and procedures that we agree are fair beforehand, so that, whatever the outcome, if the process has been followed faithfully, we can agree that the outcome was fairly obtained, even if we do not agree with the result or judge it to be unfortunate. That is, rather than focusing on a specific ethical dilemma, the focus is on coming to agreement on attributes of procedures that are fair and designing procedures to incorporate those attributes. For example, in developing policies and procedures for emergency response, there may be concerns about limited resources, determinations about quarantine, or provision of shelter. Examining alternative approaches for fairness and effectiveness, with input from ethicists and representatives of the community affected as well as from public health professionals, increases the probability that, even if there are unforeseen or unfortunate consequences, the process will be viewed as having been fair.

The use of procedural and preventive ethics approaches would, for example, contribute to creating public health programs, such as surveillance systems, that are characterized by adherence to ethical obligations and, especially with the input of community representatives as well as professionals, that reflect the values of the population under surveillance. Not everyone will agree with such a system or have a veto, but both public health practitioners and the communities where they practice can carry out programs and respond to urgent matters with greater confidence that ethical considerations will be explicitly addressed.[31,49]

Case Study: Planning for Pandemic Influenza

Emergency plans for pandemic influenza reflect the difficult choices that must be made to prepare and respond in the face of uncertainty, and show how preventive ethics and procedural ethics may be applied in the planning process. The avian influenza epidemic affecting Asia, the Pacific island nations, Europe, and Africa (2004–2008) has spurred planning efforts in many countries to respond to avian influenza outbreaks and prepare for the potential threat of a human influenza pandemic. In 2005, the World Health Organization recommended that "all countries take urgent action to prepare for a pandemic."[53] The United States initiated a major national campaign for pandemic planning and preparedness efforts in November 2005, with the release of the Department of Health and Human Services Pandemic Influenza Plan.[54]

The difficult and complex choices in pandemic influenza preparedness and response raise many ethical concerns. Health care systems will likely face a surge of patients: who will receive care? What will happen to patients with "normal" health care needs? Will standards of care be lowered? Will health care workers continue to provide care? There is likely to be a shortage of vaccines, mechanical ventilators, medications, and infection control supplies: who will receive the available supply? Containment strategies are likely to be implemented, including travel restrictions, surveillance, case investigation, isolation and quarantine, social distancing by closing workplaces, schools, and public gatherings. Any of the control measures chosen must be justified, explained, and effectively implemented. Businesses and organizations of all types face policy decisions on continuity of operations, worker attendance, compensation, customer services, and health insurance coverage.

Ethical values, science, and law should guide public health response. Decisions about disease control measures should be based on scientific knowledge of the disease characteristics and transmission; identification of population groups that may be at high risk; availability and effectiveness of vaccines for prevention and medicines for treatment; public attitudes, values, and behaviors; and community resources. Key ethical considerations for decision-making processes are: the decision process should be reasonable, based on evidence and credible information from stakeholders; it should be an open and transparent process so that decisions are offered to the scrutiny of the public; the process should be inclusive and involve stakeholders; the process should be responsive so that decisions can be revised as necessary to meet changing conditions.[55] Public health interventions are grounded in law and regulation. In recent years, many states have revised laws to expand emergency health powers of public health agencies for disease control measures such as quarantine, restrictions of travel and public meetings, providing for a surge in emergency medical care, controlling allocation of essential vaccines, medicines, and supplies, and for expanded disease surveillance and investigation. Ethical considerations for using extraordinary public health disease control measures include balancing the rational allocation of scarce resources to achieve the greatest protection for the population against the need to treat the sick and protect the most vulnerable population segments. Other key ethical considerations are intergenerational equity, social justice, and fair access to care by underserved populations.[56]

New York State Department of Health led an ethical analysis and solicited broad public input in order to develop guidelines for the allocation of ventilators in an influenza pandemic. Given that demand for mechanical ventilation will far exceed the supply available,[57] the guidelines process anticipated the ethical challenges, and proactively addressed them in voluntary guidelines for triage. The ethical framework for allocation was based on five principles: duty to care, duty to steward resources, duty to plan, distributive justice, and transparency. The guidance recommended triage criteria based on clinical patient assessment. Supervising physicians were assigned responsibility for triage decisions, not the primary care clinicians caring for patients. An appeals process was recommended so patients and physicians could request review of decisions. The process for development of these triage guidelines illustrated the value of preventive ethics and procedural ethics in planning for response to a pandemic.

Reviewing Foundational Principles

The most influential approach to bioethics at least since the Belmont Report[58] has been principlism.[6] Principlism, "or the four principles approach" developed by Beauchamp and Childress, derives a core set of guiding ethical principles from "considered judgments in the common morality and medical tradition" (p. 37).[6] The four principles are viewed as central to bioethics. They are: (1) respect for autonomy, which has to do with respecting the ability of autonomous persons to make decisions concerning themselves; (2) nonmaleficence, which calls for refraining from doing or causing harm; (3) beneficence, which literally means "do good" and has to do with creating or providing benefits, with considerations of the relative balance of benefits and costs or harms; and (4) justice, which is concerned that benefits, costs, and harms are fairly distributed or received.

Much of the material on public health ethics has relied on the four principles foundation because of its dominance and usefulness, and because it is more fully developed than alternative approaches that may be applicable. There have been recent criticisms of this approach, notably from the perspectives of communitarian ethics on the one hand and a human rights approach on the other. The foundation for ethics in public health practice presented at the beginning of this chapter relies on an understanding of the mission of public health as defining the overarching goal, the essential constitutive value, toward which public health practice is directed, thus providing an underlying unity of purpose for the broad range of disciplines, agencies, and other entities that constitute public health. Shared ends, core values, and fundamental duties internal to the practice of a profession provide the basis for the ethics of that profession. The shared values implied by public health's mission, especially related to justice and respect for persons, are central to any ethical evaluation of the means that public health practice may employ to fulfill that mission. In ethical judgments about public health practice, those shared values are joined by societal interests, especially as expressed in the values and obligations of the common morality, other more proximal ends, and scientific judgment. It is in that light that we believe the four principles should be understood and applied.

For example, among the most frequent criticisms of principlism, and bioethics in general, as a basis for public health ethics are its focus on the individual, if not individualism, and the priority given to the principle of respect for persons understood as autonomy or self-determination.[26,27,30,31,32,34,36,57,59–62] Because public health is primarily focused on the health of populations and communities, and less focused than clinical medicine on treatment of individuals, an ethics of public health practice would place relatively greater weight on public actions, programs, and policies and their impact on communities, rather than on individual patients, clinical practitioners, or caregivers. Similarly, the emerging influence of community-based participatory research is in part a reflection of the desire to demonstrate respect for the needs and wishes of communities and to provide communities a level of self-determination. These approaches are especially encouraged for vulnerable populations or those who have historically been burdened or marginalized. The community-based participatory research approach is also promoted as a means of increasing recruitment and obtaining better data.

In the U.S. the principle of respect is typically understood as self-determination or autonomy, but in the Canadian Tri-Council Policy Statement respect for the dignity of persons becomes central.[63] Though in the Kantian tradition, the dignity of the individual is derived from autonomy, the Canadian statement proposes a broader concept that "includes consideration of the human condition, cultural sensitivity by researchers, and protecting persons, not only from physical harm, but also from demeaning or disrespectful actions or situations."[64] Powers and Faden also distinguish between leading a self-determining life and having respect from others, for others, and for oneself as two distinct dimensions of well-being.[2] For them, respect is relational and has to do with treating others as "dignified moral beings deserving of equal moral concern. Respect for others requires an ability to see others as independent sources of moral worth and dignity and to view others as appropriate objects of sympathetic identification" (p. 22).[2]

For example, when conducting research or engaging in public health programs, such as vaccinations, with elderly persons, there may be limited self-determination in the sense of the ability to make an informed, competent, and autonomous decision, but the researcher or practitioner still demonstrates respect in the way he/she relates to the subject, collects the data, or administers the treatment. Even when autonomous decisions can be made, the elderly often have special needs and concerns that should be considered in order to avoid coercion, facilitate participation or treatment without undue burden or embarrassment, and provide special protection from harms.

A related area in need of further research and reflection is the potential conflict between respect for cultures and communities and public health actions deemed necessary to achieve important public health goals or to protect the health of the population. This is illustrated in the conflict between some cultural practices and what many consider basic human rights. For example, education, and especially education of women, is widely viewed as an important contributor to public health, but in some cultures women are prohibited from obtaining formal education or having access to health resources. A more extreme example is when a culture condones practices such as female genital mutilation which would be seen in other cultures as violating autonomy and threatening the life and health of the woman. It is in such conflicts that public health ethicists must make a stronger, more fully articulated case for the ethical soundness of a decision, policy, program, or action that is contrary to a prevailing cultural tradition.

The last example illustrates that the principle of beneficence plays a central role in public health ethics. We noted earlier that society's interest in the public's health implies a *prima facie* endorsement of actions to achieve public health, and constitutes an essential basis for justifying public health actions that violate other principles, such as breaches of confidentiality or mandatory (coerced) compliance, as necessary for the common good. Pursuit of the common good is central to the ethical perspective presented in this chapter and to the implementation of the beneficence principle in public health practice. Public health ethics requires an understanding of what the common good is and of the rationale or basis for its claim. We have attempted to suggest one starting point for that more extensive discussion. In coming to an understanding of common goods, we should clarify whether the goods are common in the sense of communal (for example, in the way that public schools, libraries, and parks are communal goods), or common in the sense of affecting or being enjoyed by the preponderance of people in the population (for example, in the sense that people value liberty or security). This distinction can be important in considerations of who benefits and who suffers, as well as what public health practice should pursue and how it should be pursued.

The public health ethicist should also attend to the claim of nonmaleficence, the principle that asserts a fundamental obligation not to cause harm to others, in public health practice. Public health actions do at times result in some persons involuntarily suffering harms, assuming risks, or being constrained from exercising full autonomy for the benefit of the population's health.[31,49] However, the imposition of risk or harm without consent requires justification that explicates the goods that are obtained and their value in relation to the harms suffered, along with a justification that alternatives were not feasible or effective and demonstration of conscientious efforts to minimize harm or risk.[62] The mandatory quarantine of a person with active tuberculosis serves as an example where individual autonomy is constrained to protect the community.

Much of the literature on the ethics of public health takes justice as the basic orienting principle.[2,6,35] For public health the issue goes beyond distributive justice in fair distribution of benefits and burdens. Especially when decisions are guided by analysis of cost-effectiveness, justice requires that more than a mere balance sheet approach be taken in deciding where and to whom resources should be directed. Justice also includes obligations to attend to vulnerable populations and to provide equal opportunity. Elements of compensatory (or restorative) justice may also come into play in order to address the need to compensate for past injustices.[62] Indeed, the current emphasis on addressing disparities and inequalities in health care and health outcomes is a reflection of a concern for restorative justice. This is the justification for giving greater weight to programs and policies that have the potential to enhance health and well-being of those on the margins of society, giving more attention to vulnerable populations or those previously ignored. This expansion of the concept of justice is especially important in those situations where the power of the state is employed to mandate actions or coerce persons to undergo treatment, as in directly observed treatment for tuberculosis.

The principle of justice also comes into play when determining how to target public health interventions. In that regard the seminal work of Geoffrey Rose[65] needs attention. Rose's ideas have become more influential in the United States recently, especially since the 2003 IOM report relied on his work.[25] Rose's influence is evident in three axioms of that report: (1) Disease risk exists on a continuum rather than as a dichotomy. That is, the risk of a particular disease typically ranges from zero to very high risk, with many levels of risk in between. For example, men have no risk of ovarian cancer, but they do have some risk for breast cancer, though it is very low. The degree of breast cancer risk for women varies considerably based on genetic factors, hormonal exposures, and other less-well understood behavioral and environmental factors. (2) Typically, only a small percentage of a population falls in the extremes of high or low risk, and low-cost programs with benefits for a large number of people may produce a greater impact on public health than much larger programs that benefit a small group—what Rose called the "Prevention Paradox." For example, though risk of coronary disease or stroke is higher for persons with severe uncontrolled hypertension, there are many more persons with moderately elevated blood pressure. The moderately increased risk for this larger number of people will produce more deaths than the smaller group of persons at highest risk. Quite different strategies are typically needed to reach the moderate risk group compared to the high risk group. The decision of where to direct limited resources, therefore, involves questions of both science and ethics. (3) An individual's risk of ill health cannot be isolated from the risk of his/her population, emphasizing again the importance of population-level approaches to promoting and protecting the public's health. Consideration of stewardship of scarce resources, respect for persons and communities, and expanded concepts of justice[2] are essential for public health professionals to incorporate these perspectives into practice in ethically responsible ways. Public health practitioners who take Rose's position into account should also weigh the impact that shifting resources for intervention to lower risk groups may have on groups whose higher risk status is the result of past or current injustices or disparities.

Critical Considerations for Public Health Ethics

Thus far we have presented a general foundation for ethics in public health practice and have shown connections between public health ethics and the four principles approach to bioethics, while also pointing to differences of emphasis between public health and clinical settings. These connections and distinctions have been the topic of discussion among public health and clinical ethicists.

Childress et al.[34] emphasize the importance of public justification and transparency, a component of maintaining trust. But accountability (one of the meanings of responsibility) also provides an element of mutuality in public health processes that would otherwise be entirely paternalistic. Public health actions that infringe on other moral values or rights may still be required, but the decisions are made openly and justifications are provided.

Kass raises the critically important question of "whether, or the degree to which, public health has any explicit role in righting existing injustices, especially given the strong link between poor living conditions and poor health outcomes. To what extent is there a positive responsibility on the part of public health professionals to advocate better housing, better jobs, and better access to food programs, since such advocacy might be the best route to improving the public's health?"[62] The issue of advocacy and science is yet another aspect of a core concern in this chapter, namely the inseparability of science from ethics.[3] It has to this point been cast largely in terms of the ends–means framework, that is, the importance of the values implicit in the goal (the ends) for determinations of the means to be employed. The introduction of advocacy may be seen as an additional component of concern for the centrality of ethics in public health practice. The argument for advocacy is intimately tied to the emphasis in public health circles on elimination of health disparities and, within epidemiology, on social epidemiology and the importance of the ecological model. This is consistent with the policy statement from the Association of State and Territorial Health Officials (ASTHO),[66] which asserts that public health research sponsors should "assure that programs to disseminate findings are in place for rapid translation into practical interventions that serve the public's health." The implications for researchers are that communication with practitioners and agencies is important in framing research and assuring appropriate dissemination of findings and that publication in journals not likely to reach public health agencies should be avoided when the findings have a bearing on public health practice.

Public Health Ethics and Human Rights: The Legacy of Jonathan Mann

We have referred several times to an additional consideration for public health ethics found in the work of the late Jonathan Mann, namely, his emphasis on a human rights approach to public health ethics.[25,26,35,37,39,67] In a brief 1997 article,[27] Mann proposed that, because of its individual focus, ethics is more appropriate to the domain of medicine, while human rights is the more appropriate framework for moral issues in public health. The distinction is problematic because it does not account for the ethical foundation on which human rights rests.[2] He acknowledged that public health actions and human rights are often assumed to be in conflict, though more often in theory than in practice (an indication that the theory may be deficient). He also argued that human rights violations undermine public health and that promoting human rights is integral to promoting public health, while affirming the intrinsic value of human rights in addition to their value as instrumental to public health.

Mann's argument is tied to the well-established association between well-being and social and economic status. He contended that the impact of a constellation of "societal factors," which includes more than income, education, and occupation, persists even after accounting for differences in indicators of medical care. This is yet another instance of science interfacing with ethics: the scientific study of contextual factors related to health is intimately linked to ethical questions regarding solutions to the contextual inequities, that is, means to the end of the people's health. Here again the multidimensional concept of well-being proposed by Powers and Faden[2] is helpful because their model explicitly emphasizes the interaction of health with other dimensions of well-being that are related to human rights, and they provide a discussion of the moral basis for a theory of human rights that is consistent with their view. They show that, unlike purely legal rights, basic human rights are noninstitutional, that is, "not strictly an artifact of institutional arrangements" (p. 45).[2] For them rights are grounded in fundamental human needs which are also integral to achievement of the various dimensions of well-being.

Gostin,[26] recognizing the problematic distinction between ethics and human rights perspectives, further defined the role of ethics in public health while including the contribution of the human rights perspective. He cites four critical contributions of public health ethics to public health practice: "Ethics can offer guidance on (i) the meaning of public health professionalism and the ethical practice of the profession; (ii) the moral weight and value of the community's health and well-being; (iii) the recurring themes of the field and the dilemmas faced in everyday public health practice; and (iv) the role of advocacy to achieve the goal of safer and healthier populations."[26]

Reliance on a human rights perspective to resolve ethical conflicts in public health will require a more thorough grounding of these rights in the context of public health and well-being and an examination of the ways that they are furthered or limited by public health policies, programs, and practice. One of the dangers of the human rights approach is that it may be "co-opted" by stressing individual rights, particularly individual liberty and freedom from coercion, to oppose public health actions.[68] Bayer and Fairchild[31] contend that "limitations on the rights of individuals in the face of public health threats are firmly supported by legal tradition and ethics. All legal systems, as well as international human rights, permit governments to infringe on personal liberty to prevent a significant risk to the public." Indeed, the tension between individual rights and autonomy and pursuit of the common good in the form of the public's health constitutes one of the central issues for public health ethics. Though there is no simple solution, we have sought to provide a basis for discussion in our framing of public health practice as directed toward the overarching good of the public's health, in positing that society has an interest in that end, and that society's interest constitutes a *prima facie* warrant for pursing that end and evaluating the means to achieve it in both scientific and ethical terms. The considerations outlined in the previous section indicate how ethical principles, values, and obligations are brought to bear on the determination of when some rights may be justifiably infringed in order to achieve the larger end.

Case Study: The Response to Katrina

On August 29, 2005, Hurricane Katrina made landfall as a powerful Category 3 storm near the Louisiana–Mississippi border. This hurricane devastated the region, with catastrophic wind, flooding, and storm surge effects, causing high loss of life and extensive property damage. A Congressional investigation found that governmental and private emergency response at all levels was inadequate to deal effectively with the crisis.[69] Public health departments in many coastal states have responsibility for coordinating the public health and medical response to hurricanes, including assisting health care facilities with planning and carrying out evacuations, and supporting shelter operations. Congressional findings with particular relevance for public health and medical response were

The failure of complete evacuation led to preventable deaths, great suffering, and further delays in relief (p. 2).

Medical care and evacuations suffered from a lack of advance preparations, inadequate communications, and difficulties coordinating efforts (p. 4).[69]

The impact of the Hurricane Katrina disaster fell hardest on the poor, the ill, and the aged. Medical facilities and special needs populations were not sufficiently prepared to evacuate. Many low-income residents were unprepared to evacuate or lacked the means to leave. There was inadequate evacuation transportation and sheltering. Hospitals and medical responders lacked sufficient communications capability. There were delays in post-storm rescue efforts and recovery of bodies. Confusion, uncertainty about mission assignments, and "government red tape" delayed medical care. What are the ethical issues for public health professionals and emergency managers? A human rights perspective should inform public health and emergency management with attention to both preventive and procedural ethics in planning.

Modern technology makes it possible to predict with some accuracy the landfall location, timing, and strength of hurricanes. Depending on the situation, a period of days or hours is often available for warning the public and evacuating people from the projected path of the storm. Emergency management decisions to evacuate coastal areas are made by public officials, usually state governors or city mayors, based on predictions of a storm's projected path and intensity. The purpose for evacuation is to save lives and prevent injury; this is clearly in keeping with the societal value of preserving human life. The decision to order mandatory evacuation has serious consequences, however, as evacuation is costly and inconvenient for individuals, families, and businesses; as massive traffic volumes create hazards for travelers; and as there is a period of social and economic disruption. Often, evacuations must be made before the exact path of the storm can be predicted, so some people are evacuated and inconvenienced unnecessarily. Some ethical considerations underlying evacuation decisions include the high value placed on protecting life, the responsibility of government officials who have advance knowledge of a threat to share that information with the public, and, once the decision to evacuate is made, some measure of public responsibility for providing essential supports (transportation, food, water, and shelter) for those evacuees who cannot provide for themselves. Special consideration must be given to those who lack the means for evacuation or who are unable to comply without assistance.

Even with the state or local declaration of a mandatory evacuation, the decision to evacuate is not one-sided. Individuals ultimately decide for themselves whether or not to comply with mandatory evacuation orders. In Hurricane

Katrina, as in other hurricanes, large numbers of people did not evacuate before the storm: an estimated 70,000 residents remained in New Orleans.[69] A July 2006 survey by the Harvard School of Public Health studied the opinions of adults in high hurricane risk counties in the southeast United States. In response to the question, "If government officials said that you had to evacuate the area because there was going to be a major hurricane, would you leave the area or would you stay?" 67% of coastal residents said they would leave, while 24% said they would stay and 9% were unsure.[70] Although public authorities have an obligation to warn people of impending danger, mandatory evacuation orders are rarely enforced through the coercive power of the state. Local officials may use a variety of methods to encourage compliance, such as asking for names of next of kin to notify, or shutting off utilities in advance of a storm. Rarely are people arrested or physically compelled to evacuate. In other words, some choose to place a higher value on individual freedom of choice and property than on compliance with a potentially life-saving measure. An interesting finding was that 66% of respondents were confident that they would be rescued if they did not evacuate and needed help. This implies that respondents have high expectations that public officials will value protection of life enough to take risks to rescue those facing the consequences of a poor choice. The emergency management planning process needs to include substantial input from the communities, and factor in the likelihood that some people will choose not to evacuate and require rescue.

In the case of health care facilities, including hospitals and nursing homes, evacuation itself may pose a threat to the life or health of patients. It is the responsibility of the health care facilities to comply with mandatory evacuation orders, to arrange for transportation and suitable receiving sites, and to safely conduct the evacuation. In effect, the institutions must decide on behalf of their patients, who may themselves be unable to make or act upon decisions about their own health and safety. It is very difficult and costly to evacuate a health care facility, and the danger to the frail, seriously ill, or injured patients is real. Private resources may be inadequate for evacuating health care facilities in the time available before landfall. When private resources are lacking, local, state, and federal government agencies are called on to provide additional resources. This may not be possible to achieve in time for successful evacuation. Public health and regulatory agencies are often engaged in the emergency management decisions and actions in support of health facility evacuations. Ethical issues may involve balancing the risks of evacuation against the risks posed by the imminent storm, setting priorities for patient evacuation when transportation resources are inadequate, and making allowances for lowered standards of patient care due to emergency conditions.

The experiences of health care facilities in New Orleans during and after Hurricane Katrina illustrate the consequences of the failure to evacuate. Voluntary evacuation orders were issued for a number of Louisiana parishes on Saturday, August 27, two days before landfall. Mandatory evacuation orders were issued in the City of New Orleans on Sunday, August 28, approximately 19 hours before landfall. Health care facilities were not included in mandatory evacuation orders: evacuation decisions were made on a facility by facility basis. An estimated 215 persons died in New Orleans nursing homes and hospitals.[69] There were 11 hospitals in areas that flooded and an estimated 1749 patients, with some 7600 staff, family members and others. After the storm, health care facilities operated under terrible conditions without power or water, until post-storm rescue efforts were completed. The aftermath of Katrina showed that plans for evacuation of health care facilities must be integrated into regional and state emergency plans, that evacuation plans must address the logistical challenges of evacuating frail and ill people, that public agencies must be prepared to support evacuation of health care facilities, and that arrangements must be made in advance for transportation and destination facilities.[71]

The Ethics of Scientific Decision Making

This chapter has attempted to lay a foundation for ethics in public health. We have briefly outlined some of the most common areas where public health practitioners face difficult ethical decisions. Throughout this chapter we have referred to the inseparability of science and ethics. We offer one additional example to illustrate how ethical concerns can be central to what are often considered purely scientific, methodological, or statistical decisions. These issues are especially pertinent to program evaluation and evidence-based practice, and they illustrate that there are ethical implications even of statistical issues, such as how measures are defined and used,[72] what *alpha* or *beta* levels are selected in determination of statistical significance, and what critical values are chosen for screening tests.

This issue of choosing *alpha* or *beta* levels, which determine the probability of Type I or Type II errors, has been discussed at greater length elsewhere.[73] A Type I error involves judging there is an association, effect, or difference when there is none. A Type II error means judging there is *not* an association, effect, or difference when, in fact, one exists. In the realm of hypothesis testing, Type I and Type II errors refer to decisions that are incorrect due to random error. (The probabilities associated with them do not provide information about errors resulting from bias, which is systematic or nonrandom.) In setting a very small *alpha* level, the probability level below which one rejects the null hypothesis, one can decide to reduce the probability of a Type I error, with a resulting loss of power. Or one can set a larger alpha level, reducing the probability of a Type II error, but also increasing the probability of rejecting the null hypothesis erroneously, that is, making a Type I error. The trade-off of Type I and Type II errors is not only a statistical trade-off. It requires consideration of opportunities lost because of wasted resources and needs going unaddressed or risks imposed because a Type I error results in a decision to implement a program that is ineffective or could even be harmful. Those considerations must be weighed against the risk of adverse outcomes or actual harm, unrelieved suffering, and loss of improved health because an intervention that would have been effective was not implemented due to a Type II error.

In evidence-based practice and public health program and policy development, one reaches a point when a decision must be made based on the weight of the evidence, the precision of the estimates, the relative weighting and the trade-offs of one type of error versus the other, all in light of underlying values and obligations. The adoption of *alpha* of 0.05 and *beta* of 0.2 seems too facile when we begin to probe the differences in policy and program implementation resulting from erroneous rejection of a null hypothesis or, conversely, failure to reject a null when an intervention could make a meaningful difference in the lives and well-being of people. These differences should be considered not only in terms of allocation of resources, but also in terms of the impact on the lives of the people affected and consonance with their values. Translating the principles of community-based participatory research into public health practice could mean engaging a community to factor into their risk/benefit deliberations the probability of assuming an ineffective intervention is effective, or conversely, assuming an effective intervention is not.

This issue is critical for evaluation of programs that are implemented. The ASTHO general policy statement[66] affirms the importance of evaluation for accountability and stewardship of resources, while also emphasizing responsible use of data and the need to account for variability of settings and populations. Effective evaluation considers the mission, values, and goals of programs whether in public or private agencies. Nonquantifiable goals and vocational motives may be especially difficult for usual evaluation approaches to accommodate, but failure to consider these motives and goals results in an evaluation that does not address the reasons the program was implemented. Imposition of external goals, values, and standards fails to acknowledge and respect the integrity of the community and its autonomy. Inappropriate outcomes may result in decisions concerning the effectiveness of programs that miss their actual value for accomplishing the community's desired ends. On the other hand, failing adequately to evaluate programs means that the community may be deprived of effective programs and limited resources may be wasted in programs that contribute little to the community's health.

Similar concerns arise in screening programs, where there may be several alternative tests, variations in protocol, or a range of values from which to choose in order to enhance the sensitivity or the specificity of the screening. As with the trade-offs of Type I and Type II errors, these decisions should take into account the relative importance and cost (in human terms as well as resources) of false negative versus false positive results. Receiver operating characteristic curves and other approaches to evaluating the performance of a test typically suggest a point or process that provides the optimal combination of sensitivity and specificity. These approaches may not account for the costs or values associated with the trade-off of false positive and false negative results. Though there are techniques that allow differential weighting to reflect costs or relative values, such techniques are not a substitute for careful ethical reflection. Ethical analysis becomes especially critical when the community and researchers or practitioners hold different values or have different perceptions of problems or goals.

Summary and Conclusion

We have argued in this chapter that ethics in public health practice is shaped by the mission of public health and that the ethical obligations of public health practitioners are grounded in their commitment to that mission and in their voluntary assumption of responsibility for the public's health. Society also has an interest in the public's health and that endorsement provides partial justification for infringing on certain individual rights for the sake of the common good. Though public health ethics is not as highly developed as clinical ethics, research ethics, or other subfields of bioethics, recent developments have made clear that it must make use of bioethical methods and concepts and incorporate ethical reasoning in decision-making processes. The resulting public health ethics will include expanded or modified concepts of justice and respect for persons, human rights, communitarianism, utilitarianism, and virtue ethics. Because of the multidimensional nature of public health, ethical analysis must include the perspectives of a broad range of persons, communities, agencies, and institutions. Development of preventive and procedural ethics approaches is recommended as a means of maintaining assurance of ethical approaches to urgent or emerging public health problems or disasters. Finally, we have seen that ethical considerations enter public health practice even regarding issues such as statistical decisions or design of screening programs. The case studies demonstrated how many ethical issues, concepts, values, and obligations enter public health responses, providing further evidence of the importance of ethical analysis for responsible and effective public health practice.

ACKNOWLEDGMENT

The authors gratefully acknowledge the careful reading and critique of our colleague Dr. George Khushf. His insight, probing analysis, and lucid suggestions made the chapter better than it would otherwise have been.

References

1. MacIntyre, A. C. *After Virtue: A Study in Moral Theory.* Notre Dame, IN: University of Notre Dame Press, 1984.
2. Powers, M. and Faden, R. *Social Justice: The Moral Foundations of Public Health and Health Policy.* New York: Oxford University Press, 2006.
3. Weed, D. L. and McKeown, R. E. "Science and Social Responsibility in Public Health," *Environmental Health Perspectives* 111 (2003): 1804–08.
4. Jonas, H. *The Imperative of Responsibility: In Search of an Ethics for the Technological Age* [Translation of Das Prinzip Verantwortung: Versuch einer Ethik fuer die technologishce Zivilisation, translated by H. Jonas with David Herr]. Chicago: University of Chicago Press, 1984.
5. American College of Epidemiology. "Ethics Guidelines," *Annals of Epidemiology* 10 (2000): 487–97.
6. Beauchamp, T. L. and Childress, J. F. *Principles of Biomedical Ethics* (5th ed.). New York: Oxford University Press, 2001.
7. Frankena, W. K. *Ethics.* Englewood Cliffs, NJ: Prentice-Hall, 1973.
8. Last, J. M., ed. *A Dictionary of Epidemiology.* 4th ed. New York: Oxford University Press, 2001.
9. Weed, D. and McKeown, R. E. "Glossary of Ethics in Epidemiology and Public Health: I. Technical Terms." *Journal of Epidemiology and Community Health* 55 (2001): 855–57.
10. Pellegrino, E. D. and Thomasma, D. C. *The Virtues in Medical Practice.* New York: Oxford University Press, 1993.
11. Institute of Medicine, Committee for the Study of the Future of Public Health. *The Future of Public Health.* Washington, DC: National Academy Press, 1988.
12. Winslow, C-E. A. *The Evolution and Significance of the Modern Public Health Campaign.* New Haven: Yale University Press, 1984 [Originally published 1923].
13. Sen, A. Why Health Equity? In *Public Health, Ethics, and Equity*, ed. S. Anand, F. Peter, and A. Sen. New York: Oxford University Press, 2004: 21–33.
14. Schneider, R. "Principles of Ethics for Emergency Managers," *Journal of Emergency Management* 4 (2006): 56–62.
15. World Health Organization. *Summary of Probable SARS Cases with Onset of Illness from November 1, 2002 to 31 July 2003.* Geneva: World Health Organization, 2003.
16. Centers for Disease Control and Prevention. "Update: Severe Acute Respiratory Syndrome—Toronto, Canada, 2003," *Morbidity and Mortality Weekly Report* 52 (2003): 547–50.
17. Branswell, H. "Doctors Spell Out New Fear on SARS," *Toronto Star.* Toronto, Canada, April 17, 2003.
18. Walker, D., Keon, W., Laupacis, A., Low, D., Moore, K., Kitts, J., Vincent, L., and Williams, R. "For the Public's Health: Expert Panel on SARS and Infectious Disease Control." Toronto, Canada, December 2003.
19. Monagan, K. "SARS: Down but Still a Threat," NIC ICA 2003–9. National Intelligence Council, 2003. Available at http://www.dni.gov/nic/special_sarsthreat.html
20. Blendon, R., DesRoches, C., Cetron, M., Benson, J., Meinhardt, T., and Pollard, W. "Attitudes toward the Use of Quarantine in a Public Health Emergency in Four Countries," *Health Affairs* 25 (2006): 15–25.

21. Singer, P., Benatar, S., Bernstein, M., Daar, A., Dickens, B., MacRae, S., Upshur, R., Wright, L., and Shaul, R. "Ethics and SARS: Learning Lessons from the Toronto Experience." Toronto, Canada: University of Toronto Joint Centre for Bioethics, 2003.

22. Susser, M. and Susser, E. "Choosing a Future for Epidemiology: I. Eras and Paradigms," *American Journal of Public Health* 86 (1996): 668–73.

23. Susser, M. "Epidemiology in the United States after World War II: The Evolution of Technique," *Epidemiologic Reviews* 7 (1985): 147–77.

24. Susser, M. and Susser, E. "Choosing a Future for Epidemiology: II. From Black Box to Chinese Boxes and Eco-epidemiology," *American Journal of Public Health* 86 (1996): 674–77.

25. Institute of Medicine, Committee on Assuring the Health of the Public in the 21st Century. *The Future of the Public's Health in the 21st Century.* Washington, DC: National Academy Press, 2003.

26. Gostin, L. O. "Public Health, Ethics, and Human Rights: A Tribute to The Late Jonathan Mann," *Journal of Law, Medicine, and Ethics* 29 (2001): 121–30.

27. Mann, J. M. "Medicine and Public Health, Ethics and Human Rights," *Hastings Center Report* 27 (1997): 6–13.

28. Institute of Medicine. *Healthy Communities: New Partnerships for the Future of Public Health.* Washington, DC: National Academy Press, 1996.

29. Stoto, M. A. "Sharing Responsibility for the Public's Health: A New Perspective from the Institute of Medicine," *Journal of Public Health Management and Practice* 3 (1997): 22–34.

30. Beauchamp, D. E. "Community: The Neglected Tradition of Public Health," *Hastings Center Report* 15 (1985): 28–36.

31. Bayer, R. and Fairchild, A. L. "The Genesis of Public Health Ethics," *Bioethics* 18 (2004): 473–92.

32. Roberts, M. and Reich, M. "Ethical Analysis in Public Health," *Lancet* 359 (2002): 1055–59.

33. Galarneau, C. "Health Care as a Community Good: Many Dimensions, Many Communities, Many Views of Justice," *Hastings Center Report* 32 (2002): 33–40.

34. Childress, J., Faden, R., Gaare, R., Gostin, L., Kahn, J., Bonnie, R., Kass, N., Mastroianni, A., Moreno, J., and Nieburg, P. "Public Health Ethics: Mapping the Terrain," *Journal of Law, Medicine, and Ethics* 30 (2002): 170–78.

35. Nijhuis, H. and Van der Maesen, L. "The Philosophical Foundations of Public Health: An Invitation to Debate," *Journal of Epidemiology and Community Health* 48 (1994): 1–3.

36. Ruger, J. P. "Ethics of the Social Determinants of Health," *Lancet* 364 (2004): 1092–97.

37. Khushf, G. "System Theory and The Ethics of Human Enhancement: A Framework for NBIC Convergence," *Annals of the New York Academy of Science* 1013 (2004): 124–49.

38. Burris, S. "Introduction: Merging Law, Human Rights, and Social Epidemiology," *Journal of Law, Medicine, and Ethics* 30 (2002): 498–509.

39. National Academy of Sciences, National Academy of Engineering, Institute of Medicine, Committee on Science, Engineering, and Public Policy. *On Being a Scientist: Responsible Conduct in Research.* Washington, DC: National Academy Press, 1995.

40. Ruger, J. P. "Health and Social Justice," *Lancet* 364 (2004): 1075–80.

41. Hodge, J. G., Jr., Gostin, L. O., and CSTE Advisory Committee. "Public Health Practice vs. Research: A Report for Public Health Practitioners Including Cases and Guidance for Making Distinctions." Atlanta, GA: Council of State and Territorial Epidemiologists, 2004.

42. Department of Health and Human Services. "Protection of Human Subjects," *45 CFR 46*, 1991.

43. Office of the Chief Scientific Officer, Centers for Disease Control and Prevention. Guidelines for Defining Public Health Research and Public Health Non-Research. Revised October 4, 1999, modified September 21, 2006. Available at http://www. cdc.gov/od/science/regs/hrpp/researchDefinition.htm, accessed on February 19, 2008.

44. Department of Health and Human Services. "Standards for Privacy of Individually Identifiable Health Information," *45 CFR* 160 and 164: Federal Register, August 14, 2002.

45. Pronovost, P., Needham, D., Berenholtz, S., Sinopoli, D., Chu, H., Cosgrove, S., Sexton, B., Hyzy, R., Welsh, R., Roth, G., Bander, J., Kepros, J., and Goeschel, C. An Intervention to Decrease Catheter-Related Bloodstream Infections in the ICU. *New England Journal of Medicine* 355 (2006): 2725–32.

46. Miller, F. G. and Emanuel, E. J. "Quality-Improvement Research and Informed Consent." *New England Journal of Medicine* 358 (2008): 765–67.

47. Bailey, M. A. Harming through Protection? *New England Journal of Medicine* 358 (2008): 768–69.

48. Office for Human Research Protections (OHRP). Recent announcements. February 15, 2008. OHRP Concludes Case Regarding Johns Hopkins University Research on Hospital Infections; Encourages Continuance of Work to Reduce Incidence of Catheter-Related Infections; Offers New Guidance for Future Research. Available at www.hhs.gov/ohrp/news/recentnews.html#20080215, accessed on February 21, 2008.

49. Fairchild, A. L. and Bayer, R. "Ethics and the Conduct of Public Health Surveillance," *Science* 303 (2004): 631–32.

50. MacQueen, K. and Buehler, J. "Ethics, Practice, and Research in Public Health," *American Journal of Public Health* 94 (2004): 928–31.

51. McCullough, L. B., Coverdale, J. H., and Chervenak, F. A. "Preventive Ethics for Including Women of Childbearing Potential in Clinical Trials," *American Journal of Obstetrics and Gynecology* 194 (2006): 1221–27.

52. Rawls, J. *A Theory of Justice.* Cambridge, MA: Belknap Press of Harvard University Press, 1999.

53. World Health Organization. *Responding to the Avian Influenza Pandemic Threat: Recommended Strategic Actions.* Geneva: World Health Organization Communicable Disease Surveillance and Response Global Influenza Programme, 2005.

54. U.S. Department of Health and Human Services. *HHS Pandemic Influenza Plan.* U.S. Department of Health and Human Services, 2005.

55. Upshur, R., Faith, K., Gibson, J., Thompson, A., Tracy, C., Wilson, K., and Singer, P. *Stand on Guard for Thee: Ethical Considerations in Preparedness Planning for Pandemic Influenza.* Toronto, Canada: University of Toronto Joint Centre for Bioethics, 2005.

56. Gostin, L. "Medical Countermeasures for Pandemic Influenza: Ethics and the Law," *JAMA* 295 (2006): 554–56.

57. Callahan, D. "Individual Good and Common Good: A Communitarian Approach to Bioethics," *Perspectives in Biology and Medicine* 46 (2003): 496–507.
58. The National Commission for the Protection of Human Subjects of Biomedical and Behavioral Research. *The Belmont Report: Ethical Principles and Guidelines for the Protection of Human Subjects.* Washington, DC: Government Printing Office, 1978.
59. Callahan, D. "Principlism and Communitarianism," *Journal of Medical Ethics* 29 (2003): 287–91.
60. Leeder, S. R. "Ethics and Public Health," *Internal Medicine Journal* 34 (2004): 435–39.
61. Callahan, D. and Jennings, B. "Ethics and Public Health: Forging a Strong Relationship," *American Journal of Public Health* 92 (2002): 169–76.
62. Kass, N. "An Ethics Framework for Public Health," *American Journal of Public Health* 91 (2001): 1776–82.
63. Medical Research Council of Canada. *Tri-council Policy Statement: Ethical Conduct for Research Involving Humans.* Ottawa: Medical Research Council of Canada, Natural Sciences and Engineering Research Council of Canada, Social Sciences and Humanities Research Council of Canada, 1998.
64. McKeown, R. E. and Weed, D. L. "Glossary of Ethics in Epidemiology and Public Health: II. Applied Terms," *Journal of Epidemiology and Community Health* 56 (2002): 739–41.
65. Rose, G. "Sick Individuals and Sick Populations," *International Journal of Epidemiology* 14 (1985): 32–38.
66. Association of State and Territorial Health Officials. "ASTHO General Policy." Washington, DC: Association of State and Territorial Health Officials, 2004.
67. Marks, S. P. "Jonathan Mann's Legacy to The 21st Century: The Human Rights Imperative for Public Health," *Journal of Law, Medicine, and Ethics* 29 (2001): 131–38.
68. Jacobson, P. D. and Soliman, S. "Co-opting the Health and Human Rights Movement," *Journal of Law, Medicine, and Ethics* 30 (2002): 705–15.
69. U.S. House of Representatives, and Select Bipartisan Committee to Investigate the Preparation for and Response to Hurricane Katrina. "A Failure of Initiative," U.S. Government Printing Office, 2006.
70. Blendon, R., Benson, J., Buhr, T., Weldon, K., and Herrmann, M. "High-Risk Area Hurricane Survey, July 5–11, 2006," *Project on the Public and Biological Security.* Cambridge, MA: Harvard School of Public Health, 2006.
71. Gray, B. and Hebert, K. *After Katrina: Hospitals in Hurricane Katrina – Challenges Facing Custodial Institutions in a Disaster.* The Urban Institute, 2006. Available at http://www.urban.org/url.cfm?ID=411348&renderforprint=1
72. McDowell, I., Spasoff, R. A., and Kristjansson, B. "On the Classification of Population Health Measurements," *American Journal of Public Health* 94 (2004): 388–93.
73. Weed, D. L. and McKeown, R. E. "Epidemiology: Observational Studies on Human Populations," in *The Oxford Textbook on Clinical Research Ethics,* ed. E. J. Emanuel, C. Grady, R. A. Crouch, R. K. Lie, F. G. Miller, and D. Wendler. New York: Oxford University Press, 2008: 325–35.

9

Ethical Issues in Genetic Epidemiology

LAURA M. BESKOW AND WYLIE BURKE

After amassing the nucleotide sequence of human DNA in 2001[1,2] and completing a high-quality, finished sequence in 2003—two years ahead of the original schedule—the leaders of the Human Genome Project proclaimed that "the genomic era is now a reality."[3] Together with rapid advances in technology and computational biology, achievements in genomics are expected to enrich understanding of the role of genetic factors in common, complex diseases, allow more precise definition of nongenetic factors, and provide better approaches to risk reduction, diagnosis, and treatment.[3]

Epidemiologic research is essential to realizing this potential. Key questions about the roles of genes, environmental exposures, gene–gene, and gene–environment interactions in human health can only be answered through the rigorous study of genotypic, phenotypic, and environmental data in human populations.[4] However, genetic epidemiologic research involves risks to research participants, which are primarily *informational* in nature. The main concerns are not usually about physical harms but rather about the misuse of information, including clinical and other personal data used in the research, as well as results derived from research. Responsible conduct of research includes protecting participants from these risks. At the same time, unduly restricting researchers' ability to use and generate information can add uncertainty, cost, and delay to otherwise beneficial research.[5]

Ethical issues in genetic research,[6–8] epidemiology,[9–11] and genetic epidemiology[12–15] have been explored at length. In addition, many argue that genetic information is fundamentally similar to other kinds of health information,[16–18] and thus the issues and concepts addressed elsewhere in this book are applicable to genetic epidemiology. In this chapter, we focus on three selected issues that, although not unique to genetics, are becoming increasingly important in genetic epidemiology: federal policies for widespread data sharing, the use of "race" as a variable in research involving genetics, and concepts of community engagement. These issues are interrelated and represent areas of tension between participant protection and the quality and efficiency of research.

Background

Unlocking the genomic basis of health and disease requires several study designs:

- *Family-based studies* to assess whether diseases and gene variants show correlated transmission among related individuals.[19,20]
- *Population-based studies* to determine whether diseases and gene variants show correlated occurrence among unrelated individuals.[19,21]
- *Intervention studies*, in both clinical and public health settings, to supply the evidence needed to make informed policy choices about the appropriate use of genetic information to improve health outcomes.[22,23]

The misuse of genetic information produced in these kinds of studies has the potential to lead to discrimination in insurance and employment, social stigmatization, familial disruption, and psychological distress.[24] The risk of harm occurring as a result of research participation arises primarily when individual research results are disclosed, either to participants as part of the research protocol or inadvertently to a third party, and when the information suggests serious implications for the health of the individual and his or her family. The possibility of harm is magnified when measures available for treatment or risk reduction are absent, limited, or unproven.

Some argue that the risks associated with disclosure are overstated.[25] Many of the potential harms exist primarily in the context of rare, highly penetrant gene variants that exert a strong influence on disease risk. In contrast, "susceptibility" variants that are neither necessary nor sufficient to produce disease have limited predictive power for individuals.[21,25,26] Their significance lies in what they might reveal, along with a constellation of other factors, about the molecular processes that lead to common, complex diseases in populations. Indiscriminate application of the more stringent protections called for in studies of highly penetrant gene variants can cause harm to participants if they are distracted from other more immediate risks of a study, or to the quality of the research if participation rates are reduced to a level that damages scientific validity.[21,25] Therefore, an important goal is simultaneously to protect research participants and preserve epidemiologists' ability to conduct beneficial research.

In addressing this goal, researchers need to consider the possibility of both individual and group harm. Researchers seeking to discover gene–disease associations often choose as their population a group in which the incidence of that disease or condition is high. When such groups are socially defined (e.g., by race or ethnicity), the research sometimes has implications for all members of the group, whether or not each individual decided—or was even invited—to take part.[8] One positive implication is that researchers could discover information that benefits the health of the group. However, research findings may also have the potential to be interpreted in ways that reinforce existing stereotypes and result in further stigmatization and discrimination of marginalized groups.[27]

An example of how genetic studies might reinforce negative stereotypes is a study that claimed a gene variant putatively associated with brain development had been selected for in European and Asian but not in African populations,[28] findings which erupted into contentious debates over genetics, race, and intelligence.[29] Subsequent research argued against the functional significance of the variant[30] and the evidence for evolutionary selection,[31] but these findings received less publicity than the original inflammatory claims.

The initial study, which utilized biological samples and data collected from diverse populations that were available in two biorepositories, illustrates the need for careful consideration by researchers of the issues we address here: data sharing, use of "race" in genetic epidemiological research, and community engagement.

Data Sharing

In an effort to increase the range and quantity of data available for genomic research, large-scale platforms[32-35] are being built to assemble, organize, and store data obtained from the analysis of biospecimens and to distribute these to researchers.[36] Such platforms can foster improved data quality and uniformity, and facilitate multiple secondary analyses by a wide range of investigators.[36,37]

One prominent initiative to promote broad access to data is NIH's "Policy for Sharing of Data Obtained in NIH Supported or Conducted Genome-Wide Association Studies (GWAS)."[37] This policy defines GWAS as any study of genetic variation across the entire human genome that is designed to identify genetic associations with observable traits, or the presence or absence of a disease or condition. GWAS are a powerful tool in the bid to dissect the molecular basis of common diseases.[38] GWAS require large study populations and substantial phenotypic information on research participants in addition to the genomic data generated by molecular analysis. The rationale for NIH's data sharing policy is based on the potential for societal benefit:

[T]he full value of GWAS to the public can be realized only if the genotype and phenotype datasets are made available as rapidly as possible to a wide range of scientific investigators. Rapid and broad data access is particularly important for GWAS because of the significant resources they require; the challenges of analyzing large datasets; and the extraordinary opportunities for making comparisons across multiple studies.[37]

According to this policy, all investigators who receive NIH support to conduct GWAS are expected to submit information to a central data repository. Descriptive information about the studies will be made publicly available. Detailed phenotype, exposure, genotype, and pedigree data, which have been de-identified and coded prior to submission, will be made available through a controlled-access process. ("Coded" means (1) identifying information that would enable the investigator to readily ascertain the identity of the individual to whom the data pertains has been replaced with a code, and (2) a key to decipher the code exists, enabling linkage of the identifying information back to the data, according to the Department of Health and Human Services Office for Human Research Protection's "Guidance on Research Involving Coded Private Information or Biological Specimens.")

Because data sharing platforms like the NIH GWAS repository link genotypic data with clinical and other phenotypic and social data, identifiability—the potential for such data to be associated with specific individuals—is a pivotal concern.[36] In addition, classifying the data into socially defined categories presents risks to population subgroups, even when individual identities are protected. These concerns lead to questions about the extent to which research subjects should be informed and given choices about widespread sharing of their data.[39]

Identifiability. Although identifying information is removed before data are submitted to many platforms such as the NIH GWAS repository, sequenced DNA is itself a unique identifier. Thus, even when data are "anonymized" in the traditional sense, an individual can be identified with access to as few as 75 single nucleotide polymorphisms from that person.[40] Such identification would currently require comparison to a reference sample; however, collections of reference samples (such as collections held by criminal justice systems, armed services, and health-related institutions) continue to proliferate.[36] In addition, technologies available today as well as those expected in the near future make the identification of specific individuals from raw genotype-phenotype data feasible and increasingly straightforward.[41]

Without a reference sample, an individual's identity can sometimes still be deduced by linking information from a variety of readily available sources. For example, using publicly available, de-identified hospital discharge data, census data, and voter registration data, Malin and Sweeney[42] were able to reidentify 33% of patients with cystic fibrosis, 50% of patients with Huntington's disease, 75% of patients with phenylketonuria, and 100% of patients with Refsum's disease.

Measures taken to reduce the prospect and consequences of identifiability typically include data restriction (statistical techniques to restrict the content of the data prior to release), and/or access restriction (techniques to restrict the conditions of data access).[43] Even with such measures in place, secondary users' promises that they will use the data appropriately are key. Specifically, in the case of the GWAS repository, this includes promises to use the data only for the approved research, to protect data confidentiality, to not attempt to identify individual participants, and to not sell or share any of the data elements.[41] The robustness and enforceability of such agreements will be tested by the unprecedented degree of data sharing, and new legal penalties may be needed.[36]

Group harm. With the advent of widespread data sharing, racial and ethnic labels commonly used to categorize population groups will be perpetuated across many studies. Because large-scale genomic research is expected to identify disease-associated gene variants that vary in frequency across populations, the use of such labels could exacerbate existing stereotypes and potentially stigmatize all members of a population group. (Issues surrounding the use of "race" and the possibility of group harm are explored in more detail in later sections of this chapter.)

Informed consent. Based on the ethical principle of respect for persons,[44] researchers generally cannot involve an individual as a subject of research unless they have obtained that person's informed consent. In the context of epidemiologic research, the purpose of informed consent is "to ensure that research participants fully understand the purpose and nature of the study, the identities of the investigators and sponsors, the possible benefits and risks, the scientific methods and procedures, any anticipated inconveniences or discomfort, the voluntary nature of participation, and the opportunity to withdraw at any time without penalty."[45]

The regulatory requirement to obtain consent does not apply, however, when research does not involve "human subjects." Federal Policy for the Protection of Human Research Participants, as Codified under Title 45, Part 46 of the Code of Federal Regulations, defines *human subject* as a living individual about whom an investigator obtains (1) data through intervention or interaction with the individual or (2) identifiable private information (45 CFR 46.102(f)).

Based on this definition, the U.S. Department of Health & Human Services' Office of Human Research Protections (OHRP) issued guidance that it does *not* consider research involving only coded private information or specimens to involve human subjects if both of the following conditions are met: (1) the private information or specimens were not collected specifically for the currently proposed research project through an interaction or intervention with living individuals; and (2) the investigator(s) cannot readily ascertain the identity of the individual(s) to whom the coded private information or specimens pertain.[46]

OHRP has thus advised that the GWAS repository does not involve human subjects research because the data submitted will have been collected solely for other research studies, and because the data will be coded and the identity of individuals from whom the data were obtained will not be readily ascertainable to the investigators maintaining the repository.[41] This determination means that neither IRB approval of the submission of GWAS data nor informed consent is required under the regulations. NIH's data sharing policy does, however, specify another role for local IRBs: data will only be accepted into the GWAS repository when accompanied by certain assurances from the submitting institution's IRB, including that "The submission of data to the NIH GWAS data repository and subsequent sharing for research purposes are consistent with the informed consent of study participants from whom the data were obtained."[37]

The National Bioethics Advisory Commission has recommended that evaluations of consistency with the original consent focus on the question, "Is the proposed use of the sample or data consistent with the subject's likely understanding of how it would be used?"[47] IRBs will not always find it easy to answer this question. Although some consent documents contain language that expressly restricts how samples and data can be used, more often it is unclear whether the language should be construed as consistent or not consistent with the kind of sharing contemplated by the policy. In these cases, a third option available under the Common Rule—which is for the IRB to determine that the conditions for waiver of consent (45 CFR 46.116(d)) for submission to the GWAS repository have been met—is apparently not allowed. NIH has stated that "the criteria for a waiver of consent under 45 CFR part 46 are inapplicable to such IRB considerations since the GWAS database does not currently involve human subjects research."[41] This point suggests an unintended obstacle in the NIH policy because IRBs may find an informed consent waiver the only mechanism by which the creation of a coded data set for transfer to a repository could be justified.

Responsibilities of Researchers

Large repositories provide an important resource for genetic epidemiological research, but also require researchers to be prepared to address several related concerns:

1. *To participate in decisions about whether submission of existing data to repositories can be justified.* When researchers contemplate submission of data from the analysis of existing samples to a repository, they and their IRB will need to consider whether the original consent allows submission without re-consent and if so, what types of research can be pursued with the shared data. The NIH GWAS policy[37] clearly specifies that resolution of these questions must be based on the language in the original consent form.
2. *To conduct or encourage research aimed at increasing knowledge about participants' needs and concerns related to data sharing.* Limited empiric research suggests that a substantial minority of research participants prefer re-consent for research not specified in the consent form,[48-50] that the proportion is higher for minority participants,[50,51] and that the nature of the research

influences willingness to have samples used.[49-51] These findings suggest the need for additional empiric research on participants' understanding of informed consent documents and preferences regarding uses of stored data. Genetic epidemiology offers unique opportunities for addressing these questions, through collaborative work among epidemiologists, social scientists, and bioethicists to collect data about participant understanding, views, and preferences, as added aims for studies addressing epidemiological questions.

3. *To participate in the development of model processes for prospective informed consent.* Going forward, consent processes should disclose to potential research participants any plans for widespread data sharing. Although current consent forms may contain a general statement that "data may be shared with other researchers," submission to a centralized repository and subsequent use outside the control of the original investigator is sufficiently different to merit explicit disclosure. As with data sharing for existing studies, empiric research is needed to develop consent processes and language that accurately convey the nature of large-scale data sharing efforts and its attendant risks and benefits.

Participants should also be offered the option to opt out of the data submission portion of the protocol—similar to the generally accepted notion that participants should be able to take part in a specific study without necessarily also agreeing to have their specimen stored for future research. McGuire and Gibbs have further suggested a tiered consent approach, whereby subjects are given several options for data sharing, affording them more control over whether, how, with whom, and how much of their data are shared.[52] Offering some level of choice is important not only as a matter of respect for persons and maintaining trust in the research enterprise, but also to avoid adverse effects on accrual into the original study if prospective participants are concerned about widespread data sharing.

The Use of "Race" in Research Involving Genetics

De-identification and other privacy protections such as those called for in the NIH GWAS policy limit the risks to individual research participants when samples and data are shared. However, racial/ethnic identifiers are routinely collected in genetic epidemiology studies and are retained with de-identified samples and data. In this context, the relationship between expanding scientific understanding of human genetic variation and traditional concepts of "race" and "ethnicity" raises a number of concerns. Although concerns about the use of "race" as a variable in medical and social research are neither new nor unique to genetics, there are specific concerns in the context of genetic research. One is the notion of *genetic reductionism*, which results when traits, health problems, and behaviors become attributable to genes and little attention is paid to other contributing factors.[53] Given the pattern of health disparities in the United States, research that emphasizes genetic predisposition to disease in socially defined populations could foster a tendency to attribute poor health in racial and ethnic groups to genetic makeup and to ignore alternate explanations.[54,55]

Another related concern is *genetic determinism*—the belief that one's future is fixed and predicted by genetic makeup and cannot be changed.[53] A vision of genetics that lacks perspective can foster the belief that genes are the primary and perhaps sole causal determinant of human ills and behaviors. Thus, research emphasizing genetic differences between groups could exacerbate existing ideologies of race that already distort, exaggerate, and maximize human differences,[56] and could help reify racial categories as though they are immutable in nature and society.[57]

Given the gravity and magnitude of these concerns about linking "race" and genetics, why might genetic epidemiologists use racial variables in their research? As an administrative matter, current practices for the use of such variables are shaped by federal policies aimed at ensuring the inclusion of racial/ethnic minorities and other underrepresented populations.[58] Researchers are required to categorize participants into the five race categories (American Indian or Alaska Native, Asian, Black or African American, Native Hawaiian or Other Pacific Islander, and White) and two ethnicity categories (Hispanic or Latino and Not Hispanic or Latino) specified by the Office of Management and Budget (OMB) (62 FR 58781) and used in the U.S. census.

From a scientific point of view, unraveling the complex interplay between multiple genetic and nongenetic factors requires a comprehensive description of the genetic variation found in the human genome.[3] Although the genetic sequence of any person is estimated to be 99.9% identical to that of any other unrelated person,[1] the remaining 0.1% still represents millions of differences in the DNA sequence between individuals. Because of evolutionary forces such as genetic drift, founder effects, and natural selection, the *frequencies* of some of these gene variants are not constant in populations throughout the world.[59] Therefore, to the extent that geographical ancestry corresponds to notions of race, patterns of genetic variation also co-vary with notions of race.[60] Accounting for such nonrandom patterns of genetic variation may be important to avoid confounding due to population stratification, that is, the possibility that one or more subgroups within a population has both a higher risk for the disease of interest and a higher prevalence of a gene variant unrelated to outcome status.[61]

The problem is that social conceptions of race often used to define populations and categorize study subjects do not neatly correspond to genetic ancestry. According to Smedley and Smedley,[56] "The consensus among most scholars in fields such as evolutionary biology, anthropology, and other disciplines is that racial distinctions... are not genetically discrete, are not reliably measured, and are not scientifically meaningful." In other words,

- *Racial distinctions are not genetically discrete* because no sharp boundaries can be drawn between human groups; there are no gene variants present in all individuals in one population group and in no individuals of another.[59]
- *Race cannot be reliably measured* because concepts of race can be highly variable and arbitrary, changing as a function of time, history, law, politics, social context, and emotions.[59,62,63]
- Finally, *race is not scientifically meaningful* because it is a social construct, not a biologic reality. A person's self-reported identity incorporates a complex mixture of biological, cultural, psychological, and behavioral factors.[64]

Problems created by reliance on the limited correlation between race and genetic ancestry are compounded by the fact that genes, culture, and environment are strongly confounded.[65] Although "race" may be an appropriate variable to include in describing and monitoring disparities between social groups, it provides little help in elucidating the underlying causal pathways of disease when it is used as a proxy in lieu of direct measurement of environmental contributors.[65,66] Overfocusing on associations among race, genetics, and disease could divert attention from what considerable evidence already suggests are the central causes of health disparities in the United States, which include discrimination, differences in treatment, poverty, lack of access to health care, health-related behaviors, racism, stress, and other socially mediated factors.[54,67]

Responsibilities of Researchers

Ideally, populations for future genetic research will be stratified based on the presence or absence of particular polymorphisms, rather than current imprecise classifications such as "race."[62] If successful, such stratification could contribute to the deconstruction of "race" and other ill-defined group definitions.[62] Until that time, scholars have suggested steps researchers can take to reduce the potential for negative effects from the use of racial categories:

1. *Assess the need for using "race" as a research variable.* As noted by Rivara and Finberg,[68] "Analysis by race and ethnicity has become an analytical knee-jerk reflex, accompanying every table that examines demographic differences in groups, such as age and sex." Researchers should state the relevance of "race" to their particular study[55,69,70] and not use it "when there is no biological, scientific, or sociological reason for doing so."[68] With regard to the use of race as a proxy, many have urged researchers to explain the rationale for doing so and attempt to measure directly as many variables as possible.[67,69,71]

2. *When "race" is used as a research variable, define it clearly and completely.* Use of broad labels without careful definitions can impair scientific understanding, weaken the ability to make valid comparisons across studies, and imply that distinctions between socially defined populations are genetically well established.[67,69] As with any variable, researchers should explain how "race" was defined, how the categories were selected, and how descriptors were assigned to individuals.[63,69,70,72]

3. *Approach data analyses with intentionality and care.* Mandatory requirements to recruit and describe human subjects using OMB categories do not mean the same categorization scheme must be used in the statistical analyses of genetic variation.[66] The OMB itself stated that its categories "represent a social-political construct designed for collecting data on the race and ethnicity of broad population groups in this country, and are not anthropologically or scientifically based" (62 FR 58781). Researchers should explore multifactorial research designs that accommodate complex interactions, avoid giving undue emphasis to the post hoc interpretation of differential findings by race, and, because of the de facto biological presumption conferred on independent variables, consider models that instead use race as a moderating and/or mediating variable.[63,73]

4. *Be mindful of ethical implications in the interpretation and dissemination of findings.* Researchers have a responsibility to examine carefully their use of racial and ethnic categories—including how research results are framed and how they are likely to be interpreted and understood.[66,67] Researchers must recognize and provide explicit caveats with regard to the imprecision of racial and ethnic labels and their connection to human genetic variation.[59,66] Specificity is also important in summarizing and interpreting research results: a study showing a difference in allele frequency in subjects recruited in Helsinki and Lagos should not, for example, be assumed to document a difference between Europeans and Africans.

Community Engagement

Despite general agreement that research on human genetic variation can present collective risks to members of socially identifiable populations,[74] there is debate about how these risks should be addressed. Existing regulations and ethical principles governing human subjects research focus on the individual, with an emphasis on the informed consent process.[75] The landmark *Belmont Report* includes discussion of vulnerable groups, noting that "Even if individual subjects are selected fairly by investigators and treated fairly in the course of research, injustice can appear in the selection of subjects due to social, racial, sexual, and cultural biases institutionalized in society."[44] However, this discussion is focused on avoiding coercion in recruitment, as in the case of prisoners or gravely ill patients, and assuring appropriate surrogacy, as when an individual is unable to provide informed consent by virtue of cognitive impairment or other disabling condition. No clear theory of group protection has emerged that would encompass the risks posed by research investigating group differences in socially charged areas such as intellectual ability or criminal behavior, or by the use of shared samples and data to investigate questions considered culturally offensive by some groups (as in the use of samples collected from the Havasupai tribe for diabetes research to study migration patterns and endogamy[76]).[75]

One suggestion has been that researchers should facilitate the capacity of individuals to consider the interests of other group members as part of their own decision making. As Juengst[27] stated, "If potential DNA donors were informed of the risks that their donation would impose on all others who share their broadest social identities (and not just on their local community), they could incorporate those collateral risks into their decisions, just as individuals now incorporate the interests of their nuclear families into decisions to pursue clinical genetic testing."

Others have criticized current policies for overemphasizing individual rights and failing to consider family and community relationships.[77] Regarding genomic research, Knoppers and Chadwick[78] argue for a shift in emphasis toward the ethical principles of reciprocity, mutuality, solidarity, citizenry, and universality, and note that these represent a trend away from autonomy as the ultimate arbiter and toward an appreciation of the need for a participatory approach. This analysis implies a social duty to participate in research beneficial to society. Such a duty is already embodied in certain public health surveillance measures, such as state-mandated reporting of cancer diagnoses[79] and infectious diseases.[80] However, the relevance of such a duty to most biomedical research is not clear. Some would argue that widespread sharing of samples and data represents a circumstance in which the social benefits of the research are sufficiently high to justify these uses even when not contemplated in the original consent form.[81] The potential for group harm resulting from the retention of racial or other demographic labels represents a strong counterargument to this position. This concern has led to an increasing interest in engaging representatives of the proposed study population directly in the research process in order to gain group perspectives.

Community engagement offers a number of important advantages: first, it can identify risks that members of the study population deem important, so that any negative implications for the group can be both minimized and factored into risk–benefit evaluations of the research.[82] In particular, input from the community can be used to address risks to unique, population-specific beliefs, values, and social arrangements that outsiders might otherwise fail to identify.[77] Second, community engagement can highlight areas of shared interest, helping to ensure that the research topic reflects local concerns and promoting genuine collaborations.[82]

Community input can provide information about social context that helps to frame research questions and may identify secondary research topics that yield a more complex picture of disease risk, thereby increasing the practical and policy relevance of the research compared to observational studies at the individual level.[83] Third, engaging community representatives demonstrates respect for that community's social and cultural structures, thereby helping establish trust between researchers and study populations—especially in research projects undertaken in communities of color or in populations that are "other" to the researchers.[82–84] Fourth, achieving community buy-in may increase recruitment and retention, as well as the quantity and quality of data collected.[74,83] It may also facilitate the translation of research results into locally relevant policy or action.[83,84]

However, community engagement can also present significant challenges and concerns. Several ethical and moral questions have also been raised about community engagement, including whether scientists should censor their inquiries to avoid disrupting the world views of a particular group,[85] whether it is paternalistic to suggest that individuals lack the capacity to decide and need a special layer of protection,[85] and whether implementing community engagement could in fact harm socially identifiable groups by reinforcing the idea that biological differences underlie race, ethnicity, and other socially constructed categories.[27]

The heterogeneity in the formation and structure of communities provides a starting point for considering these concerns. The word *community* is used to describe a wide variety of human associations (e.g., cultural, political, religious, sexual, geographical, professional) and every individual is a member of multiple communities, which may be nested within larger social categories.[27,77,82,85] Further, if the population of interest is a group thought to be genetically related, then the study population is unlikely to coincide with geographic boundaries—a problem exacerbated by the increasing tendency of individuals to migrate and be adopted by other cultures.[86] Once a community is defined, the next challenge is to identify individuals within the community who are socially empowered to speak for the rest.[85] These and other operational concerns have led some to posit that community engagement models are workable only with small groups that have a well-defined leadership structure—for example, among Native American tribes[74,87–91]—and that efforts to proceed in a similar fashion elsewhere could lead to expense, delays, and a chilling effect on research.[85]

A more robust approach is suggested by the work of others. Emanuel and Weijer[75] propose a typology of different kinds of communities, incorporating salient characteristics such as geographic localization, the presence of a legitimate political authority or representative group that speaks for and is accountable to the community, shared culture, shared resources, and self-identification as a community. This typology allows researchers to match the form of community engagement and protection efforts to be undertaken to the characteristics of the community.[75]

Hausman[92] provides additional perspectives concerning the nature of the potential group harms arising in research. Harms to members of a group may occur as a consequence of the research process, for example, when participants are subjected to injustices as in the Tuskegee syphilis studies, or as a consequence of interpreting research results in ways that exacerbate existing stigma or stereotypes. Because the latter harm, which is more relevant for epidemiological research, can occur not just to research participants but also to members of the group who are not participants, informed consent disclosures do not provide an adequate solution. Community engagement can reduce the risk of such harms by promoting dialogue between group members and researchers, providing researchers with guidance about the perspectives and experiences of individuals within the group, and potentially framing questions and reporting results in ways that reduce the likelihood of harm. Research involving structurally defined groups also has the potential to harm the group itself, as contrasted with harm to individuals mediated by group membership.[92] Research that challenges land claims or group stability could pose this kind of harm.[93] When a highly organized group is involved in the research process, researchers arguably have an obligation to engage with group leadership in a process appropriate to the governmental or representative structure of the group, in part to avoid this kind of harm.[94]

Researchers sometimes face situations in which protection of the rights of individual participants appears to be in conflict with cultural practices, as when social structures or practices limit participants' opportunity to make voluntary decisions about research participation.[95] In these circumstance, researchers need to balance the respect due to a legitimate political authority with the obligation to ensure just treatment to individuals.[75,94] Hausman identifies a prima facie obligation to recognize structured groups potentially harmed by the research process, accord them value, and engage with group leadership. He notes, however, that these are

only *prima facie* obligations. Since structured groups that are very important to their members can be oppressive, the disrespect one shows to those who are committed to oppressive groups may be minor compared to the harm one condones or encourages by recognizing such groups and interacting respectfully with their leaders.[94]

With these considerations in mind, researchers need to consider different forms of community engagement:[82]

- *Community dialogue*: Formal and informal discussion of the proposed study and potential implications for socially identifiable groups
- *Community consultation*: Documentation of community concerns through interaction with a representative subset of individual members and organizations

- *Formal community approval (or disapproval)*: Negotiation of a formal contractual agreement between researchers and the study population
- *Community partnership*: Involvement of community members as partners in the research

Community partnership, or community-based participatory research (CBPR)[83,84,96,97] is among the most intensive forms of community engagement. CBPR has been defined as[97]

a collaborative process that equitably involves all partners in the research process and recognizes the unique strengths that each brings. CBPR begins with a research topic of importance to the community with the aim of combining knowledge and action for social change to improve health and human welfare.

In other words, CBPR involves three overlapping components—participatory research, education, and social action—and engages community members and researchers in a joint process to which each contributes equally.[83,97] Although CBPR itself can take many forms, this research model emphasizes participation by the community of interest in all aspects of a project, including definition of the research problem, study design and implementation, collection and analysis of data, formulation of conclusions and recommendations, identification of future areas of research, and publication and application of the findings.

CBPR is increasingly being recognized as a powerful approach to researching complex health problems, such as racial disparities in health and health care.[98] When successful at promoting open communication with affected communities, CBPR offers the opportunity to ensure that research addresses problems the community considers important and utilizes methods the community deems acceptable. It may also generate more robust research, informed by epistemological understandings of the community. For example, a successful study related to alcohol use in certain Alaska Native communities was conducted as a partnership between village leaders and researchers.[99] In the research planning phase, the partners agreed that the focus of the study should be "sobriety" rather than "alcoholism" and worked out differences regarding the study of individuals with moderate alcohol intake. Subsequently, both partners worked together to address the requirements of the funding agency; the result was a study that met both partners' needs for valid study design and results that were informative for the community.[100,101]

One common aspect of CBPR and other community engagement approaches is the use of a community advisory board or comparable structure for community input. Advisory boards, comprising community members who share a common identity, history, symbols, language, and culture, can facilitate research by serving as a liaison between participants and researchers.[102] If an advisory board is to be effective in influencing and guiding research, however, researchers must be willing to listen to the concerns of the board, and there must be adequate resources for its development and management.[102]

Responsibilities of Researchers

The inclusion of diverse populations strengthens genetic epidemiologic research. Both research quality and the potential for group harm point to the need for epidemiologists to consider incorporating some form of community engagement as part of the research process. In addition to promoting participation by community members, engagement may play a crucial role in ensuring that research questions address the needs of the community and that acceptable procedures are followed. Researchers should:

1. *Be knowledgeable about the communities in which they do research.* The ethics guidelines of the American College of Epidemiology [45] stress that

   Epidemiologists should be well informed about the history, circumstances, and perspectives of groups within the community. They should form relationships with formal or informal leaders in the community and consider the relevance of the epidemiologic research agenda to perceived community needs.

2. *Use methods of participatory research when appropriate.* The Guidelines further state that, in order to maintain public trust, epidemiologists should consider adopting a participatory approach to the extent possible and whenever appropriate, although care should be taken to ensure that community participation does not adversely affect scientific objectivity. These sentiments are echoed in guidelines issued by the National Institutes of Health.[103,104]

3. *Incorporate respect for groups with a commitment to the principles of beneficence, justice, and respect for persons.* When a research setting appears to pose a conflict between respect for group leadership and just treatment of individual participants, the latter concern is overriding. Judgments about conflicts of this kind must be made carefully, however, with respect for a community's cultural traditions and concern for the well-being of the group.[95]

Conclusion

Genetic epidemiology addresses questions of significance to families, communities, and population groups. It is therefore not surprising that social tensions have the potential to raise ethical questions for epidemiologists. In considering the issues raised by current genetic epidemiologic research, three concerns are especially pressing: protecting privacy and confidentiality, particularly in the context of widespread data sharing, the risk of oversimplifying the complex construct of "race," and the possibility of group harm. These issues must be approached with awareness and caution.

With regard to data sharing, it is important to strive for a balance between protecting individuals and groups from harm and overprotecting them in ways that impair the conduct of beneficial research. Removing identifying information and replacing it with a code prior to sharing reduces but does not eliminate the risk of harm. Thus, OHRP's guidance on the use of coded specimens and data raises some ambiguities with regard to the integrity of the consent process which are reflected in NIH's GWAS policy. Careful deliberation is needed on the role of waivers of consent, an issue that remains to be resolved in the context of large-scale data sharing. Further empiric work is urgently needed to understand participants' attitudes and opinions about data sharing, and to develop model consent documents and processes.

"Race" has long been used as a basis for discrimination, prejudice, marginalization, and subjugation,[105] but as Francis Collins[106] has stated, " 'Race' and 'ethnicity' are poorly defined terms that serve as flawed surrogates for multiple environmental and genetic factors in disease causation, including ancestral geographic origins, socioeconomic status, education, and access to health care. Research must move beyond these weak and imperfect proxy relationships to define the more proximate factors that influence health." When "race" is used as a variable in genetic epidemiologic research, it is essential that it be assiduously defined, justified, and interpreted.

The possibility of group harm is of particular concern in research that involves socially defined groups. Even when risks to individual participants are small, research results can have negative consequences for the entire group—including nonparticipants. Epidemiologists must be well aware of group-level perspectives and the relevance of their research to the needs of the community. One way to gain and incorporate these insights is through community engagement, with the form and intensity of engagement tailored to the characteristics of the study and the nature of the community and study population.

References

1. Lander, E. S., Linton, L. M., Birren, B., Nusbaum, C., Zody, M. C., Baldwin, J., et al. "Initial Sequencing and Analysis of the Human Genome," *Nature* 409 (2001): 860–921.
2. Venter, J. C., Adams, M. D., Myers, E. W., Li, P. W., Mural, R. J., Sutton, G. G., et al. "The Sequence of the Human Genome," *Science* 291 (2001): 1304–51.
3. Collins, F. S., Green, E. D., Guttmacher, A. E., and Guyer, M. S. "A Vision for the Future of Genomics Research," *Nature* 422 (2003): 835–47.
4. National Human Genome Research Institute. "Design Considerations for a Potential United States Population-Based Cohort to Determine the Relationships Among Genes, Environment, and Health: Recommendations of an Expert Panel."

Available at http://www.genome.gov/Pages/About/OD/ReportsPublications/ PotentialUSCohort.pdf, accessed January 9, 2008.

5. Ness, R. B. " Influence of the HIPAA Privacy Rule on Health Research," *JAMA* 298 (2007): 2164–70.

6. Reilly, P. R., Boshar, M. F., and Holtzman, S. H. "Ethical Issues in Genetic Research: Disclosure and Informed Consent," *Nature Genetics* 15 (1997): 16–20.

7. Fuller, B. P., Ellis Kahn, M. J., Barr, P. A., Biesecker, L., Crowley, E., Garber, J., et al. "Privacy in Genetics Research," *Science* 285 (1999): 1359–61.

8. Greely, H. T. "Human Genomics Research. New Challenges for Research Ethics," *Perspect Biochemical Medicine* 44 (2001): 221–29.

9. Capron, A. M. "Protection of Research Subjects: Do Special Rules Apply in Epidemiology?" *Journal of Clinical Epidemiology* 44 Suppl 1 (1991): 81S–89S.

10. Feinleib, M. "The Epidemiologist's Responsibilities to Study Participants," *Journal of Clinical Epidemiology* 44 Suppl 1 (1991): 73S–79S.

11. Coughlin, S. S. "Ethics in Epidemiology at the End of the 20th Century: Ethics, Values, and Mission Statements," *Epidemiologic Reviews* 22 (2000): 169–75.

12. Bondy, M. and Mastromarino, C. "Ethical Issues of Genetic Testing and Their Implications in Epidemiologic Studies," *Annals of Epidemiology* 7 (1997): 363–66.

13. Holtzman, N. A. and Andrews, L. B. "Ethical and Legal Issues in Genetic Epidemiology," *Epidemiologic Reviews* 19 (1997): 163–74.

14. Austin, M. A. "Ethical Issues in Human Genome Epidemiology: a Case Study Based on the Japanese American Family Study in Seattle, Washington," *American Journal of Epidemiology* 155 (2002): 585–92.

15. Beskow, L. M. "Ethical, Legal, and Social Issues in the Design and Conduct of Human Genome Epidemiology Studies." In *Human Genome Epidemiology: A Scientific Foundation for Using Genetic Information to Improve Health and Prevent Disease,* ed. M. J. Khoury, J. Little, and W. Burke. New York, NY: Oxford University Press, 2004: 58–76.

16. Gostin, L. O. and Hodge, J. G. "Genetic Privacy and the Law: an End to Genetics Exceptionalism," *Jurimetrics* (1999): 21–58.

17. Green, M. J. and Botkin, J. R. " 'Genetic Exceptionalism' in Medicine: Clarifying the Differences Between Genetic and Nongenetic Tests," *Annals of Internal Medicine* 138 (2003): 571–75.

18. Rothstein, M. A. "Genetic Exceptionalism and Legislative Pragmatism,"*Journal of Law, Medicine & Ethics* 35 (2007): 59–65.

19. Lander, E. S. and Schork, N. J. "Genetic Dissection of Complex Traits," *Science* 265 (1994): 2037–48.

20. Beskow, L. M., Botkin, J. R., Daly, M., Juengst, E. T., Lehmann, L. S., Merz, J. F., et al. "Ethical Issues in Identifying and Recruiting Participants for Familial Genetic Research," *American Journal of Medical Genetics A* 130A (2004): 424–31.

21. Beskow, L. M., Burke, W., Merz, J. F., Barr, P. A., Terry, S., Penchaszadeh, V. B., et al. "Informed Consent for Population-Based Research Involving Genetics," *JAMA* 286 (2001): 2315–21.

22. Tunis, S. R., Stryer, D. B., and Clancy, C. M. "Practical Clinical Trials: Increasing the Value of Clinical Research for Decision Making in Clinical and Health Policy," *JAMA* 290 (2003): 1624–32.

23. Spitz, M. R., Wu, X., and Mills, G. "Integrative Epidemiology: From Risk Assessment to Outcome Prediction," *Journal of Clinical Oncology* 23 (2005): 267–75.

24. American Society of Human Genetics. "Statement on Informed Consent for Genetic Research," *American Journal of Human Genetics* 59 (1996): 471–74.

25. Wilcox, A. J., Taylor, J. A., Sharp, R. R., and London, S. J. "Genetic Determinism and the Overprotection of Human Subjects," *Nat Genet* 21 (1999): 362.

26. Clayton, E. W., Steinberg, K. K., Khoury, M. J., Thomson, E., Andrews, L., Kahn, M. J., et al. "Informed Consent for Genetic Research on Stored Tissue Samples," *JAMA* 274 (1995): 1786–92.

27. Juengst, E. T. "Group Identity and Human Diversity: Keeping Biology Straight From Culture," *American Journal of Human Genetics* 63 (1998): 673–77.

28. Evans, P. D., Gilbert, S. L., Mekel-Bobrov, N., Vallender, E. J., Anderson, J. R., Vaez-Azizi, L.M., et al. "Microcephalin, a Gene Regulating Brain Size, Continues to Evolve Adaptively in Humans," *Science* 309 (2005): 1717–20.

29. Balter, M. "Bruce Lahn Profile. Brain Man Makes Waves with Claims of Recent Human Evolution," *Science* 314 (2006): 1871–73.

30. Mekel-Bobrov, N. D., Posthuma, D., Gilbert, S. L., Lind, P., Gosso, M. F., Luciano, M., et al. "The Ongoing Adaptive Evolution of ASPM and Microcephalin Is Not Explained by Increased Intelligence," *Human Molecular Genetics* 16 (2007): 600–08.

31. Currat, M. L., Excoffier, L., Maddison, W., Otto, S. P., Ray, N., Whitlock, M. C., et al. "Comment on 'Ongoing Adaptive Evolution of ASPM, a Brain Size Determinant in Homo Sapiens' and 'Microcephalin, a Gene Regulating Brain Size, Continues to Evolve Adaptively in Humans'," *Science* 313 (2006): 172; author reply 172.

32. National Cancer Institute. "The Cancer Genome Atlas (TCGA)." Available at http://cancergenome.nih.gov/index.asp, accessed January 19, 2008.

33. Foundation for the National Institutes of Health. "Genetic Association Information Network (GAIN)." Available at http://www.fnih.org/GAIN2/home_new.shtml, accessed January 19, 2008.

34. National Institutes of Health. "Genes, Environment and Health Initiative (GEI)." Available at http://www.gei.nih.gov/, accessed January19, 2008.

35. Wellcome Trust. "The Wellcome Trust Case Control Consortium (WTCCC)." Available at http://www.wtccc.org.uk/, accessed January 19, 2008.

36. Lowrance, W. W. and Collins, F. S. "Ethics. Identifiability in Genomic Research," *Science* 317 (2007): 600–02.

37. National Institutes of Health. "Policy for Sharing of Data Obtained in NIH Supported or Conducted Genome-Wide Association Studies (GWAS)." Available at http://grants.nih.gov/grants/guide/notice-files/NOT-OD-07–088.html, accessed January 20, 2008.

38. Wellcome Trust Case Control Consortium. "Genome-Wide Association Study of 14,000 Cases of Seven Common Diseases and 3,000 Shared Controls," *Nature* 447 (2007): 661–78.

39. McGuire, A. L. and Gibbs, R. A. "Genetics. No Longer De-Identified," *Science* 312 (2006): 370–71.

40. Lin, Z., Owen, A. B., and Altman, R. B. "Genetics. Genomic Research and Human Subject Privacy," *Science* 305 (2004): 183.

41. National Institutes of Health. "Genome-Wide Association Studies (GWAS). NIH Points to Consider for IRBs and Institutions." Available at http://grants.nih.gov/grants/gwas/gwas_ptc.pdf, accessed January 19, 2008.

42. Malin, B. and Sweeney, L. "How (Not) to Protect Genomic Data Privacy in a Distributed Network: Using Trail Re-Identification to Evaluate and Design

Anonymity Protection Systems," *Journal of Biomedical Informatics* 37 (2004): 179–92.

43. de Wolf, V. A., Sieber, J. E., Steel, P. M., Zarate, A. O. "Part III: Meeting the Challenge When Data Sharing Is Required," *IRB* 28 (2006): 10–5.

44. National Commission for the Protection of Human Subjects of Biomedical and Behavioral Research. *The Belmont Report: Ethical Principles and Guidelines for the Protection of Human Subjects of Research.* Washington DC: US Government Printing Office, 1978.

45. American College of Epidemiology. "Ethics Guidelines," *Annals of Epidemiology* 10 (2000): 487–97.

46. Department of Health and Human Services. "Office for Human Research Protections. Guidance on Research Involving Coded Private Information or Biological Specimens." Available at http://www.hhs.gov/ohrp/humansubjects/guidance/cdebiol.htm, accessed January 19, 2008.

47. National Bioethics Advisory Commission. *Research Involving Human Biological Materials: Ethical Issues and Policy Guidance*, Volume 1. Rockville, MD: National Bioethics Advisory Commission, 1999.

48. Pulley, J. M., Brace, M. M., Bernard, G. R., and Masys, D. R. "Attitudes and Perceptions of Patients Towards Methods of Establishing a DNA Biobank," *Cell Tissue Bank* 9 (2008): 55–65.

49. Wendler, D. and Emanuel, E. "The Debate Over Research on Stored Biological Samples: What Do Sources Think?" *Archives of Internal Medicine* 162 (2002): 1457–62.

50. Fong, M., Braun, K. L., and Chang, R. M. "Native Hawaiian Preferences for Informed Consent and Disclosure of Results From Genetic Research," *Journal of Cancer Education* 21 (2006): S47–S52.

51. Schwartz, M. D., Rothenberg, K., Joseph, L., Benkendorf, J., and Lerman, C. "Consent to the Use of Stored DNA for Genetics Research: a Survey of Attitudes in the Jewish Population," *American Journal of Medical Genetics* 98 (2001): 336–42.

52. McGuire, A. L. and Gibbs, R. A. "Meeting the Growing Demands of Genetic Research," *Journal of Law, Medicine & Ethics* 34 (2006): 809–12.

53. Rothenberg, K. H. "Breast Cancer, the Genetic 'Quick Fix,' and the Jewish Community. Ethical, Legal, and Social Challenges," *Health matrix (Cleveland, Ohio)* 7 (1997): 97–124.

54. Sankar, P., Cho, M. K., Condit, C. M., Hunt, L. M., Koenig, B., Marshall, P., et al. "Genetic Research and Health Disparities," *JAMA* 291 (2004): 2985–89.

55. Rebbeck, T. R. and Sankar, P. "Ethnicity, Ancestry, and Race in Molecular Epidemiologic Research," *Cancer Epidemiology, Biomarkers & Prevention* 14 (2005): 2467–71.

56. Smedley, A. and Smedley, B. D. "Race As Biology Is Fiction, Racism As a Social Problem Is Real: Anthropological and Historical Perspectives on the Social Construction of Race," *The American Psychologist* 60 (2005): 16–26.

57. Duster, T. "Race and Reification in Science," *Science* 307 (2005): 1050–51.

58. Kahn, J. "Genes, Race, and Population: Avoiding a Collision of Categories," *American Journal of Public Health* 96 (2006): 1965–70.

59. Bonham, V. L., Warshauer-Baker, E., and Collins, F. S. "Race and Ethnicity in the Genome Era: the Complexity of the Constructs," *The American Psychologist* 60 (2005): 9–15.

60. Bamshad, M., Wooding, S., Salisbury, B. A., Stephens, J. C. "Deconstructing the Relationship between Genetics and Race," *Nature Reviews. Genetics* 5 (2004): 598–609.

61. Cardon, L. R. and Palmer, L. J. "Population Stratification and Spurious Allelic Association," *Lancet* 361 (2003): 598–604.
62. Rotimi, C. N. "Are Medical and Nonmedical Uses of Large-Scale Genomic Markers Conflating Genetics and 'Race'?" *Nature Genetics* 36 (2004): S43–S47.
63. Wang, V. O. and S. Sue. "In the Eye of the Storm: Race and Genomics in Research and Practice," *The American Psychologist* 60 (2005): 37–45.
64. Kittles, R. A. and Weiss, K. M. "Race, Ancestry, and Genes: Implications for Defining Disease Risk," *Annual Review of Genomics and Human Genetics* 4 (2003): 33–67.
65. Kaufman, J. S. and Cooper, R. S. "Considerations for Use of Racial/Ethnic Classification in Etiologic Research," *American Journal of Epidemiology* 154 (2001): 291–98.
66. Shields, A. E., Fortun, M., Hammonds, E. M., King, P. A., Lerman, C., Rapp, R., et al. "The Use of Race Variables in Genetic Studies of Complex Traits and the Goal of Reducing Health Disparities: A Transdisciplinary Perspective," *Am Psychol* 60 (2005): 77–103.
67. Race, Ethnicity, and Genetics Working Group. "The Use of Racial, Ethnic, and Ancestral Categories in Human Genetics Research," *American Journal of Human Genetics* 77 (2005): 519–32.
68. Rivara, F. and Finberg, L. "Use of the Terms Race and Ethnicity," *Archives of Pediatrics & Adolescent Medicine* 155 (2001): 119.
69. Winker, M. A. "Measuring Race and Ethnicity: Why and How?" *JAMA* 292 (2004): 1612–14.
70. Bamshad, M. "Lost in Translation: Meaningful Policies for Writing about Genetics and Race," *American Journal of Medical Genetics A* 143 (2007): 971–72.
71. Wacholder, S., Rothman, N., and Caporaso, N. "Counterpoint: Bias From Population Stratification Is Not a Major Threat to the Validity of Conclusions from Epidemiological Studies of Common Polymorphisms and Cancer," *Cancer Epidemiology, Biomarkers & Prevention* 11 (2002): 513–20.
72. International Committee of Medical Journal Editors. "Uniform Requirements for Manuscripts Submitted to Biomedical Journals: Writing and Editing for Biomedical Publication." Available at http://www.icmje.org/, accessed January 9, 2008.
73. Cooper, R. S. and Psaty, B. M. "Diversity and Inclusiveness Should Remain the Guiding Principles for Clinical Trials," *Circulation* 112 (2005): 3660–65; discussion 3665–66.
74. Foster, M. W., Sharp, R. R., Freeman, W. L., Chino, M., Bernsten, D., Carter, T. H. "The Role of Community Review in Evaluating the Risks of Human Genetic Variation Research," *American Journal of Human Genetics* 64 (1999): 1719–27.
75. Emanuel, E. J. and Weijer, C. "Protecting Communities From Research." In *Belmont Re-Visited*, ed. J. F. Childress, E. M. Meslin, and H. T. Shapiro. Washington, DC: Georgetown University Press, 2005.
76. Shaffer, M. "Havasupai Blood Samples Misused." Available at http://www.indiancountry.com/content.cfm?id=1078833203, accessed March 28, 2008.
77. Weijer, C. "Protecting Communities in Research: Philosophical and Pragmatic Challenges," *Cambridge Quarterly of Healthcare Ethics* 8 (1999): 501–13.
78. Knoppers, B. M. and Chadwick, R. "Human Genetic Research: Emerging Trends in Ethics," *Nature Reviews. Genetics* 6 (2005): 75–79.

79. Beskow, L. M., Sandler, R. S., and Weinberger, M. "Research Recruitment through US Central Cancer Registries: Balancing Privacy and Scientific Issues," *American Journal of Public Health* 96 (2006): 1920–26.

80. Centers for Disease Control and Prevention. "National Notifiable Diseases Surveillance System." Available at http://www.cdc.gov/ncphi/disss/nndss/nndsshis.htm, accessed March 28, 2008.

81. Helgesson, G., Dillner, J., Carlson, J., Bartram, C. R., Hansson, M. G. "Ethical Framework for Previously Collected Biobank Samples," *Nature Biotechnology* 25 (2007): 973–76.

82. Sharp, R. R. and Foster, M. W. "Involving Study Populations in the Review of Genetic Research," *Journal of Law, Medicine & Ethics* 28 (2000): 41–51, 3.

83. Leung, M. W., Yen, I. H., and Minkler, M. "Community Based Participatory Research: a Promising Approach for Increasing Epidemiology's Relevance in the 21st Century," *International Journal of Epidemiology* 33 (2004): 499–506.

84. Israel, B. A., Parker, E. A., Rowe, Z., Salvatore, A., Minkler, M., López, J., et al. "Community-Based Participatory Research: Lessons Learned From the Centers for Children's Environmental Health and Disease Prevention Research," *Environmental Health Perspectives* 113 (2005): 1463–71.

85. Reilly, P. R. "Rethinking Risks to Human Subjects in Genetic Research," *American Journal of Human Genetics* 63 (1998): 682–85.

86. Juengst, E. T. "Commentary: What 'Community Review' Can and Cannot Do," *Journal of Law, Medicine & Ethics* 28 (2000): 52–54, 3.

87. Foster, M. W., Eisenbraun, A. J., and Carter, T. H. "Communal Discourse As a Supplement to Informed Consent for Genetic Research," *Nature Genetics* 17 (1997): 277–79.

88. Foster, M. W., Bernsten, D., and Carter, T. H. "A Model Agreement for Genetic Research in Socially Identifiable Populations," *American Journal of Human Genetics* 63 (1998): 696–702.

89. Sharp, R. R. and Foster, M. W. "Community Involvement in the Ethical Review of Genetic Research: Lessons from American Indian and Alaska Native Populations," *Environmental Health Perspectives* 110 Suppl 2 (2002): 145–48.

90. Holkup, P. A., Tripp-Reimer, T., Salois, E. M., and Weinert, C. "Community-Based Participatory Research: an Approach to Intervention Research with a Native American Community," *Advances in Nursing Science* 27 (2004): 162–75.

91. Burhansstipanov, L., Christopher, S., and Schumacher, S. A. "Lessons Learned from Community-Based Participatory Research in Indian Country," *Cancer Control* 12, Suppl 2 (2005): 70–76.

92. Hausman, D. "Protecting Groups From Genetic Research," *Bioethics* 22 (2008): 157–65.

93. Foulks, E. F. "Misalliances in the Barrow Alcohol Study," *American Indian and Alaska Native Mental Health Research* 2 (1989): 7–17.

94. Hausman, D. "Group Risks, Risks to Groups, and Group Engagement in Genetics Research," *Kennedy Institute of Ethics Journal* 17 (2007): 351–69.

95. Marshall, P. A. "Human Rights, Cultural Pluralism, and International Health Research," *Theoretical Medicine and Bioethics* 26 (2005): 529–57.

96. Green, L. W. and Mercer, S. L. "Can Public Health Researchers and Agencies Reconcile the Push From Funding Bodies and the Pull From Communities?" *American Journal of Public Health* 91 (2001): 1926–29.

97. Minkler, M. "Ethical Challenges for the 'Outside' Researcher in Community-Based Participatory Research," *Health Education & Behavior* 31 (2004): 684–97.

98. Potvin, L., Cargo, M., McComber, A. M., Delormier, T., Macaulay, A. C. "Implementing Participatory Intervention and Research in Communities: Lessons From the Kahnawake Schools Diabetes Prevention Project in Canada," *Social Science & Medicine (1982)* 56 (2003): 1295–1305.

99. Mohatt, G. V., Hazel, K. L., Allen, J., Stachelrodt, M., Hensel, C., Fath, R. "Unheard Alaska: Culturally Anchored Participatory Action Research on Sobriety With Alaska Natives," *American Journal of Community Psychology* 33 (2004): 263–73.

100. Mohatt, G. V., Rasmus, S. M., Thomas, L., Allen, J., Hazel, K., Hensel, C. " 'Tied Together Like a Woven Hat': Protective Pathways to Alaska Native Sobriety," *Harm Reduction Journal* [Electronic Resource] 1 (2004): 10.

101. Mohatt, G. V., Rasmus, S. M., Thomas, L., Allen, J., Hazel, K., Marlatt, G. A. "Risk, Resilience, and Natural Recovery: a Model of Recovery From Alcohol Abuse for Alaska Natives," *Addiction* 103 (2008): 205–15.

102. Strauss, R. P., Sengupta, S., Quinn, S. C., Goeppinger, J., Spaulding, C., Kegeles, S. M., et al. "The Role of Community Advisory Boards: Involving Communities in the Informed Consent Process," *American Journal of Public Health* 91 (2001): 1938–43.

103. National Institute of General Medical Sciences. "Report of the First Community Consultation on the Responsible Collection and Use of Samples for Genetic Research." Available at http://www.nigms.nih.gov/news/reports/community_consultation.html, accessed January 9, 2008.

104. National Institutes of Health. "Points to Consider When Planning a Genetic Study That Involves Members of Named Populations." Available at http://bioethics.od.nih.gov/named_populations.html, accessed January 9, 2008.

105. Burchard, E. G., Ziv, E., Coyle, N., Gomez, S. L., Tang, H., Karter, A. J., et al. "The Importance of Race and Ethnic Background in Biomedical Research and Clinical Practice," *The New England Journal of Medicine* 348 (2003): 1170–75.

106. Collins, F. S. "What We Do and Don't Know About 'Race', 'Ethnicity', Genetics and Health at the Dawn of the Genome Era," *Nature Genetics* 36 (2004): S13–S15.

10

Ethics and Epidemiology in the Age of AIDS

CAROL LEVINE

AIDS (acquired immunodeficiency syndrome) now commands a global army of specialists and subspecialists in nearly every field of medicine and science, as well as in ethics, law, psychology, sociology, education, economics, journalism, and politics. However, 25 years ago AIDS was relatively unknown. It was epidemiologists who first gave this new disease its name and defined its modes of transmission. These epidemiologists now monitor its spread, natural history, and its effect on public health and clinical interventions. Each step and misstep in this process has had far-reaching consequences, many of which will be described in this chapter. (More specific accounts of the early years of the epidemic and the role played by epidemiologists have been chronicled elsewhere.[1,2,3])

Epidemiology deals with disease processes and trends in populations. However, as Gerald Oppenheimer points out, "Epidemiology, unlike virology, has a strong social dimension. His assertion that epidemiology *explicitly* "incorporates perceptions of a population's social relations, behavioral patterns, and experiences into its explanations"[4] may be an overstatement, but it is true that epidemiology frequently *encounters* such social dimensions. When, as in the case of AIDS, those perceptions involve a lethal disease, stigmatizing behaviors such as drug use and homosexual sex, and a suspicious and fearful public, the potential for moral implications soars.

After some general discussion of ethics and epidemiology, this chapter focuses on five examples, mostly drawn from my experience and research, which illustrate the interrelationship of ethics and epidemiology in the case of AIDS. These examples are presented in roughly chronological order. The first describes the conflict during the early years of the epidemic between the need for valid data about a new disease of unknown etiology and subjects' fears of confidentiality breaches. The second details the conflict between the scientific definitions of the term "disease" and the economic and regulatory uses of these definitions, as well as their impact on individuals. The third pits the epidemiologic value of anonymous serological surveillance techniques against the clinical value of identifying seropositivity in individuals as it played out in the case of pregnant women and newborns. The fourth example concerns the global impact of HIV/AIDS on children whose parents are either ill or dead, and the ethical implications of various definitions of orphanhood. The fifth example relates the story back to the outset of the epidemic, describing the announcement of a new and rapidly progressing HIV variant to a highly sexually active gay man.

These examples are neither comprehensive nor the end of the story. The epidemic is global—ravaging sub-Saharan Africa and parts of Asia, spreading in Asia and Eastern Europe, and continuing to take a terrible toll in communities of color and among gay men in the United States. Lacking a cure and with a vaccine only a distant promise, we will be dealing with AIDS and its social impact for decades. Furthermore, AIDS was not an aberration, as originally surmised, but a harbinger. In a world where global travel is commonplace, other infectious diseases—SARS and avian flu being the best known examples—pose new threats.

The examples described in this chapter demonstrate how the relationship between ethics and epidemiology has evolved over time. Ethical principles are timeless but their emphasis and interpretation may vary as new knowledge becomes available. Questions that appear to be resolved may reappear in a different context, as has occurred in discussions of HIV testing. Questions that did not appear at the beginning, such as just allocation of resources, emerge when therapies became available. Populations once thought immune—non-drug-using women—are now vulnerable.

Before AIDS, epidemiology was mostly a concern for specialists who defined disease, identified risk factors, and established potential associations. After AIDS, and for future epidemics, advocates for the affected populations will insist on being part of the process. For epidemiologists and ethicists alike, their presence can be both helpful and challenging.

Ethical Issues in Epidemiologic Studies

Although all the ethical principles that govern research apply to both clinical and noninterventional epidemiologic research, the weight given to one principle or another varies according to the context. Clinical research focuses on the individual as part of a study population. Ethical principles that predominate in clinical research also focus on individuals: Respect for autonomous decision making, beneficence (enhancing the welfare of the individual), and nonmaleficence (avoiding the causation of harm to individuals). These principles weigh heavily in considerations of the ratio of risks to benefits in medical decision making, informed consent, and privacy and protection of confidentiality.

Epidemiologic studies, on the other hand, focus on populations but may involve identified individuals. The predominant ethical values include the importance of knowledge to be gained and the potential benefit to groups, including future patients or society in general. Questions of justice concerning fairness between the subjects who are selected to bear the burdens of research and the eventual recipients of any benefits derived from the research also arise in epidemiologic studies. For example, in some studies of environmental toxins, subjects may want to be included and may not perceive participation as a burden or a risk. Some of the ethical problems common in epidemiology are invasion of privacy, violation of confidentiality, conflict of interest, and tension between a researcher's values and those of the communities studied.[5]

Clinical trials and noninterventional epidemiologic research present different types of risks or harms. Risks in clinical trials typically involve adverse physical effects or, less commonly, psychological harm. However, as Alexander Morgan Capron[6] points out,

Epidemiologic research can also involve the risk of harm, but it is typically of a different sort. Since, in most cases, investigators do not physically intervene with the subject and do not even have direct contact of any sort, physical and psychological injuries are unlikely. Yet other sorts of harm may occur. First, if data dealing with sensitive matters, either raw data or final results, can be linked to subjects, they may suffer social harm, such as ostracism or loss of employment. Second, even when individuals cannot be linked to information that is embarrassing (or worse), findings that paint an adverse picture of an entire population may eventuate in harm to that group, either directly or as a result of the adoption of laws or policies that have a negative impact on the welfare of group members.

Furthermore, Capron continues, even when subjects are not physically or psychologically harmed, they may be wronged by invasion of privacy without consent or by treating people solely as a means to an end. This possibility, he rightly maintains, explains why ethical guidelines are important, even if the risk of direct harm to subjects is negligible.

For these reasons and others, epidemiologic studies are governed by special regulatory requirements. Examples of these exemptions include research involving the collection or study of existing data, records, pathologic specimens, or diagnostic specimens as long as there are no identifiers linking the data to the subjects. IRBs accustomed to reviewing clinical studies may have difficulty in devising appropriate standards for epidemiologic studies.[7] The following section illustrates some of the problems during the initial attempts to track the then-unknown disease.

Confidentiality and the Wary Subject

In 1981 Michael Gottlieb, a Los Angeles physician, reported to the federal Centers for Disease Control and Prevention (CDC) the unexpected occurrence of the rare *Pneumocystis carinii* pneumonia (PCP) in five previously healthy homosexual men he had treated in 1980 and 1981. An editorial note in the *Morbidity and Mortality Weekly Report (MMWR)* suggested that some aspect of a "homosexual lifestyle" might be involved.[8] Soon afterwards, a second MMWR report described a finding of Kaposi's sarcoma, a cancer rarely seen in the United States, in 26 gay men treated in the previous 30 months in California and New York City.[9] Although it is now known that cases of AIDS had been seen as early as 1977, these MMWR reports marked the official start of the epidemic.

In mid-1981 the CDC formed a surveillance task force, which contacted state and local health departments to identify suspected cases of what was soon to be called AIDS. (An earlier designation, Gay-Related Immunodeficiency, or GRID, was used until late 1982.[10]) Although the case of a heterosexual woman with AIDS had been reported to the CDC by August 1981, and a New York City investigation of eleven men with PCP included seven drug users, five of them heterosexual, the focus remained on men who had sex with men as the defining characteristic of the population at risk. By 1983, several investigations were under way involving gay men as subjects. To gather valid data on the sexual, drug-using, and other behavior of gay men, epidemiologists sought to obtain highly detailed and accurate descriptions of these aspects of subjects' lives. The researchers focused on the numbers of sex partners, following the "promiscuity" theory, and on the use of amyl nitrates, commonly known as "poppers," during sex. In these interviews the subjects might have revealed information about homosexual behaviors, which were illegal in many states, sometimes with severe penalties, including 5 years to life (Idaho), 20 years (Oklahoma), and 15 years (Michigan). In its decision in *Lawrence* v. *Texas* (539 U.S. 558 [2003]), the U.S. Supreme Court held that sodomy laws were unconstitutional and unenforceable. However, 14 states and Puerto Rico still had these laws on the books as of late 2007. Even if not illegal, homosexuality was stigmatized everywhere. Subjects might have revealed drug use, criminal activities such as prostitution, or illegal entry into the United States. They also might have named other individuals involved in these activities. Many subjects, however, were unwilling to trust government researchers with such potentially damaging information, and either refused to cooperate or gave inaccurate or incomplete answers, rendering the data questionable.

Although some epidemiologists were sensitive to the subjects' concerns, others failed to see why they should treat information about this disease or the people who had it with any special protections. Public health departments were proud of their record of maintaining confidentiality of information about other diseases. Nevertheless, in some instances at least, internal procedures were less than strict with AIDS information. Case folders with identifying names were sometimes left on desks or given to other researchers or agency employees. Local health departments reported cases with identifiers to the CDC. At that time the modes of transmission of this deadly disease were still under investigation. Considering the fact that police departments, fire departments, and others were calling for lists of people with AIDS and considering the demands that people with AIDS be isolated, the subjects' concerns were understandable.

At this point ethicists became involved in the issue. Early in 1983, a physician treating gay men with AIDS involved in epidemiologic research asked the staff of The Hastings Center to help stress the importance of confidentiality in AIDS research. These advocates specifically sought to bolster their views, which were regarded as biased by some health department officials, by using the professional standing of ethicists. The Center's staff subsequently decided to convene a working group to develop guidelines on this subject. The proposal to the Charles A. Dana Foundation, which funded the project, stated:

There is an inherent tension between the needs of researchers who want access to a maximum of information with a minimum of hindrance and the desires of AIDS patients who want sensitive and identifiable information about themselves given the maximum protection and the most restricted distribution. This tension need not pose an insuperable difficulty. While the legitimate interests of researchers and patients can be accommodated, it will require a serious examination of the contexts in which disclosure takes place, the purposes for which the information may be used, and the people who will have access to it.

The proposal warned that "the future integrity of epidemiological research on AIDS" depended on reaching a mutual understanding. Given adversarial positions that were hardening, the staff judged that the composition of the working group would be a determining factor in the acceptance of the guidelines. No matter how ethically justifiable or well argued the guidelines were, if they did not have the support of the parties whose interests were at stake, they would have no impact.

Many gay men believed that quarantine in "concentration camps" was a distinct possibility. They were, they believed, facing a hostile, angry, and irrational public. Researchers and health department officials, on the other hand, feared a rapidly spreading and uncontrollable epidemic. These perceptions made the issues emotionally explosive. For these reasons, the working group included government and academic researchers, epidemiologists, lawyers, privacy specialists, ethicists, physicians, and representatives of gay and AIDS organizations. Most of the professionals had never talked with the subject representatives of the target population, who were extremely wary of researchers and government officials of any kind. Interestingly, the way epidemiologists had framed the epidemic to that date helped determine the composition of the group. There were no participants representing drug users or women, because these groups or their behaviors had not been formally linked with the disease. However, there were representatives of the Haitian community, which had been officially termed a "risk group," a designation later dropped because of protests.[11]

The overall question addressed in the guidelines dealt with the procedures and policies that would protect the privacy of research subjects as well as enable research to proceed effectively. In the grant proposal the ethical challenge was described as "striking a balance between the principle of respect for the autonomy of persons (which requires that individuals be treated as autonomous agents who have the right to control their own destinies) and the pursuit of the common good (which requires maximizing possible benefits as well as minimizing possible harms, to society as well as to individuals)."

Despite their different perspectives, members of the working group reached a consensus on all but one of the proposed guidelines. The guidelines covered descriptive issues such as what identifiers are necessary, when they are needed, and what precautions should be taken to protect identifiable data; who should and who should not have access to personally identifiable information, the rather severe limitations of relevant legal protections, the steps that should be taken to enhance the legal protections for both research subjects and researchers whose data might be subpoenaed, the standards for institutional review boards, and questions of consent.

The single issue on which the working group could not agree was the use of the Social Security Number (SSN) as an identifier. The guidelines pointed out that SSNs offer the greatest potential for matching data sets but that they also pose the greatest threat to confidentiality: "Some researchers believe that Social Security numbers are indispensable in longitudinal studies, where it is important to be able to recognize that different sets of data have come from a single person. Those who oppose the use of Social Security numbers stress that these numbers are assigned and held by the federal government. Potential misuse of information by government agencies is one of the strongest fears expressed by subjects in AIDS research."[12]

This question recurred in 1994 in the debate over national health reform, and in 1996 the Health Insurance Privacy and Accountability Act of 1996 (HIPAA) addressed the increasing concern about the privacy of data collected electronically under a regional or national system. Lawrence O. Gostin and colleagues assert that, "Perhaps the most critical single decision regarding privacy and security in a reformed health care system is whether to use the Social Security Number...as the individual identifier."[13] Pointing out that the SSN currently is not a completely reliable identifier and that this identifier is used extensively for a variety of non-health-related purposes, Gostin et al. instead recommended a personal health security number, which would serve no purpose except as a health record itself. Despite the importance of this issue, at the time it seemed a minor matter in the face of the overwhelming consensus on other issues that the confidentiality guidelines were written by the AIDS working group.

The guidelines had no official weight, but they were cited repeatedly in the course of negotiations over epidemiologic research. The process of their formulation set important precedents. At this early stage of the epidemic, ethics was firmly established as integral to public health decision making. Affected communities were involved in recommendations about their interests. Finally, consensus could be achieved on most thorny issues. Even when agreement could not be reached, the dissenting positions could be articulated and clarified. Since then, this collaborative model has been used many times, with varying success, in developing AIDS policy and programs. The rallying cry of disability activists —"Nothing about me without me"—has at least some roots in AIDS activism. On a less confrontational level, there is scarcely a public health or disease group that does not have a "consumer" representative. In hindsight, the process of inclusion in this early effort seems as important as the outcome.

What Counts as an "AIDS Case" and Who Decides?

Ethical dimensions of epidemiology come into play even before the design and implementation of specific studies. Before diseases can be tracked and studied they must be defined and classified. Disease classification systems and surveillance definitions are ordinarily tools for epidemiologists and clinicians, not matters for political debate and patient advocacy. It is hard to imagine a street demonstration protesting the classification system for stages of colon cancer. But when it comes to AIDS, nothing is ordinary.

Disease surveillance is a major public health activity. Case reporting is the primary, although not the only, surveillance tool in monitoring the incidence and prevalence of disease. The surveillance case definition is intended to provide consistent statistical data for public health purposes.

The CDC first defined AIDS in 1981 and established criteria for public health reporting. By 1983, all U.S. states required name reporting of AIDS cases but not of HIV infection. In addition, the CDC developed an alternative, comprehensive "classification" system for HIV infection for adults and adolescents, with a separate classification system for children. The classification system covered the broad spectrum of HIV disease, from initial infection, asymptomatic infection, and persistent generalized lymphadenopathy through serious opportunistic infections and cancers. The primary purpose was to provide a framework for categorizing HIV-related morbidity and immunosuppression.

In the early 1990s controversy erupted over the CDC's proposed revision of the existing surveillance case definition of AIDS.[14] The surveillance case definition was the primary focus of the controversy discussed in this section, although the classification system was also involved by virtue of its reliance on the surveillance case definition for criteria for the end stage of AIDS. Public health officials, researchers, clinicians, hospital administrators, disability specialists, insurance administrators, health economists, legislators, social workers, psychologists, policy makers, and the media all used the CDC's surveillance case definition of AIDS. It influenced the way the epidemic was perceived, managed, and funded. An AIDS diagnosis triggered a series of benefits and services generally not available to a person with HIV infection. It is not surprising, then, that the CDC's surveillance case definition of AIDS transcended epidemiology to become a symbol for the inadequacies of the U.S. government's response to the HIV epidemic. It also symbolized the failure to address adequately the needs of HIV-infected women.

Since the first version in 1981, the CDC's surveillance case definition of AIDS has been changed four times—in 1985, 1987, 1993, and, most recently, in 1999. The CDC's initial surveillance case definition required the diagnosis of one of eleven opportunistic infections, or of two cancers that were considered "at least moderately predictive of a defect in cell-mediated immunity, occurring in a person with no known cause for diminished resistance to that disease."[15] In 1984, when HIV-1 was discovered, various laboratory tests were developed to measure and confirm the presence of HIV antibodies. Using these tests as diagnostic indicators, the CDC broadened the surveillance case definition of AIDS in 1985 to include additional opportunistic infections or cancers that would be indicative of AIDS in persons with positive HIV antibody test results.[16] The surveillance case definition was further expanded in 1987 to include several severe nonmalignant HIV-associated conditions, including HIV wasting syndrome and neurological manifestations, and to permit "presumptive" diagnoses, such as diagnoses of AIDS based on the presence of one of seven indicator diseases without confirmatory laboratory evidence of HIV.[17]

In 1991, the CDC proposed still another revision of the surveillance case definition and the disease classification system. Under this scheme there would be three categories of HIV disease: asymptomatic, symptomatic, and AIDS. There would also be three categorical levels of CD4+ cells (also called T cells) per cubic millimeter of blood, which would guide clinicians in recommending therapeutic actions in disease management. Because declining CD4+ cell counts have been shown to be reliable indicators of disease progression, individuals with less than 200 CD4+ cells would be considered to have AIDS, regardless of their symptoms. No new opportunistic infections or other conditions would be added to the already long list of 23 AIDS-defining conditions in the surveillance case definition.[18]

This proposal was greeted with intense and often acrimonious debate. Virtually everyone agreed that the surveillance case definition should be revised, but many disagreed with the CDC's approach. Advocates argued that the "outdated" surveillance case definition artificially lowered the number of cases of AIDS, which led to inadequate federal funding and attention. Officials in states with large numbers of women and drug users with HIV-related illnesses, the groups most likely to fall outside the CDC's 1987 surveillance case definition for AIDS, were concerned that funding formulas based on case reports of CDC-defined AIDS were inequitable. Women's advocates claimed that many women with HIV-related illnesses were improperly diagnosed and treated because the surveillance case definition was developed from data on clinical manifestations in gay men. Moreover, community-based organizations that provided services to individuals, especially women who were disabled by HIV illness but did not meet the criteria for AIDS, found it difficult to obtain various federal, state, and local entitlements and benefits for their clients. A full-page advertisement in *The New York Times* (June 19, 1991), initiated by the AIDS Coalition to Unleash Power (ACT UP) and signed by over 200 individuals and organizations, protested: "Women don't get AIDS. They just die from it."

One ad hoc group went even further, forcibly handcuffing selected participants who were all well-known AIDS advocates, including some physicians, at a meeting at the offices of the American Public Health Association held with CDC officials to discuss the controversy. During the several hours that followed, the group protested that the meeting should not have been held, that AIDS advocates by their very presence were betraying their constituents, that the proposed revisions failed to include conditions specific to women, and that the government was to blame for just about everything connected to the epidemic.

The CDC claimed that there was insufficient evidence to include specific gynecological conditions. By strict research standards, the evidence was indeed scant, but the studies that would have provided more adequate evidence one way or the other had not been conducted or had not been initiated early enough during the onset of the epidemic to provide reliable data. In the end, the advocates won a small victory. The CDC's final revision of the HIV infection classification system and the surveillance case definition for AIDS contained all of the CDC's original proposals, but it also included pulmonary tuberculosis, recurrent pneumonia, and one female-specific condition: invasive cervical cancer.[19]

As a result of the expanded surveillance case definition, 1993, AIDS cases increased 111% over cases reported in 1992 (103,500 compared with 49,016),[20] significantly surpassing the 75% rise the CDC had predicted.[21] Of the cases reported in 1993, 54% were based on conditions added to the definition in that year, and the increase was greater among females (151%) than males (105%). The largest increases were among racial/ethnic minorities, adolescents and young adults, and cases attributed to heterosexual transmission. As expected, the rate of increase declined in subsequent reporting periods.

In 1999 the CDC recommended that all states and territories conduct case surveillance for HIV as an extension of their AIDS surveillance.[21] The new definition combined reporting criteria for HIV and AIDS into a single case definition and reflected new laboratory techniques that were not available in 1993. With the advent of Highly Active Antiretroviral Therapy (HAART), which slowed the progression of HIV to AIDS, it became especially important to identify HIV-infected individuals early in order to offer treatment and to monitor the epidemic's course more accurately. The CDC also pointed to the opportunities for public health prevention efforts and the targeting of resources. By February 2007, all states except Hawaii, Maryland, and Vermont had instituted HIV reporting by name. These three states use code-based reporting.[22]

The acrimonious controversy over the 1993 case definition demonstrated that surveillance case definitions, disease classification systems, and the CDC's role in both were poorly understood. The public's comprehension of the current state of the epidemic (actually a series of smaller epidemics, which began in different cities at different times and have followed different courses) suffered from the initial, almost single-minded focus on gay men. The controversy also showed how secondary uses of surveillance information—in this case, formulas for funding or benefits—can have a far greater impact than its primary epidemiologic purpose.

HIV Surveillance and Mother-to-Child Transmission

As the previous section discussed, women with HIV/AIDS were clearly neglected in surveillance and prevention during the outset of the epidemic. When HIV/AIDS was identified in infants and young children, "AIDS babies" as the media called them, the public image of their mothers was largely negative. The public saw hemophiliacs and tainted blood transfusion recipients and newborns as "innocent victims," but gay men and HIV-infected mothers who gave birth to these babies were seen as "guilty." It is ironic that, given the persistent perception that the disease in the United States primarily affects gay men, several of the major debates around HIV testing have concerned pregnant women and newborns.

During the evolution into today's practice, which began in the mid-1990s, two issues were most contentious: whether testing in clinical care should be mandatory, voluntary, or routine; and whether blinded seroprevalence surveys should be unblinded to inform those who were HIV-positive of their status. These dilemmas have social and bioethical implications beyond mother-to-child transmission.

HIV testing. Discussions about HIV counseling and testing policies for pregnant women and newborns have taken place in the context of a broader debate over whether testing should be voluntary with informed consent, mandatory (legally required), or routine (usually interpreted to mean that clinicians will test for HIV as they do for other conditions unless patients refuse or "opt out"). With some exceptions of mandatory screening, such as blood donors, military personnel, and immigrants, for example, the debate was resolved in favor of voluntary testing. With the advent of effective therapy and faster, more accurate laboratory techniques, many public health officials and physicians now advocate routine testing as being cost-effective and an important way to identify and to treat HIV-infected people who are unaware of their status.[23,24,25,26]

In the early 1990s, however, all the major organizations and groups that specifically examined testing policies for pregnant women concluded that voluntary screening with informed consent was the course most likely to produce the desired effects of education, prevention, and appropriate medical and social service follow-up. For example, the Institute of Medicine (IOM) asserted that "individuals (or their legally recognized representatives) should have the right to consent to or refuse HIV testing (except when such testing is conducted anonymously for epidemiologic purposes)." By opposing mandatory newborn or prenatal screening programs, the IOM found "no compelling evidence that women and children should constitute an exception to this principle."[27] Similarly, a working group from Johns Hopkins University and Georgetown University rejected mandatory screening and recommended a range of voluntary policies.[28]

This consensus began to erode, however, following announcement in February 1994 of the results of AIDS Clinical Trial Group Study 076, which showed that transmission from mother to fetus was reduced dramatically (from 25% to 4.3%) in a group of pregnant women treated with zidovudine (AZT).[29] Pediatricians were also seeing the benefits for HIV-infected children of antiretroviral therapy and prevention of opportunistic infections.[30] In addition, the risk of HIV transmission from breast milk, while small, can be avoided if an HIV-infected mother does not breast-feed. These benefits, while no panacea, had a significant impact on the ethics of the screening calculus. In April 2003, Julie Gerberding and Harold Jaffe of the CDC sent a "Dear Colleague" letter recommending that "clinicians routinely screen all pregnant women for HIV infection, using an 'opt out' approach and that jurisdictions with statutory barriers to such routine prenatal screening consider revising them."[31] In November 2004, the American College of Obstetrics and Gynecology similarly recommended that "pregnant women universally should be tested as part of the routine battery of prenatal blood tests unless they decline the test."[32]

In one of the epidemic's few clear-cut successes, mother-to-child HIV transmission has been drastically reduced in the United States and Europe. In Africa, where the prevalence of HIV infection is very high and the availability of antiretroviral treatment for pregnant women is low but increasing, HIV mother-to-child transmission remains a serious problem. According to the CDC, the number of mother-to-child HIV transmissions peaked in 1991, when 1650 such cases were reported, and declined to an estimated range of 100 to 200 in 2005.[33] In New York State, the epicenter of the U.S. epidemic, the transmission rate declined from 10.9% in 1997 to 2.4% in 2002.[34] Major medical centers that once were home to "boarder babies" with AIDS now seldom see a new case of an HIV-infected newborn. Although only two states (New York and Connecticut) have mandatory newborn HIV testing, voluntary counseling and testing of pregnant women has become standard in most jurisdictions. In a paradoxical result, a pregnant woman may refuse testing for herself but not for her baby. Although the baby's test is inconclusive for the newborn, it definitively reveals the mother's HIV status. Her refusal to learn her HIV status only postpones being told. Obtaining consent for testing and counseling, however, is still valuable in encouraging follow-up.[35,36] The availability of a highly successful method of preventing transmission changed the public health and clinical emphasis from one of voluntary testing to required testing—or at least vigorously recommended testing. It also changed the emphasis for women, the vast majority of whom would not want to transmit HIV to their babies. It did not eliminate, however, the need for counseling and services.

Blinded seroprevalence studies. The potential conflict between the values that predominate in epidemiologic studies and those that weigh most heavily in clinical practice became real in the case of HIV seroprevalence surveys conducted in newborns. Under these circumstances the importance of obtaining accurate knowledge about the course of the epidemic, in a way that does not present any risk to the individuals, came into conflict with the importance of identifying and treating individual patients. This was not an instance of one goal being more valuable than the other, it was a case of seroprevalence surveys being unable to serve the goals of obtaining accurate knowledge and identifying named individuals.

To estimate the prevalence of HIV infection in sentinel areas and groups throughout the country, in 1988 the CDC developed what it called a "family" of serological surveys, which were anonymous unlinked HIV surveys in sentinel sites, including STD clinics and drug treatment centers, in selected metropolitan areas.[37] In 1987, New York State initiated blinded serosurveys of newborns to estimate HIV prevalence among pregnant women. In June 1999, the New York State Department of Health proposed to "modify its on-going blind newborn HIV antibody testing program to permit voluntary notification of mothers whose infants test positive." Under the proposal, new mothers would have the option of learning their baby's test results and, as a consequence, their own HIV status.

Several objections were raised to the proposal by community-based healthcare providers and others. These objections primarily concerned (1) the confusing and psychologically traumatic impact on new mothers of learning about their own HIV infection and the possible infection of their babies at a time when they are physically and emotionally vulnerable; (2) the potential for manipulation or coercion by health-care providers who might not understand or accept a mother's unwillingness to learn the test results at that time, and (3) the lack of health care and support services for women and their children, once identified as seropositive.

Because of these objections, the state Department of Health agreed to postpone the implementation of this proposal in favor of a much more aggressive but still voluntary program, called the Obstetrical HIV Counseling/Testing/Care Initiative. Instead of a "take it or leave it" approach to testing, practitioners in this program advocated for testing. It was designed to increase rates of voluntary testing for women who had given birth without access to prenatal care.[38] In addition, New York City's child welfare administration revised its policy on HIV testing for infants and children entering foster care.[39] Because newborns in foster care were much more likely to be HIV-positive than newborns going home with their mothers, the agency took several steps to ensure that they receive appropriate evaluation and follow-up. Infected children and their foster parents became eligible for special medical and social services.

Despite these two initiatives aimed at increasing the numbers of HIV-infected infants identified at birth, the controversy over newborn testing erupted in the New York State Legislature in 1993–94. Nettie Mayersohn, an assemblywoman from Queens, introduced legislation that required the State Department of Health to notify parents if their infant showed positive results on the HIV test that was being done anonymously. The debate quickly polarized and raged not only in the legislative halls but also in the media.

To deflect the furor and to table action on the Mayersohn bill, the New York State Assembly's Ad Hoc Task Force on AIDS asked the Governor's AIDS Advisory Council to study the issue. After several months of hearings and debate, in February 1994 a subcommittee convened in 1994 by the Advisory Council recommended a policy of "mandatory counseling and strongly encouraged voluntary testing for all pregnant and postpartum women," as well as other measures to strengthen counseling, testing, and the availability of services.[40] Pediatricians have been vigorous advocates for their HIV-infected patients. A group of pediatricians dissented from the report, declaring that this policy was "insufficient to offer the protection which every infant deserves" and that voluntary testing has an "unacceptably high failure rate.[41]

A legislative compromise that would have mandated counseling and encouraged voluntary testing failed on the last day of the session. The New York State Task Force on Life and the Law, another executive branch body, was then asked to restudy the entire issue. In May 1995 the CDC suspended funding of the blinded newborn seroprevalence studies. The CDC had already discontinued the unlinked "family" of seroprevalence studies in 1999.[42]

Although name-based or coded HIV reporting has become standard in most of the United States, it is still important to distinguish this kind of monitoring from blinded seroprevalence surveys. In the acrimonious debate about unblinding the newborn studies, the value of anonymous surveillance as an epidemiologic tool was hardly mentioned, and when it was, it was often misunderstood.

Anonymous unlinked surveys test blood samples already collected for other medical purposes and are stripped of all personal identifiers. Blinded surveys conversely can generate less-biased estimates of HIV prevalence because individuals do not have the opportunity to select whether or not to participate in serological testing. Blinded surveys are simpler, quicker, and less costly than nonblinded surveys. Ethically, blinded surveys do not place any participant at risk of identification, and thus issues of privacy and confidentiality are not raised.[43] Since they are a matter of public health *practice* rather than human studies *research*, survey protocols are exempt from IRB review. Even so, the CDC IRB reviewed and approved the protocol for the HIV seroprevalence surveys. As Fairchild and Bayer point out, in public health, there is an ethical mandate to "undertake surveillance that enhances the well-being of populations." At the same time, they urge, ethical oversight of surveillance "can serve as a means of avoiding inadvertent breaches in confidentiality and stigma; it can help to ensure that the public understands that surveillance will occur and what purposes it serves; and it can protect politically sensitive surveillance efforts."[44]

Generally, blinded seroprevalence surveys have been remarkably uncontroversial and free of political influence. However, blinded HIV serological surveys on adults or children have been very controversial in England[45] and the Netherlands.[46] One commentator in the United States has claimed that "surreptitious testing is deceitful" and that "in the quest to eliminate self-selection bias, epidemiologists are ignoring the difference between human subjects and laboratory animals."[47]

One of the purposes of blinded serological surveys is to pinpoint precisely where resources and services, such as counseling and testing, are needed. However, as the Public Health Service pointed out, "The surveillance activity, in the case of an HIV prevalence survey, must not be confused with the public health intervention for which the survey may indicate a need."[48] In this view, the use of blinded surveys seems to be compatible with a parallel system of voluntary counseling and testing in settings in which individuals likely to be at risk of HIV infection are treated.

More recent international discussions of surveillance focus on "second-generation surveillance." According to UNAIDS and WHO, this includes "biological surveillance of HIV and other sexually transmitted infections (STIs) as well as systematic surveillance of the behaviour that spreads them. It aims to use these data together to build up a comprehensive picture of the HIV/AIDS epidemic."[49] The Working Group warns, however, "second-generation surveillance for HIV is an intrusive business. It involves collecting specimens of people's body fluids and asking them questions about some of the most intimate aspects of their lives. Continuing to do this over time is morally unacceptable unless the data are actively used to improve life for the people from whom they are collected and their communities." This statement takes a strong moral stance that could equally be and often is applied to clinical research. Although I agree with the principle, the implementation in practice is often difficult because of resource constraints and a lack of health infrastructure. The agencies that conduct the surveillance are not usually the agencies that make resource decisions. Nevertheless, public health officials should advocate for positive actions based on the knowledge they obtain.

Defining Orphanhood

If the low rates of HIV testing in the United States—even among populations at greatest risk—are a good indicator,[50] public fears about the HIV/AIDS epidemic have waned. However, international efforts, such as the U.S. President's Emergency Plan for AIDS Relief (PEPFAR), Unicef's campaigns on behalf of children, and private foundation funding, have increased awareness about the global epidemic. Media stories frequently catalog the crises in these far-off places, perhaps displacing Americans' concern about their own HIV status. Because of the vast scale of the epidemic in Africa and Asia and the poverty of the countries where it has killed millions and wreaked devastation on fragile economies and medical and social infrastructures, there are daunting ethical and economic issues. The controversy over the use of placebo-controlled trials to prevent mother-to-child transmission in countries where the Western standard of care cannot or will not be provided is the best known example.[51] Debates about who will receive the growing but still inadequate supplies of antiretroviral therapy accompany the efforts to provide treatment.[52,53]

In the United States, the relationship between children and HIV was considered almost exclusively in the context of mother-to-child transmission. That these inaptly termed "AIDS babies" had uninfected siblings who would become orphans when their mother died was neither recognized, studied, nor addressed. Since the mid-1990s, however, significant efforts have been made to provide services for all these children and their new guardians.[54] In sub-Saharan Africa, however, the situation was quite different. In the context of a heterosexually transmitted disease, the growing number of orphans and the strain placed on extended families caring for them was recognized, but not addressed, in the late 1980s. The first survey of orphan prevalence was conducted in Uganda in 1989. Some of these orphans were HIV-infected; most were not.

In 2004 Unicef estimated that 14 million children had been orphaned (lost at least one parent) by AIDS, 12.3 million of them in sub-Saharan Africa. By 2010 the global figure is estimated to reach 25 million orphans, with 18 million in sub-Saharan Africa.[55] More than one-third (36.8%) of all orphans in this region are due to AIDS. In the past few years, international organizations such as Unicef and UNAIDS and international nongovernmental organizations like Save the Children and World Vision have made the care of orphans, a term now usually linked with "other vulnerable children" (OVC), a priority.

Despite the apparent simplicity of the term "orphan," it is conceptually and logistically complex to conduct epidemiologic studies that define the population, monitor changes, and identify areas of particular need. Yet it is essential to do so to target limited resources in a way that does not stigmatize these children or deprive others in similarly dire circumstances of assistance.

In Biblical times and patriarchal societies, orphans were defined by their fathers' death; numerous references in both the Old and New Testaments, Islamic texts, and in other religious writing cite the obligation to care for "widows and orphans." This phrase was further immortalized in Lincoln's Second Inaugural Address. The phrase continues to be used in modern times to denote typographic infelicities (widows being short lines at the ends of paragraphs and orphans being short lines at the top of a page). In another example, the Widows and Orphans Act of 2005 (S. 644) was introduced in the U.S. Senate to create new immigration categories for "certain women and children at risk of harm," even though these individuals are not necessarily either widows or orphans.

Despite the history and persistence of this metaphor, when it comes to real children today, the death of a mother has come to be seen as the primary loss, since mothers are presumed to be the nurturing parent. In U.S. epidemiologic studies, the category of "orphan" does not exist; "motherless child" is the relevant category.[56] Since there are no epidemiologic data on the number of children men father analogous to women's fertility rates, there is no way to calculate the number of fatherless children, if "fatherless" means that the male parent has died and is not simply absent from the family.[57]

In international epidemiologic usage, a child whose mother has died is a "maternal orphan"; if the dead parent is the father, the child is a "paternal orphan." In either case, that child is a "single orphan." If both parents are dead, the child is a "double orphan." Until 2004, UNAIDS and Unicef used the cutoff age of 15.[58] In the 2004 report, these agencies extended the age to 18,[59] which is the age cutoff for a "child" in the 1989 UN Convention on the Rights of the Child. (In reporting cases of AIDS, however, the age of adulthood is 15.)

From a child rights perspective, Gruskin and Tarantola argue that "the inconsistency of age groupings is further compounded by the different age cut-offs at which countries recognize the legal 'age of consent' for consensual sex, as these may affect the degree to which children feel comfortable coming forward for needed services."[60] Since orphaning is more common in Africa than in the West in general, because of war, civil unrest, and tropical diseases, it is important to understand the contribution of HIV/AIDS to the total orphan population. All studies indicate that AIDS has contributed significantly to increasing the number of orphans, especially double orphans, since HIV is sexually transmitted.[61] One study comparing household-survey estimates with projections of mortality and orphan numbers in sub-Saharan Africa concluded that the fraction of orphans attributable to AIDS may be greater than previously estimated.[62]

The numbers of orphans can be estimated based on the number of children born to women who have died from AIDS over the preceding 17 years using country- and age-specific fertility rates, as well as rates of mother-to-child transmission that would result in the death of an HIV-infected child. Declining fertility rates in the year preceding death are also included in the equation. These estimates vary according to the reliability of the data on which they are based.

Using a more direct method, investigators can conduct censuses asking about the number of orphans in households and communities. This method also has limitations of both under- and over-counting. Children may not be identified as orphans to avoid stigmatization or because they may have been living with the family prior to the parent's illness and death. Family members may be reluctant to mention disabled and sick children. On the other hand, families seeking to obtain benefits that are designed for orphans may misrepresent their number. Children may be miscategorized based on the death of one or both parents. The phenomenon of "orphan clustering" as parents migrate or send their children to relatives may affect censuses.

Programs developed to serve orphans in a particular community generally try not to single out orphans due to AIDS, because this causes resentment and increases stigma. (Donor agencies and the public, however, are more likely to support programs if they are "helping orphans.") If the definition of "orphan" is elastic, the definition of "vulnerable child" or "child in especially difficult circumstances" is even more so. The World Bank Toolkit on orphans and vulnerable children defines them as "children who are more exposed to risks than their peers . . . and most likely to fall through the cracks of regular programs."[63]

As Webb points out,

While acknowledging international epidemiological definitions, practitioners must also investigate local definitions of orphanhood and vulnerability more generally, which may include abandoned children (as in Romania), children living in destitute households, or those whose parents are sick or unemployed or whose caregivers are elderly.[64]

Although it is important to understand local definitions in targeting resources, Webb continues, they will be "less amenable to cross-cultural comparisons" and "introduce a subjective aspect to meta-analyses."

Among the more problematic consequences of defining orphans as age 15 and under is the assumption that adolescents of 16 are fully adult and able to take care of themselves, as well as their younger siblings. Members of this group have particularly urgent psychological and material needs and are at risk of becoming HIV-infected themselves through early sexual activity. Teenage girls are particularly vulnerable to sexual exploitation, HIV infection, and pregnancy. The phenomenon of "orphans of orphans" is already occurring.

For all these reasons, Webb says,

A consensus on definitions is urgently needed and . . . would facilitate better learning between projects, allow uniformity in policy design, and ease the establishment of systematic surveillance. (p. 248)

Such a consensus would only be the first step; the ethical challenge of using the data in the most effective and just way would remain.

Back to the Future: The HIV "Superbug"

After nearly 30 years, women and children are clearly on the AIDS agenda. But the epidemic's impact on gay men, the first population identified, continues even after the introduction of HAART. The past remains vivid for those who survived and those who have taken on advocacy roles.

On February 11, 2005, Thomas Frieden, the New York City Health Commissioner, took the unusual step of calling a press conference to announce that a particularly virulent strain of HIV had been identified.[65] This "HIV superbug," as it was quickly named, was resistant to nearly all AIDS drugs and induced an unusually rapid course of illness—weeks or months, not years—from infection to full-blown AIDS. The one patient in whom the virus had been identified is a gay man who had multiple unprotected sexual encounters while using the street drug crystal methamphetamine. Flanking Dr. Frieden at the press conference were the scientists who had identified the virus strain and representatives of several leading gay service organizations.

Given the criticism of government officials that they had not done enough in the 1980s to warn gay men about the spreading disease, this announcement might be seen as a prudent step and as a reminder that HIV is still a serious threat. Some gay leaders, however, dissented, claiming that the announcement was premature and unfairly stigmatized the gay community, hearkening back to the demonization of "Patient Zero," the gay airline employee singled out as the source of the epidemic in North America in the early 1980s.

Some scientists also criticized the announcement, recalling other instances of mutant viral strains that did not spread. Stephen Smith, a New Jersey infectious disease specialist, wrote: "The reason for the NYC Department of Health press release at this early point in the investigation is unclear. In the absence of a documented cluster of patients, should the entire health system react? No, we should wait for more information...."[66] Paul Volberding, one of the earliest AIDS physicians, said: "Clearly rigorous epidemiologic investigation is preferred over public alerts that cause only fear. But we should just as firmly insist that the true crises of HIV transmission—failure to use condoms, poor case finding of acute infection, and control of epidemic methamphetamine abuse—are the real issues in cases like this patient."[67] In response, Dr. Frieden reiterated that "the goal of public health is to prevent, not describe, outbreaks."[68] Since the initial announcement no additional cases have been reported.

This incident shows the continuing link between the problems faced by epidemiology (in this case, the presumed occurrence of a new and virulent strain of HIV) and problems of ethics (here primarily the obligation to prevent harm while avoiding stigmatizing individuals or groups). Arguing that AIDS has never been and is not now "ordinary," epidemiologist Philip Alcabes says, "When one case of AIDS can claim headlines for days in a city as large and AIDS-experienced as New York, ordinariness seems far away." [69]

Although the definitive history is yet to be written, Oppenheimer has given an astute preliminary assessment:

From the beginning of the epidemic, epidemiologists conceptualized HIV infection as a complex social phenomenon, with dimensions that derived from the social relations, behavioral patterns, and past experiences of the population at risk. On the one hand, the epidemiologists' approach may have skewed the choice of models and the hypotheses pursued and may have offered some justification for homophobia. On the other, by defining HIV infection as a multifactorial phenomenon, with both behavioral and microbial determinants, epidemiologists offered the possibility of primary prevention, a traditional epidemiological response to infectious and chronic diseases. Epidemiologists, in effect, established the basis for an effective public health campaign and—through publications, conferences, and the continuous collection of surveillance data—helped make AIDS a concern of policymakers and the public [4] (p. 76).

Ethics provides a reasoned and principled approach to some of the conflicts that have arisen. Ethical considerations have provided models for resolutions of controversies, an emphasis on values of confidentiality and respect for individuals, and recognition of the social context of disease in designing prevention and treatment programs. Unfortunately, the end of the epidemic is nowhere in sight, and the ethical issues are likely to evolve in the future as they have done in the past. Some questions will have been adequately answered; others are still debated; and the future may still hold surprises.

References

1. Shilts, R. *And the Band Played On: Politics, People and the AIDS Epidemic.* New York: St. Martin's Press, 1987.
2. Fee, E. and Fox, D. M. *AIDS: The Making of a Chronic Disease.* Berkeley, CA: University of California Press, 1992.
3. Bayer, R. *Private Acts, Social Consequences: AIDS and the Politics of Public Health.* New York: The Free Press, 1989.
4. Oppenheimer, G. M. "In the Eye of the Storm: The Epidemiological Construction of AIDS." In *AIDS: The Burdens of History,* ed. E. Fee and D. M. Fox. Berkeley, CA: University of California Press, 1988.
5. Last, J. M. "Epidemiology and Ethics," *Law, Medicine & Health Care* 19 (1991): 166–74.
6. Capron, A. M. "Protection of Research Subjects: Do Special Rules Apply to Epidemiology?" *Law, Medicine & Health Care* 19 (1991): 184–90.
7. Cann, C. I. and Rothman, K. J. "IRBs and Epidemiological Research: How Inappropriate Restrictions Hamper Studies," *IRB* 6 (1984): 5–7.
8. Centers for Disease Control. "*Pneumocystis* Pneumonia—Los Angeles," *Morbidity and Mortality Weekly Report* 30 (1981): 250–52.

9. Centers for Disease Control. "Kaposi's Sarcoma and *Pneumocystis* Pneumonia among Homosexual Men—New York City and California," *Morbidity and Mortality Weekly Report* 30 (1981): 305–07.

10. Oppenheimer, G. M. "Causes, Cases, and Cohorts: The Role of Epidemiology in the Historical Construction of AIDS." In *AIDS: The Making of a Chronic Disease*, ed. E. Fee and D. M. Fox. Berkeley, CA: University of California Press, 1992.

11. Farmer, P. *AIDS and Accusation: Haiti and the Geography of Blame*. Berkeley, CA: University of California Press, 1992.

12. Bayer, R., Levine, C., and Murray, T. H. "Guidelines for Confidentiality in Research on AIDS," *IRB: A Review of Human Subjects Research* 6 (November/December 1984): 1–3.

13. Gostin, L. O., Turek-Brezina, J., Powers, M., Kozloff, R., Faden, R., and Steinauer, D. D. "Privacy and Security of Personal Information in a New Health Care System," *Journal of the American Medical Association* 270 (1993): 2488.

14. Levine, C. and Stein, G. L. "What's in a Name? The Policy Implications of the CDC Definition of AIDS," *Law, Medicine, and Health Care* 19 (1991):278–90.

15. Centers for Disease Control. "Update on Acquired Immune Deficiency Syndrome (AIDS)—United States," *Morbidity and Mortality Weekly Report* 31 (1982): 507–14.

16. Centers for Disease Control. "Revision of Case Definition of Acquired Immunodeficiency Syndrome for National Reporting—United States," *Morbidity and Mortality Weekly Report* 34 (1985): 373–75.

17. Centers for Disease Control. "Revision of the CDC Surveillance Case Definition for Acquired Immunodeficiency Syndrome," *Morbidity and Mortality Weekly Report* 36 (1987) (Suppl.): 1S–15S.

18. Centers for Disease Control. "1992 Revised Classification System for HIV Infection and Expanded Case Definition for Adolescents and Adults," Draft, November 15, 1991.

19. Centers for Disease Control. "1993 Revised Classification System for HIV Infection and Expanded Surveillance Case Definition for AIDS among Adolescents and Adults," *Morbidity and Mortality Weekly Report* 41, no. RR-17 (1992): 1–5.

20. Centers for Disease Control and Prevention. "Update: Impact of the Expanded AIDS Surveillance Case Definition for Adolescents and Adults on Case Reporting United States, 1993," *Morbidity and Mortality Weekly Report* 43 (1994): 160–61, 167–70.

21. Centers for Disease Control and Prevention. "HIV Infection Reporting." Available at http://www.cdc.gov/hiv/topics/surveillance/reporting.htm, accessed October 29, 2007.

22. Kaiser Family Foundation State Health Facts. "HIV Name/Code-Based Reporting Policies, 2005." Available at http://www.statehealthfacts.kff.org, accessed May 30, 2005.

23. Sanders, G.D., Bayoumi, A.M., Sundaram, V., Biir, S. P., Neukermans, A. B., Ryzdak, C. E. et al. "Cost-Effectiveness of Screening for HIV in the Era of Highly Active Antiretroviral Therapy," *New England Journal of Medicine* 352, no. 6 (2005): 570–85.

24. Paltiel, A. D., Weinstein, M. C., Kimmel, A. D., Seage, G. R., Losina, E., Zhang, H. et al. "Expanded Screening for HIV in the United States–An Analysis of Cost-Effectiveness," *New England Journal of Medicine* 352, no. 6 (2005): 586–95.

25. Bozzette, S. A. "Routine Screening for HIV Infection – Timely and Cost-Effective," *New England Journal of Medicine* 352, no. 6 (2005):620–21.

26. Paltiel, A. D., Weinstein, M. C., Kimmel, A. D., Seage, G. R. III, Zhang, H. et al. Expanded Screening for HIV in the United States—An Analysis of Cost-Effectiveness. *New England Journal of Medicine* 352(6) (2005): 586–95.

27. Institute of Medicine. *HIV Screening of Pregnant Women and Newborns*. Washington, DC: Institute of Medicine, 1991: 2–3.

28. Faden, R., Geller, G., and Powers, M. *AIDS, Women and the Next Generation*. New York: Oxford University Press, 1992: 333–34.

29. Centers for Disease Control and Prevention. "Zidovudine for the Prevention of HIV Transmission from Mother to Infant," *Morbidity and Mortality Weekly Report* 43 (1994): 285–87.

30. Brogly, S., Williams, P., Seage, G. R., Oleske, J. M., Van Dyke, R., and McIntosh, K., for the PACTG 219C Team. "Antiretroviral Treatment in Pediatric HIV Infection in the United States: From Clinical Trials to Clinical Practice," *Journal of the American Medical Association* 293 (18) (2005): 2213–20.

31. Gerberding, J. L. and Jaffe, H. W. "Dear Colleague" letter, April 23, 2003. Atlanta: Centers for Disease Control and Prevention.

32. American College of Obstetrics and Gynecology. "ACOG Committee Opinion Number 304, November 2004. Prenatal and perinatal human immunodeficiency virus testing: Expanding Recommendations," *Obstetrics and Gynecology* 104, no. 5, Pt 1 (2004): 1119–24.

33. Centers for Disease Control and Prevention. "Mother-to-Child (Perinatal) HIV Transmission and Prevention," *CDC HIV/AIDS Fact Sheet*, October 2007.

34. Warren, B. "Pediatric HIV Infection in New York State." Presentation April 14, 2005, New York City, to Doctors of the World training session for Russian health-care workers.

35. Webber, D. W. "HIV Testing during Pregnancy: The Value of Optimizing Consent," *AIDS & Public Policy Journal* 18, no. 3 (2004): 83–97.

36. Kelly, K. "Obtaining Consent Prior to Prenatal HIV Testing: The Value of Persuasion and the Threat of Coercion," *AIDS & Public Policy Journal* 18 (2004): 98–111.

37. Pappaloanou, M., Dondero, Jr., T. J., Peterson, L. R., Onorato, I. M., Sanchez, C. D., and Curran, J. W. "The Family of HIV Seroprevalence Surveys: Objectives, Methods, and Uses of Sentinel Surveillance for HIV in the United States," *Public Health Reports* 105 (1990): 113–19.

38. New York State Department of Health, AIDS Institute. "Women and Children with HIV Infection in New York State: 1990–92 AIDS Institute Program Review." Albany, NY: New York State Department of Health, 1992.

39. New York City, Human Resources Administration, Child Welfare Administration. Draft Bulletin: HIV Testing of Children in Foster Care, April 23, 1993.

40. New York State AIDS Advisory Council. Report of the Subcommittee on Newborn HIV Screening of the New York State AIDS Advisory Council. Albany, NY. February 10, 1994: 17, iii.

41. Dissenting Comments on the January 31, 1994 Report of the Subcommittee on Newborn Screening to the AIDS Advisory Council, February 4, 1994. New York State Department of Health, AIDS Institute, Albany, NY.

42. Centers for Disease Control and Prevention. *HIV Prevalence Trends in Selected Populations in the United States: Results from National Serosurveillance, 1993–1997*. Atlanta, GA: Centers for Disease Control and Prevention, 2001: 2.

43. Bayer, R., Levine, C., and Wolf, S. M. "HIV Antibody Screening: An Ethical Framework for Evaluating Proposed Programs," *Journal of the American Medical Association* 256 (1986): 1768–74.
44. Fairchild, A. L. and Bayer, R. "Ethics and the Conduct of Public Health Surveillance," *Science* 303 (2004):631–32.
45. Zulueta, P. "The Ethics of Anonymised HIV Testing of Pregnant Women: A Reappraisal," *Journal of Medical Ethics* 26 (2000): 25–26.
46. Bayer, R., Lumey, L. H., and Wan, L. "The American and Dutch Responses to Unlinked Anonymous HIV Seroprevalence Studies: An International Comparison" [Letter], *AIDS* 4 (1992): 4283–90.
47. Isaacman, S. I. "HIV Surveillance Testing: Taking Advantage of the Disadvantaged" [Letter], A*merican Journal of Public Health* 83 (1993): 597.
48. Dondero, T. J., Pappaioanou, M., and Curran, J. W. "Monitoring the Levels and Trends of HIV Infection: The Public Health Service's HIV Surveillance Program," *Public Health Reports* 103 (1998): 213–20.
49. UNAIDS/WHO Working Group on Global HIV/AIDS/STI Surveillance. *Guidelines for Effective Use of Data from HIV Surveillance Systems.* Geneva: World Health Organization, 2004: 5, 46. Available at www.unaids.org, accessed October 20, 2008.
50. Ostoermann, J., Kumar, V., Pence, B. W., and Whetten, K. "Trends in HIV Testing and Differences between Planned and Actual Testing in the United States, 2000–2005," *Archives of Internal Medicine* 267 (2007): 2128–35.
51. Macklin, R. *Double Standards in Medical Research in Developing Countries.* New York: Cambridge University Press, 2004.
52. UNAIDS and WHO. *Guidance on Ethics and Equitable Access to HIV Treatment and Care.* Geneva: UNAIDS and WHO, 2004.
53. Rennic, S. and Behets, F. "AIDS Care and Treatment in Sub-Saharan Africa: Implementation Ethics." *Hastings Center Report* 36 (2006): 23–31.
54. Draimin, B. H. and Reich, W. A. "Troubled Tapestries: Children, Families, and the HIV/AIDS Epidemic in the United States." In *A Generation At Risk: The Global Impact of HIV/AIDS on Orphans and Vulnerable Children,* ed.,G. Foster, C. Levine, and J. Williamson. New York: Cambridge University Press, 2005: 213—32.
55. UNAIDS, Unicef, and USAID. *Children on the Brink 2004: A Joint Report of New Orphan Estimates and a Framework for Action.* Washington, DC, 2004.
56. Lee, L. M. and Fleming, P. L. "Estimated Number of Children Left Motherless by AIDS in the United States, 1978–1998," *Journal of the Acquired Immune Deficiency Syndrome* 34 (2003): 231–36.
57. Michaels, D. and Levine, C. "Estimates of the Number of Motherless Youth Orphaned by AIDS in the United States," *Journal of the American Medical Association* 268 (1992): 3456–61.
58. UNAIDS, USAID, and UNICEF. *Children on the Brink 2002: A Joint Report on Orphan Estimates and Program Strategies.* Geneva, 2003.
59. UNAIDS, UNICEF, and USAID. *Children on the Brink 2004: A Joint Report of New Orphan Estimates and a Framework for Action.* Geneva, 2004: 4, 33–35.
60. Gruskin, S. and Tarantola, D. "Human Rights and Children Affected by HIV/AIDS." In *A Generation at Risk: The Impact of HIV/AIDS on Orphans and Vulnerable Children,* ed. G. Foster, C. Levine, and J. Williamson. New York: Cambridge University Press, 2005: 134–58, p. 148.

61. Monasch, R. and Boerma, J. T. "Orphanhood and Childcare Patterns in Sub-Saharan Africa: An Analysis of National Surveys from 40 Countries," *AIDS* 18 (Suppl. 2, 2004): S55–S65.

62. Grassly, N. C., Lewis, J. J. C., Mahy, M., Walker, N., and Timaeus, I. M. "Comparison of Household-Survey Estimates with Projections of Mortality and Orphan Numbers in Sub-Saharan Africa in the era of HIV/AIDS," *Population Studies* 58 (2004): 207–17.

63. World Bank OVC Toolkit. "Defining OVC." Available at http://www.worldbank.org/ wbi/childrenandyouth/toolkit, accessed June 1, 2005.

64. Webb, D. "Interventions to Support Children Affected by HIV/AIDS: Priority Areas for Research." In *A Generation at Risk: The Impact of HIV/AIDS on Orphans and Vulnerable Children,* ed. G. Foster, C. Levine, and J. Williamson. New York: Cambridge University Press, 2005: 233.

65. Santora, M. and Altman, L. K. "Health Alert in New York: Rare and Aggressive H.I.V. Reported in New York," *The New York Times*, February 12, 2005, p. A:1.

66. Smith, S. M. "Commentary: New York City HIV Superbug: Fear or Fear Not?" *Retrovirology* 2 (2005): 14.

67. Volberding, P. "The New York Case: Lessons Being Learned," *Annals of Internal Medicine* 142 (2005): 866–68, p. 868.

68. Frieden, T. R. "The New York Case: Lessons Being Learned," *Annals of Internal Medicine* 143 (2005): 760.

69. Alcalbe, P. "The Ordinariness of AIDS," *American Scholar* 75 (2006): 18–32, p. 20.

11

Ethical Issues in International Health Research and Epidemiology

JOHN D. H. PORTER, CAROLYN STEPHENS, AND ANTHONY KESSEL

In this chapter we look at our divided world and explore issues such as the poverty of resources, health care infrastructure, research capability in developing countries, and the potential for exploitation that is inherent in this context and can occur through international research collaborations. We do not aim to repeat the well-rehearsed lists of ethical issues that can arise in international health research, but instead endeavor to grapple with these issues through the lens of the divided world, with an emphasis on the central role of the researcher.

In investigating research as we currently conduct it, we engage in descriptive ethics. But we also need to ask how we ought to be acting, which requires exploring systematically developed moral theories or normative ethics. Through the latter, research ethics may provide a guide toward changes in behavior, which may help us understand better the nature of our individual and collective roles in international health research. The Nuffield Institute of Bioethics has recognized that we have a great deal to do in this area:

Many people in the developing world suffer from poor health and reduced life expectancy. The role of research that contributes to the development of appropriate treatments and disease prevention measures is vital. However, lack of resources and weak infrastructure mean that many researchers in developing countries have very limited capacity to conduct their own clinical research. A sound ethical framework is a crucial safeguard to avoid possible exploitation of research participants in these circumstances (Quote from the Executive Summary of Nuffield Institute of Bioethics report on "The Ethics of Research Related to Healthcare in Developing Countries," 2005: p. xi).[1]

We argue here that ethics in international public health research needs to combine use of international understandings and guidelines with a close examination of how humans actually function in societies—both their own societies and in other peoples.

Science itself is cultural and therefore embedded in a particular historical and social milieu.[2] Part of the current historical and social milieu is the phenomenon of globalization, which has been defined as "the process of increasing economic, political and social interdependence and global integration that takes place as capital, traded goods, persons, concepts, images, ideas and values diffuse across state boundaries."[3] This is particularly true in health, where social, political, and economic forces are widening global inequalities in health leading to decreasing equity in resources, health protection, and health care.[4]

Often values are being traded, not integrated, and different value systems are coming into conflict. This conflict is often linked to the global inequities and social injustice. These divisions and differences need to be taken into account when creating research collaborations. Although globalization provides different ways of communicating in order to develop research proposals, how each of us should develop these collaborations continues to be an ethical question in international research. The creation of successful research collaborations and partnerships itself affects both how research subjects and communities are treated and how research teams operate.[5]

Although low-income countries are gradually developing their own guidelines and ways of institutionalizing ethics, most of the international research guidelines are currently presented within a Western framework. [6,7,8] We will discuss these changing value systems within international research after first looking briefly at international developments in research ethics.

History of International Research and Ethical Issues

Interest in the ethics of international health research accelerated in the early 1990s with the growth of international collaborations, led by the CIOMS guidelines and changes to the Declaration of Helsinki.[9] From an international perspective, it is important to understand the history of the development of such guidelines.

Current regulations and guidelines are a direct consequence of research atrocities during World War II, and have evolved over the past 60 years. The history of research ethics shows the importance of remaining conscious to the problems of unethical research. By the beginning of the 20th century the medical codes created by Thomas Percival *circa* 1800[10] that consisted of the moral virtues of physicians with some mention of moral rules, rules of etiquette, and rules of professional conduct[11,12,13] had become the dominant basis of professional ethics in the United States.[13,14,15] In 1947 the British Medical Association (BMA) published its code of ethics, which essentially summarized the previous half-century's work.[11] The Nuremberg and Geneva Codes then expressed a new agenda based on the concept of human rights,[16] and in 1964 the World Medical Association (WMA) published the Helsinki Declaration.[7]

The Belmont Report of 1978, issued by the National Commission for the Protection of Human Subjects of Biomedical and Behavioral Research, went beyond the Nuremberg Code [17] and the Helsinki Declaration to focus on informed consent, favorable risk–benefit ratios, and the need to ensure that vulnerable populations are not targeted for risky research.[13] The report established the three main ethical principles in clinical research: respect for persons, beneficence, and justice.[18]

In the 1980s there was an increase in international health research activity. In the early 1990s, the Council for International Organization of Medical Sciences (CIOMS) worked with the World Health Organization (WHO) to develop two sets of international guidelines for international medical research.[6,19] Controversies in the late 1990s around international HIV and TB trials [20,21] resulted in changes in the Helsinki Declaration and the CIOMS guidelines, and led to a working party report from the Nuffield Council of Bioethics in London.[1,8]

This section outlines the emergence of the field of research ethics within epidemiology and other health sciences in the late 20th century. It shows the domi nance of guidelines developed in wealthy Western societies. This links strongly to the dominant models of health research conducted internationally, which we discuss in the next section.

Types of Research Being Conducted Internationally

Research is "the systematic investigation into and study of materials, sources . . . in order to establish facts and reach new conclusions" (*Oxford English Dictionary*), and science is "the systematic study and knowledge of natural and physical phenomena" (*Collins English Dictionary*). Epidemiology is a core discipline within public health research, whose aim has been defined as "to generate organized community effort to address the public interest in health by applying scientific and technical knowledge to prevent disease and promote health." [22] Epidemiology has further been described as "the study of the distribution and determinants of health related states or events in specified populations." [23] It is a quantitative science that is considered by many to be among the most important disciplines in public health.[22] Examples of classical epidemiological research include cohort studies and case-control studies. In addition to epidemiology, public health research contains many different disciplines and research approaches that includes clinical research (e.g., drug and vaccine trials), laboratory research, social science research (qualitative studies), health systems research (interdisciplinary), and policy research (transdisciplinary). All these disciplines may be used in the creation of intervention studies, including clinical trials and community-based trials, health services, and operational research. Operational research has been defined as "the application of scientific methods of investigation to the study of complex human organisations and services."[24]

For some, the most important aspect of research is not the "type of research" being conducted but "how" it is conducted and with whom. For example, some believe that epidemiology is becoming increasingly divorced from its important role in public health policy and practice.[25] One reason is the lack of involvement of communities in the research process.[26] These shifting sands have led to the creation of the term "popular epidemiology," a process that highlights social structural factors and involves social movements.[27,28] Popular epidemiology seeks to return the knowledge creation process to ordinary people and is committed to assuring that the problem defined arises from within the community and that local people function as cornerstones in the research process.[29,30] The essence of popular epidemiology is its commitment to the sharing of power with the people with and for whom researchers work.[27] Popular epidemiology is about how we interact as researchers and the importance of the management of research studies. The emergence of popular epidemiology may in part be derived from some moral problems encountered in international research.

How We Develop Research Internationally

Many research materials report the stages involved in the creation of a research project, such as introduction (study plan and ethical considerations), definition of study objectives, selection of interventions (if any), allocation of interventions (e.g., randomized or not), choice of outcome measure(s), study population (criteria for selection, inclusion, exclusion criteria, size, and compliance), implementation (community acceptance, staff recruitment and training, and field organization), data handling, quality control, and, finally, analysis and reporting.[31] In addition to these stages, there is also the search for funding, discussions with funding bodies, and the creation of links and partnerships with local communities and other organizations.

Although some research disciplines (principally qualitative ones) study the process of the creation and management of research, little information on this subject had been published until recently.[32] However, social scientists are now providing important insights into research processes in developing countries.[33,34,35] Their studies highlight the different perspectives, approaches, and beliefs that distinguish international researchers and local populations. Little is also known about how Research Ethics Committees (RECs) function. A recent group of studies from Mexico, using both qualitative and quantitative methods, highlights the importance of structures, actions, and processes of Mexican RECs and suggest a need for audit of committees.[36,37]

This section outlines very briefly a growing debate within international health research: there is now evidence suggesting that researchers are often very distant from research subjects—both culturally and in terms of interaction in the research process. But what does this mean for the development of ethics guidelines in international health research and how do researchers use the guidelines that exist? The following section outlines some of the current issues in ethical guideline development and implementation.

Guidelines

When planning research in developing countries, there are now many regulations and ethics guidelines for researchers to consult.[38] Those available include international guidelines and conventions, directives, national laws or guidelines, regulations and guidelines for research sponsored by the pharmaceutical industry, guidelines produced by funding agencies, institutional guidelines, and guidelines relating to a specific disease.[1] These sources highlight the groups of stakeholders involved, which include lawyers, sponsors, researchers, civil servants, insurance brokers, study subjects, and communities.

Every researcher is responsible for understanding the research process and what is required to create, undertake, manage, and disseminate information to those people who can benefit from the research findings. Guidelines and regulations do not provide a simple rational basis for decision making, but highlight the complexity and difficulty of ethical decision making. For example, the executive summary from the Nuffield Council on Bioethics meeting on research in developing countries in 2004 indicates how difficult it was for the committee involved to apply the ethics guidelines:

Delegates emphasised that applying guidance in practice is often fraught with difficulty. When the different guidelines are compared, they are markedly inconsistent in some areas. For example, the guidelines vary with regard to the scope and level of detail of information to be provided in the consent process, the obligation to provide a universal standard of care to control groups, the use of placebos, and the extent to which research participants are owed access to successful therapeutics after research is complete. There is also variation with the degree of involvement of the host country in the review process.[1]

Guidelines need to be interpreted and specified for each research context, and the role and the integrity of the researcher is key in the process. Each researcher needs to ensure, on a minimal level, that the formalities required are completed in the host country as well as in the collaborating overseas country. Researchers need to ask themselves constantly whether they believe the research maneuver being employed is ethical. Regulations and guidelines will provide assistance in this iterative process, but the decision making ultimately is every party's responsibility. Although research ethics are important in every context, they become particularly crucial when the balance of power between the researcher and the researched is skewed to the extent that we see in international research undertaken in low-income countries. The next section discusses this.

Ethical Issues in International Research
in Low-income Countries

This section identifies and presents some key ethical issues that arise in international research. The controversy over the role of the drug Tenofovir in the prevention of HIV provides a story, which illustrates some of the current controversies inherent in international health research projects. It highlights the centrality of power dynamics within the milieu of different stakeholders and interests that come together in research collaborations that link rich with poor.

On Wednesday February 23, 2005 Andrew Jack of the *Financial Times* wrote: "Testing Tenofovir on Cameroon prostitutes has landed researchers in a storm of criticism...." The aim of the trial was to test whether Tenofovir could be used to stop AIDS infection. Such findings could revolutionize AIDS prevention. But attacks on the Cameroon study—and on similar research in half a dozen more countries—have raised broader issues about the economics and ethics of clinical trials in developing countries while the main beneficiaries are often in richer countries.[39]

Tenofovir is a powerful antiretroviral (ARV) drug (marketed by Gilead) and approved for human use in 2001. A number of human studies were planned to investigate the drug for pre-exposure prophylaxis against HIV infection (PREP). The countries involved included Botswana, Cambodia, Cameroon, Ghana, Malawi, Nigeria, Thailand, and the United States. The study was funded by the U.S. National Institutes of Health and the Gates Foundation, and planned to recruit 1000 sex workers to the trial. The trial was suspended in February 2005 because of Cameroon Government concerns about the future support of trial participants, particularly if they were infected with HIV during the trial.

Nongovernment organizations (NGOs) were also involved in the debate, and a representative from Médecins sans Frontiéres (MSF) reportedly said: "Our concern is that these women who become infected receive adequate treatment. They must be guaranteed treatment by the trials sponsors."[39] Following the suspension of the trial, the Global Campaign for Microbicides and the AIDS Vaccines Advocacy Coalition (AVAC) made its own statement: "Recently clinical trials have been launched in Africa, Asia and the United States to explore the potential use of oral Tenofovir as a 'once a day' pill to prevent HIV in uninfected individuals—an intervention known as pre-exposure prophylaxis (PREP). Yet concerns from a few activists opposed to these efforts have resulted in government decisions to halt the trial in Cambodia and the Cameroon." [40]

The statement from AVAC later invokes assorted beliefs, assumptions, and ethical imperatives. In a list of five points, AVAC states that the HIV pandemic is creating an urgent demand for safe and effective tools to treat HIV infection and to stop transmission; that this can only be achieved through responsible credible scientific studies; that the rights of vulnerable populations need to be protected; that communities need to be involved in the conceptualization and implementation of scientific studies; that rights of trial subjects need to be respected and that "they should be admired for their contribution to helping others." Finally the AVAC statement indicated that researchers, and the organizations for whom they work, need to be held accountable for their studies. [40]

The Tenofovir story demonstrates the different perspectives of the stakeholders involved (study subjects, research groups, NGOs, advocacy groups, governments, international agencies) and the overall complexity of the international research context. The use of ethics debate in international research collaborations provides a tool for presenting different positions, for debating particular research processes, while at the same time engaging with the individuals and groups involved in the research.

What are the general themes we can derive from the Tenofovir story? They include: social and cultural issues; priority-setting and equity; consent; ethical review of research; and standards of care. Each of these is discussed in turn in the following subsections.

Social and Cultural Issues

By the nature of much work in international health, many researchers move across cultures. A society is made up of all the skills, feelings, values, and beliefs that are learned, shared, and taught by its members from one generation to the next. [41] This applies to the local culture of the population to be studied but also to the culture of the research team and of the sponsoring agency or national government. Researchers need to be asking themselves the following kinds of questions: How much consideration has there been in the process of developing a protocol on social and cultural issues within the particular countries involved? Whose perspectives have been respected and considered unimportant? Whose perspective has ultimately been felt to be most important? Which group has funded the project, and for whom is the work to be conducted?

Crossing social and cultural boundaries challenges our norms, lifestyles, and ways of seeing the world. A globalized world requires us to come to grips with the huge disparities between the rich and poor. This is an important theme within all international health research.[4] Is scientific research the most appropriate way to address the health problems in a particular country? In the north we often (though not always) think it is, and if we have collaborators in the south, then they also may think that it is an appropriate approach. At the same time, they may have different processes and methods for conducting the work, which may include different priorities.[26]

Priority and Equity

Research in developing countries should be responsive to the health needs and the priorities of the community in which it is to be carried out.[6] Ninety percent of all medical research conducted is on those diseases that cause ten percent of the global burden of disease.[4,42] Our task as researchers is to ally ourselves with approaches that help reduce these inequities because a reduction of inequity produces better health.[4,43] Health related research needs to be allied to each country's health priorities. International organizations such as the United Nations (UN), the World Health Organization (WHO), and the World Bank identify international health priorities. Currently the focus is on the Millennium Development Goals (MDGs) and the reduction of poverty,[44] but each country and each research group creates its own priorities within these goals and tries to ensure that the goals themselves do not impede creative work.

Although we can speak meaningfully of setting priorities internationally, international priorities cannot and should not be the same for each country. Each country has its own unique context, its own unique identity, and ways of working. Health priorities are ultimately created in each country through the government and its relationships with international organizations and other stakeholders. However, international research groups also influence decision making within countries. The researcher should be asking how these priorities are created and who influences these decisions.

Consent

Research subjects need to understand and give consent to participation in research studies, as is discussed by Jeffrey Kahn and Anna Mastroianni in Chapter 4. This is affected by social and cultural issues.[34,45] Guidance from the different bodies agrees that each research participant must be adequately informed about the "nature, significance, implications and risks associated with a research trial," and that in the majority of cases, informed consent should be sought from each potential research participant. Some guidelines stress the importance of respecting cultural beliefs and norms, which means that in certain situations community consent may be appropriate, though it is important not to assume that individual consent is thereby not required.[8] The default position should always be individual-subject consent.

International guidelines published by the Council for International Organisations of Medical Sciences (CIOMS) 2002, World Medical Association (WMA) 2000, Council of Europe (CoE) 2004, European Union (EU) 2001, European Group on Ethics in Science and New Technologies (EGE) 2003, and Nuffield Council on Bioethics (NCOB) 2002 all address the issue of consent in international research. The areas they cover include who should give consent, how it should be recorded, provision of information, inducements, and concepts of "genuine consent."[1] These documents supply a significant body of good advice, though it cannot always be taken as authoritative for epidemiology.

The degree of detail of information required varies between the guidelines and indicates the increasing bureaucracy around international trials. For example, the Helsinki Declaration of 2000 states that each potential subject must be adequately informed about "the aim of the study and methods to be used, the sources of funding and possible conflicts of interest, the institutional affiliations of the researchers; the anticipated benefits and potential risks and the follow-up of the study, the discomfort it might entail, and the right to abstain from taking part in the study, or to withdraw from it at any time without any reprisals."[7] As consent becomes an increasingly bureaucratic process, there is a potential to completely miss the point of consent, which is the creation of relationship and understanding.

Ethical Review of Research

If countries want to be involved in the funds that come through international research collaborations they must have functioning RECs. For those of us living in wealthy industrialized countries, it is important to remember the long historical process that led to the creation of ethics committees in North America and Europe, as discussed by Robert Levine in Chapter 12. RECs have huge responsibilities that are often compromised of their ability to act due to competing interests. As Figure 11.1 shows, ethical decision making involves different tensions that include power equalization, reflection on ethics, reconciliation between personal interest and values, and democratic dialogue.[13,46] An inappropriate balance in any of these areas will lead to poor decision making and unethical research. It is also clear that local and national RECs are being increasingly directed by outside influences, including international regulations as well as international research collaborations.[47] There is a need to keep this process under review and not to assume that ethics committees are able to do the job they were established to perform. Sometimes, the process or structure of the committee needs to change, and there have been suggestions that regular audit may be needed.[36,37]

International guidelines help to clarify the role of RECs. For example, the Helsinki Declaration and the International Guidelines for Biomedical Research (CIOMS) have established that RECs exist to ensure that proposed research will not expose participants to unacceptable risks and practices. Also, they must ensure

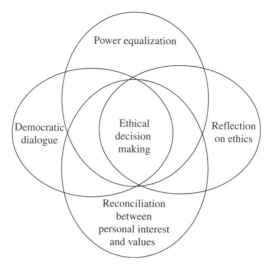

Figure 11–1. Tensions in ethical decision making.[13,46]

that the potential participants can evaluate the expected consequences of their involvement and decide for themselves whether to participate.[6,7,36] These guidelines state that a REC should operate inside a defined framework that includes "membership and size of committee, working rules, and ethical, legal and regulatory requirements for research on human subjects in the country where it is situated as well as applicable international requirements."[6,7] International guidelines stress the importance of the review of scientific research,[1] but some countries have no established system for review, rendering the maintenance of an ethical review process expensive. There is currently a lack of information in many countries about the processes and standards of their ethics committees.[48,49]

The working party from the Nuffield Council on Bioethics recommended that all countries establish an effective system for the ethical review of research that is independent of government and sponsors of research.[8] Adequate provision should be made for training all professionals involved in the ethics of research. This recommendation brings with it a responsibility on the part of industrialized countries to help train ethics committees in poorer countries. It also emphasizes the importance of the independence of impartially constructed committees.

Standards of Care

In the late 1990s the issue of standards of care was highlighted through the publication of clinical trials investigating the prevention of the transmission of HIV from mother to child.[20,21] This issue relates to the treatment that participants in a control group should receive as part of a trial. Some would argue that participants in trials should receive the same standard of care as those people in countries sponsoring the research.[8] But who determines the best standard of care, and which criteria are to be used? In deciding which standard of care is best, the context of the research is critical. As the Nuffield Report indicates "The context of the research in different countries must be critically assessed to establish whether or not it provides a morally relevant reason for offering a different standard of care."[8] In the quest for equality and equity, it is important to realize that people and countries are different and that local socio-political, financial, infrastructural, and cultural circumstances are important.[9] Equality does not mean that people must always be treated identically but that "for every difference in the way men are treated, a reason should be given that is relevant."[8,50]

Guidelines have continued to adapt following the revision of the Helsinki Declaration. The debate has proved productive and led to several new perspectives. In 2002 the Nuffield Council recommended the following: "The minimum standard of care that should be offered is the best intervention available as part of the national public health system."[1]

Externally Sponsored Research

In many cases funding for international research comes from outside a low-income country in which the research is to be carried out. For example, the Tenofovir study was conducted in several different countries and funded by the National Institutes of Health (NIH) and the Gates Foundation. This leads to conflicts and tensions around control of the processes of research. The ethics review process attempts to deal with some of these issues, but each research group and funding agency has a responsibility to ensure that individual research subjects are not compromised in the process. Respect for difference means that sponsoring agencies need to accept and negotiate various possible approaches to the research process.

The Declaration of Helsinki (Clause 13) stresses the importance of ethics review, but does not recognize a special responsibility for ethics review in the host country.[9] In contrast, the Nuffield Council on Bioethics Report of 2002 recommends that externally sponsored research projects be subject to independent ethical review in the sponsor's country in addition to the host country. This ensures that all countries are represented in the research ethics discussions.

Current international guidelines provide differing information and stimulate debate without providing a solution to various conflicting approaches. A main point of disagreement in the guidelines and regulations concerns the degree of involvement of the host country in the review process. The CIOMS guidelines call for representation from host countries, whereas the Council of Europe requires ethical review by an independent ethics committee "in each State in which any research activity is to take place" (CoE 2004 Article 9).

There is little information available on how these processes actually work. The Nuffield Guidelines are useful in providing scenarios to help the reader address the issues in particular contexts, but more work is needed to support the research and better understand the differing processes.

What Happens When the Research Is Over?

"Wherever possible, the results of trials where the interventions prove to be effective must be translated to improve health care for communities in which they were undertaken."[1] It is no longer appropriate to conduct research in a particular setting and then simply leave with the data. The process of conducting ethical research is about the creation of relationships with each of the stakeholders involved including study subjects and communities. At the completion of the study there needs to be a clear understanding of how the community involved will benefit from the research conducted. For example, in the case of Tenofovir,[39] important questions include: Will the community receive the drug if it is found to be efficacious? Will the placebo group receive the intervention and for how long? Who should pay for and supply the treatment or intervention?

As part of the preparation of the protocol there needs to be close collaboration between the researcher and the stakeholders, particularly with the communities that are receiving the intervention. These discussions need to be linked to national health priorities and the local priorities of those communities. The research needs to be seen as part of a larger public health agenda for improving the health of the population. A critical part of the engagement must include a precise understanding of investigator responsibility once the research is finished. Consideration of what happens when the research is over is not limited to provision of drugs or other interventions after the study has ceased. Thought must be given to the impact of the research on issues of equity of health-care provision and ongoing issues of capacity building and the training and support of staff.

Conclusions

When crossing international borders and boundaries it is important to understand that particular ways of thinking are not present in all countries. Each context, like each individual, is unique. If we are from a developed country, we may be projecting our values onto countries that may have different beliefs and values. In international health research, guidelines and declarations provide us with some information, but each researcher and each institution sponsoring research needs to reflect morally on the often conflicting advice in order to find his or her own way through the plethora of codes, guidelines, and recommendations. The whole process of research, from the idea of the study, through the development of the protocol, discussions with stakeholders, ethics committees, funding activities, the research itself, and the results and the dissemination are all points of reflection for each researcher. Each of us needs to be satisfied that our contribution, the contribution of our team of researchers, and ultimately the impact of the work on the communities involved can be morally justified. The Nuffield Council highlights four principles to use when considering research work related to health care in developing countries: (1) the duty to alleviate suffering; (2) the duty to show respect for persons; (3) the duty to be sensitive to cultural differences; and (4) the duty not to exploit the vulnerable.[8]

Benatar and Singer[4] also suggest a list of requirements to consider for making moral progress in international health research. These include educating researchers and members of RECs about research ethics; ensuring that international researchers understand and are sensitive to the social, economic, and political milieu that frames the context in which their research is taking place; involving members of the host country in the design and conduct of the trial; ensuring that trials are of direct relevance to the health needs of the host country and that the balance of benefits and burdens of the project are fairly distributed; conducting prior evaluation by a local committee or governing body of whether the study findings can, and will, be incorporated into the local health-care system; providing subjects with care or treatment they would not ordinarily get in the country where the trial is carried out; ensuring existing disparities are not more deeply entrenched by inappropriate deflection of local human or material resources away from the health-care system in the host country toward the research project; and ensuring that research produces benefits for the practice setting and builds the capacity of health-care professionals in the host country.

These requirements stress the importance of connecting with the values that underpin local communities, which are often far from obvious. The roots of communities are essential to understand in the creation of a morally appropriate relationship. We need to respect differences and find a way of actively encouraging dialogue, group discussion, and ultimately translation of information. If we are unable to listen, learn, translate, and respect, we will fail to be ethical researchers. We should go beyond our current research ethics approach. As Benatar and Singer note, "There is a need to go beyond the reactive research ethics of the past. A new, proactive research ethic must be concerned with the greatest ethical challenge – the huge inequities in global health."[4]

In this chapter we have explored the ethical issues that arise in the course of undertaking epidemiological and international health research. At the outset we explained that it was not our intention to provide another set of ethics guidelines or benchmarks for researchers. Already, a number of such documents exist, and we have signposted the reader toward these, as well as outlining milestones in the historical development of key guidelines.

The chapter has instead focused on ethical issues that the researcher inevitably has to grapple with during the conduct of research. These include how to plan and develop international research, the value systems of different cultures and countries, particular issues in low-income countries such as those around priority-setting, equity, and consent, external sponsorship and ethical review of research, and what happens when the research is over.

Most significantly, however, we have tried to convey that, although following guidelines and adhering to the law are both important, what is perhaps critical is that the researcher approaches the research with an open mind and willing heart. There is no replacement whatsoever for thoughtfulness, sensitivity, and treating people with respect and dignity.

References

1. Nuffield Council on Bioethics. *The Ethics of Research Related to Healthcare in Developing Countries — A Follow Up Discussion Paper.* London: Nuffield Council on Bioethics, 2005.

2. Parker, M. and Harper, A. "The Anthropology of Public Health," *Journal of Biosocial Science* 38 (2006): 1–5.

3. Hurrell, A. and Woods, N. "Globalisation and Inequality," *Millennium Journal of International Studies* 24 (1995): 3.

4. Benatar, S. R. and Singer, P. A. "A New Look at International Research Ethics," *British Medical Journal* 321 (2000): 824–26.

5. Ogden, J. and Porter, J. D. H. "The Politics of Partnership in Tropical Public Health: Researching Tuberculosis Control in India," *Social Policy and Administration* 34 (2000): 377–91.

6. CIOMS. *International Ethical Guidelines for Biomedical Research Involving Human Subjects.* Geneva, Switzerland: Council for International Organisations of Medical Science (CIOMS), 1993.

7. "Helsinki Declaration. Revising the Declaration — A Fresh Start," *Bulletin of Medical Ethics.* ABS Print Services 1999 and World Medical Association, Declaration of Helsinki 1, June 1964. Available at http:www.augsburg.edu/irb/helsinki/html accessed June 2006.

8. Nuffield Council on Bioethics. *The Ethics of Research Related to Healthcare in Developing Countries.* London: Nuffield Council on Bioethics, 2002.

9. Tolman, S. M. "What are the Effects of the Fifth Revision of the Declaration of Helsinki? Fair Partnerships Support Ethical Research," *British Medical Journal* 323 (2001): 1417–19.

10. Percival, T. *Medical Ethics or a Code of Institutes and Precepts Adapted to the Professional Conduct of Physicians and Surgeons.* Manchester: Johnson, J., Bickerstaff, R., 1803.

11. Jonsen, A. R. *A Short History of Medical Ethics.* New York: Oxford University Press, 2000.

12. Engelhardt, H. T. "The Philosophy of Medicine and Bioethics: An Introduction to the Framing of a Field." In *The Philosophy of Medicine,* ed. H. T. Engelhardt. London: Kluwer Academic Publishers 2000: 1–15.

13. Valdez-Martinez, E. *Medical Research Committees in Mexico: Their Role in the Ethics of Scientific Research.* DrPH thesis. London School of Hygiene and Tropical Medicine. Faculty of Medicine, London University, 2004.

14. American Medical Association. *History of AMA Ethics, 1847-1999.* Chicago: AMA, 2006. Available at http://www.ama-assn.org/ama/pub/category/1931.html. Accessed June 2006).

15. Baker, R. B., Caplan, A. L., Emmanuel, L. L., Latham, S. R.. *The American Medical Ethics Revolution.* Baltimore: Johns Hopkins University Press, 1999.

16. Alexander, L. "Medical Science under Dictatorship," *New England Journal of Medicine* 241 (1949): 39–47.

17. "Nuremberg Code," *Journal of the American Medical Association* 276 (1996): 1691.

18. The National Commission for the Protection of Human Subjects of Biomedical and Behavioral Research. *The Belmont Report. Ethical Principles and Guidelines for the Protection of Human Subjects of Research.* Washington, DC: U.S. Government Printing Office, 1978.

19. CIOMS. *International Ethical Guidelines for Ethical Review of Epidemiological Studies.* Geneva, Switzerland: Council for International Organisations of Medical Science (CIOMS), 1991.

20. Lurie, P. and Wolfe, S. M. "Unethical Trials of Interventions to Reduce Peri-natal Transmission of the Human Immunodeficiency Virus in Developing Countries," *New England Journal of Medicine* 337 (1997): 853–56.

21. Angell, M. "The Ethics of Clinical Research in the Third World," *New England Journal of Medicine* 337 (1997): 847–49.

22. Institute of Medicine. *Future of Public Health.* Washington, DC: National Academy Press, 1988: 1–7.

23. Last, J. M. *Dictionary of Epidemiology.* Oxford: Oxford University Press, 1988: 42.

24. Parks, K. *Textbook of Preventive and Social Medicine.* Jabalpur, India: Banarsidas Bhanot Publishers, 1997.

25. Beaglehole, R. and Bonita, R. *Public Health at the Cross Roads: Achievements and Prospects.* Cambridge: Cambridge University Press, 1997.

26. Wing, S. "Whose Epidemiology, Whose Health?" *International Journal of Health Services* 28 (1998): 241–52.

27. Brown, P. "Popular Epidemiology and Toxic Waste Contamination: Lay and Professional Ways of Knowing," *Journal of Health and Social Behavior* 33 (1992): 267–81.

28. Watterson, A. "Whither Lay Epidemiology in UK Public Health Policy and Practice? Some Reflections on Occupational and Environmental Health Opportunities," *Journal of Public Health Medicine* 16 (1994): 270–74.

29. Matsunaga, D. S., Enos, R., Gotay, C. C., Banner, R. O., DeCambra, H., Hammond, O.W., et al. "Participatory Research in a Native Hawaiian Community: The Wai'anae Cancer Research Project," *Cancer* 78 (1996): 1582–86.

30. San Sebastian, M. and Hurtig, A. K. "Oil Development and Health in the Amazon Basin of Ecuador: the Popular Epidemiology Process," *Social Science & Medicine* 60 (2005): 799–807.

31. Smith, P. G. and Morrow R. H. *Methods for Field Trials of Interventions against Tropical Diseases: A Toolbox.* Oxford: Oxford University Press, 1991.

32. Fairhead, J., Leach, M., and Small, M. "Public Engagement with Science? Local Understandings of a Vaccine Trial in the Gambia," *Journal of Biosocial Science* 38 (2006): 103–16.

33. Molyneux, C. S., Wassenaar, D., and Marsh, K. "Even if They Ask You to Stand by a Tree All Day, You Will Have to Do It (laughter)!" *Social Science & Medicine* 61 (2005): 443–54.

34. Molyneux, C. S., Mutemi, W., and Marsh, K. "Trust and Informed Consent: Insights from Community Members on the Kenyan coast," *Social Science and Medicine* 61 (2005): 1463–73.

35. Geissler, P. W. "Kachinja Are Coming! Encounters around a Medical Research Project in a Kenyan Village," *Africa* 75 (2005): 173–202.

36. Valdez-Martinez, E., Garduno-Espinosa, J., Porter, J. D. H. "Understanding the Structure and Practices of Research Ethics Committees through Research and Audit: A Study from Mexico," *Health Policy* 74 (2005): 56–68.

37. Valdez-Martinez, E., Turnbull, B., Garduno-Espinosa, J., Porter, J. D. H.. "Descriptive Ethics: A Qualitative Study of Local Research Ethics Committees in Mexico," *Developing World Bioethics* 6 (2006): 96–105.

38. Eckstein, S. *Manual for Research Ethics Committees*. Cambridge: Cambridge University Press, 2003.

39. Jack, A. "Testing of Tenofovir on Cameroon Prostitutes Has Landed Researchers in a Storm of Criticism." *Financial Times*, London. Wednesday, February 23, 2005: 15.

40. AIDS Vaccine Advocacy Coalition (AVAC). A Public Statement from the Global Campaign for Microbicides and the AIDS Vaccines Advocacy Coalition on the Impact of Stopping PREP Trials in Cambodia and Cameroon. February 18, 2005. Available at http://www.avac.org/ accessed May 2005.

41. Lonergan, B. *Understanding Being: An Introduction and Companion to Insight*. New York: Edwin Mellen Press, 1987.

42. Commission on Health Research for Development. *Health Research: Essential Link to Equity in Development*. Oxford: Oxford University Press, 1990.

43. Pronyk, P. and Porter, J. D. H. "Public Health and Human Rights." In *Tuberculosis — An Interdisciplinary Perspective*, ed. J. D. H. Porter and J. M. Grange. London: Imperial College Press, 1999.

44. United Nations Millennium Development Goals. Available at www.un.org/ millenniumgoals/, accessed April 2006.

45. Leach, A., Hilton, S., Greenwood, B. M., Manneh, E., Dibba, B., Wilkins, A., et al. "An Evaluation of the Informed Consent Procedure Used During a Trial of Haemophilus Influenzae Type B Conjugate Vaccine Undertaken in the Gambia, West Africa," *Social Science & Medicine* 48 (1999): 139–48.

46. Prilleltensky, I. "Applied Ethics in Mental Health in Cuba: Part 11 — Power Differentials, Dilemmas, Resources, and Limitations," *Ethics and Behavior* 12 (2002): 243–60.

47. Lavery, J. V. "A Culture of Ethical Conduct in Research: The Proper Goal of Capacity Building in International Research Ethics." In: *Macroeconomics and Health: Investing in Health for Economic Development*. Report of the Commission on Macroeconomics and Health. Geneva: World Health Organization, 2001.

48. Hyder, A. A., Wali, S. A., Khan, A.N., Teok, N. B., Kass, N. E., Dawson, L. "Ethical Review of Health Research: A Perspective from Developing Country Researchers," *Journal of Medical Ethics* 30 (2004): 68–72.

49. Gambia Government, Medical Research Council Joint Ethical Committee. "Ethical Issues Facing Medical Research in Developing Countries," *Lancet* 351 (1998): 286–87.

50. Williams, B. "The Idea of Equality." In his *Problems of the Self*. New York: Cambridge University Press, 1973.

IV

THE REGULATORY CONTEXT AND PROFESSIONAL EDUCATION

12

The Institutional Review Board

ROBERT J. LEVINE

This chapter describes the committees that have the responsibility to review proposals to conduct research involving humans as subjects to determine whether they include adequate safeguards of the rights and welfare of the research subjects. These committees, generally called institutional review boards (IRBs), but sometimes called by other names (e.g., ethical review committees) now exist in many locales in most countries. National regulations in an increasing number of countries and the leading international codes of research ethics establish the requirement that research involving humans as subjects, with few exceptions, may not be carried out without review and approval of these committees; hence their importance to epidemiologists. This article presents a detailed introduction to the history, composition, organizational settings and purposes of these committees and major themes in contemporary controversies about them.

In 1975, the Tokyo revision of the Declaration of Helsinki[1] established as the international standard for biomedical research involving human subjects the requirement that "each experimental procedure involving human subjects should be clearly formulated in an experimental protocol which should be transmitted for consideration, comment and guidance to a specially appointed committee independent of the investigator and sponsor" (Article I.2). In the United States, federal law assigns to these committees the name Institutional Review Board (IRB) and the authority and responsibility to approve or disapprove proposals to conduct research involving human subjects.[2,3] In Canada, Research Ethics Boards have similar authority to approve or disapprove research proposals, not merely to offer "consideration, comment and guidance."[4] In most of the world such committees were, until recently, called Research Ethics Committees; many are now changing their names to IRBs.

The Council for International Organizations of Medical Sciences (CIOMS), in its *International Ethical Guidelines for Biomedical Research Involving Human Subjects*, assigns to the research ethics committee the authority and responsibility for review and approval of research proposals before their initiation.[5] In the *International Guidelines for Ethical Review of Epidemiological Studies*, CIOMS extends the requirement for committee review and approval to research in the field of epidemiology.[6] The Declaration of Helsinki, in its most recent revision (2000), states that committee approval should be sought, but only "when appropriate."[7]

History

The Nuremberg Code (1949) and the original Declaration of Helsinki (1964) made no mention of committee review. These documents placed on the investigator all responsibility for safeguarding the rights and welfare of research subjects. The first mention of committee review in an international document was in the Tokyo revision of the Declaration of Helsinki (1975). The first international document to require review *and approval* by an independent committee was the *Proposed International Guidelines for Biomedical Research Involving Human Subjects*, promulgated by CIOMS in 1982.[8] It is worth noticing that the CIOMS document states that its purpose is to indicate how the ethical principles embodied in the Declaration of Helsinki can be effectively applied, particularly in developing countries. This point notwithstanding, it goes beyond Helsinki in several substantive respects including the requirement for committee approval.

In the United States, the first federal document requiring committee review was issued November 17, 1953. Entitled "Group Consideration for Clinical Research Procedures Deviating from Accepted Medical Practice or Involving Unusual Hazard," its guidelines applied only to research conducted at the newly opened Clinical Center at the National Institutes of Health (NIH).[9] Little is known about peer review in other institutions in the 1950s other than that it existed at least in some medical schools. In 1961 and again in 1962, questionnaires were sent to American university departments of medicine. Approximately one-third of those responding reported that they had committees and one-quarter either had or were developing procedural documents.[10]

On February 8, 1966, the Surgeon General of the United States Public Health Service (USPHS) issued the first federal policy statement requiring research institutions to establish the committees that subsequently came to be known as IRBs.[10] This policy required recipients of USPHS grants in support of research involving human subjects to specify that "the grantee institution will provide prior review of the judgment of the principal investigator or program director by a committee of his institutional associates. This review shall assure an independent determination: (1) Of the rights and welfare of the... individuals involved, (2) Of the appropriateness of the methods used to secure informed consent, and (3) Of the risks and potential medical benefits of the investigation."

The evolution of the federal government's charges to the committee and of its recognition of the need for diversity of its membership were reflected in several revisions of its policy between 1966 and 1969;[2,11] these are discussed subsequently.

The Purpose of the IRB

The purpose of the IRB is to assure that research involving human subjects is designed to conform to relevant ethical standards. Historically, the IRB's primary focus has been on safeguarding the rights and welfare of individual research subjects, concentrating on the plans for informed consent and the assessment of risks and anticipated benefits. In 1978, the National Commission for the Protection of Human Subjects of Biomedical and Behavioral Research (National Commission) added a requirement that the IRB assure equitableness in the selection of research subjects.[2] The National Commission was concerned primarily with protecting vulnerable subjects from involvement in unjustifiably risky research and from bearing a disproportionately large share of the burdens of research. Subsequently, as participation in some types of research became widely perceived as a benefit, IRBs also assumed responsibility for assuring disadvantaged persons' equitable access to such benefits.[12,13]

The authority and responsibility of the IRB is limited to review and approval of research involving human subjects. The IRB's domain is customarily identified by defining "research" and distinguishing it from other seemingly similar activities that are outside its province. The following definitions are provided by the National Commission in its *Belmont Report*:[14]

For the most part, the term "practice" refers to interventions that are designed solely to enhance the well-being of an individual patient or client and that have a reasonable expectation of success. The purpose of medical or behavioral practice is to provide diagnosis, preventive treatment or therapy to particular individuals. By contrast, the term "research" designates an activity designed to test an hypothesis, permit conclusions to be drawn, and thereby to develop or contribute to generalizable knowledge (expressed, for example, in theories, principles, and statements of relationships). Research is usually described in a formal protocol that sets forth an objective and a set of procedures designed to reach that objective.

Although the IRB has neither the responsibility nor the authority to review activities that conform to the definition of "practice," it often is properly called upon to review research designed to evaluate the safety and efficacy of various "practices" including diagnostic, therapeutic and preventive modalities. Because the activities of some epidemiologists and public health professionals (e.g., emergency responses, outbreak investigations, surveillance) involve methods characteristic of scientific research, they may be difficult to classify as either "research," "program evaluation," or "practice." Consequently, disputes arise over which professional activities should be reviewed by IRBs. Definitions of the terms "research," "practice," and "human subject" as well as the regulatory implications of such definitions have been debated extensively.[2,15]

According to CIOMS International Guidelines for Ethical Review of Epidemiological Studies,[6]

It may at times be difficult to decide whether a particular proposal is for an epidemiological study or for evaluation of a programme on the part of a health-care institution or department. The defining attribute of research is that it is designed to produce new, generalizable knowledge as distinct from knowledge pertaining only to a particular individual or programme.

For instance, a governmental or hospital department may want to examine patients' records to determine the safety and efficacy of a facility, unit or procedure. If the examination is for research purposes, the proposal should be submitted to [an IRB]. However, if it is for the purpose of programme evaluation... the proposal may not need to be submitted to ethical review; on the contrary, it could be considered poor practice and unethical not to undertake this type of quality assurance....

If it is not clear whether a proposal involves epidemiological study or routine practice, it should be submitted to the [IRB] responsible for epidemiological protocols for its opinion on whether the proposal falls within its mandate.

Epidemiologists and members of IRBs that review their research activities should also be aware of the Ethical Guidelines of the American College of Epidemiology.[16]

A source of continuing controversy is whether the IRB has an obligation to approve, disapprove or require revision of the *scientific* design of research protocols for reasons other than those of ethical flaws.[2] Those who argue that they do or should have such an obligation point out that each of the leading international codes for research involving human subjects establishes an ethical requirement for good scientific design. As noted in the CIOMS *International Ethical Guidelines*, "scientifically unsound research involving humans as subjects is *ipso facto* unethical." Moreover, they argue that the IRB's obligation to determine that risks to subjects are reasonable in relation to anticipated benefits necessarily relies on a prior determination that the scientific design is adequate, for if it is not, there will be no benefits and any risk must be considered unreasonable.

Opponents to assigning such an obligation to the IRB, while conceding these two points, argue that the typical IRB is not designed to make expert judgments about the scientific merits of research proposals. Such judgments require evaluation of two different features of the protocol—value and validity.[17] Evaluation of the value entails an appraisal of what the Principle 6 of the Nuremberg Code calls "the humanitarian importance of the problem to be solved." Some commentators, myself included, believe that the properly constructed IRB has the capacity and authority to make reasonably reliable assessments of scientific value in this sense. However, others point to the numerical dominance on most IRBs by scientists and health professionals, suggesting that such persons value things differently than does the majority of the population. Almost certainly, for example, health professionals and scientists typically place a higher value on the pursuit of knowledge for its own sake than do persons outside the health professions or academia.

Moreover, most IRBs do not have the competence to provide more than a superficial assessment of the validity of the scientific methods or the results. In most cases, scientists in the institution who are most qualified to evaluate the scientific validity of a research plan are the investigators who have proposed the research. Federal regulations require that they be excluded from the IRB's discussion of their own protocol even if they are members of the IRB. In general, responsibility for assessment of scientific validity is and ought to be delegated to committees designed to have such competence—for example, scientific review committees either within the institution or at funding agencies such as the National Institutes of Health.[2]

According to the CIOMS *International Ethical Guidelines*, the basic responsibilities of the ethical review committee include inter alia "to determine that the proposed research is scientifically sound or to verify that another competent expert body has done so."

Peer Review and the Membership of the IRB

The Surgeon General's 1966 memo called for prior review by "a committee of [the investigator's] associates," commonly called "peer review." In 1968, 73% of committees were limited in membership to immediate peer groups of scientists and physicians.[10] However, on May 1, 1969, USPHS Guidelines were revised to indicate that a committee constituted exclusively of biomedical scientists would be inadequate to perform the functions now expected of such a committee: "The membership should possess ... competencies necessary in the judgment as to the acceptability of the research in terms of institutional regulations, relevant law, standards of professional practice and community acceptance."

Regulations of the U.S. Department of Health and Human Services (DHHS), first promulgated in 1974 and since revised several times, maintain the spirit of the 1969 policy and in addition require gender diversity. They also require at least one nonscientist (e.g., lawyer, ethicist, member of the clergy) and at least one member who is not otherwise affiliated with the institution (commonly, but incorrectly, called a "community representative"). Persons having conflicting interests are to be excluded; this concern for independence from the sponsor and investigators is also reflected in both the Declaration of Helsinki and CIOMS.

International Ethical Guidelines

According to Robert Veatch, the IRB is an intermediate case between two models of the review committee:[11] The "interdisciplinary professional review model," made up of diverse professionals such as doctors, lawyers, scientists, and clergy, brings professional expertise to the review process, while the "jury model... reflects the common sense of the reasonable person." In the jury model "expertise relevant to the case at hand is not only not necessary, it often disqualifies one from serving on the jury." Veatch concedes that in order to perform all of its functions the IRB requires both professional and jury skills. However, he argues that the presence of professionals makes it more difficult for the IRB to be responsive to the informational needs of the reasonable person or to be adept at anticipating community acceptance. John Robertson[18] would correct the "structural bias" of professional domination by introducing a "subject surrogate," an expert advocate for the subjects' interests. According to federal regulations, "If an IRB regularly reviews research that involves a vulnerable category of subjects,...consideration shall be given to the inclusion of one or more individuals who are knowledgeable about and experienced in working with these subjects" (45 CFR 46.107a). For research involving prisoners, for example, regulations require that at least one member of the IRB be either a prisoner or a prisoner representative. There is unresolved controversy over whether persons with AIDS should be appointed to membership on all IRBs that review research in the field of HIV infection.[19]

If representatives of the various populations of prospective research subjects were to be added to the IRB, the committee would become much too large to be an effective deliberative body. In the typical university hospital, it would be necessary to include patients with cancer, heart disease, diabetes, strokes and hypertension, to name just a few categories of diseases having a far greater incidence and prevalence than HIV infection. Moreover, if it were decided to include as a committee member a person with HIV infection, should this person be a gay white male, a user of illicit intravenous drugs, or a heterosexual sex partner of one, a male or female sex worker, a person with hemophilia, or a representative of any of the other subsets of the population with HIV infection? Members of each of these subsets may have vastly different perspectives on matters relevant to the design and conduct of research.

IRBs must have access to accurate information about the various populations of prospective research subjects of potential interest to their institutions. Gaining such access, which is essential for the IRB to take effective action, may be accomplished with the aid of consultants or through such means as community consultation,[2,19] surrogate consultation,[2] establishment of advisory committees,[19] and other means that are discussed elsewhere in this book.

The Institute of Medicine (IOM), citing concerns similar to those expressed by Robertson and Veatch, recommended that each "research organization should...assemble a board with at least 25 percent of its membership not affiliated with the institution, not trained as scientists, and able to represent the local community and/or the [subject] perspective."[20]

Location and Independence of the IRB

In the United States the first IRBs were established in the institutions in which research was conducted. The 1966 Surgeon General's policy statement required a committee of "institutional associates." In 1971 the FDA promulgated regulations that required committee review only when regulated research was conducted in institutions, known as Institutional Review Committees (IRC). Regulations proposed in 1973 by the Department of Health, Education and Welfare, which was the forerunner of the Department of Health and Human Services, also reflected a local setting in their term, Organizational Review Board (ORB). In 1974 the National Research Act established a statutory requirement for review by a committee to which it assigned the name Institutional Review Board (IRB), a compromise between the two names then extant.

IRBs are required to comply with federal regulations when reviewing activities involving FDA-regulated "test articles" such as investigational drugs and devices, and when reviewing research supported by federal funds.[3] Moreover, all institutions that receive federal research grants and contracts are required to file "statements of assurance" of compliance with federal regulations. The names given to assurances have changed over the years. In 1966 the Surgeon General required that each application to secure USPHS funding for research involving human subjects include a statement of assurance of compliance with USPHS policy for the protection of human subjects. Subsequently, policy was changed to permit institutions with multiple grants and contracts to file "general statements of assurance." With time the names of these documents were changed to "single project assurances" and "multiple project assurances." At the time of this writing, all institutions receiving funds from any agency of the federal government must file "federal-wide assurances" to indicate their commitment to comply with the requirements of the "common rule" and the Office for Human Research Protection (OHRP). In these assurances most institutions voluntarily promise to apply the principles of federal regulations to all research they conduct regardless of the source of funding.

These points notwithstanding, each IRB has a decidedly local character. Most have local names such as Human Investigation Committee or Committee for the Protection of Human Subjects. Each is appointed by its own institution and each lends its own interpretation to the requirements of federal regulations. For example, at one university medical students were forbidden to serve as research subjects, whereas at another, involvement of medical students as research subjects was sometimes required as a condition of approval.[2] The National Commission recommended that IRBs be "located in institutions where research...is conducted. Compared to the possible alternatives of a regional or national review...local committees have the advantage of greater familiarity with the actual conditions."[21] The National Commission envisioned the local IRB as an ally of the investigator in safeguarding the rights and welfare of research subjects and a contributor to the education of both the research community and the public.

The FDA's change in regulations in 1981 to require IRB review of all regulated research regardless of where it was done created a problem for the numerous physicians who were conducting investigations in their private offices, many of whom had no ready access to IRBs. In response, private corporations developed "noninstitutional review boards" (NRBs).[22] There are reasons to question the validity of NRB review. For example, they do not (in the words of the National Commission) "have the advantage of familiarity with" local conditions. This point notwithstanding, many of them appear to be performing satisfactorily.[2,23]

In 1986, FDA began to waive the requirement for local IRB review for some protocols designed to evaluate, or to make available for therapeutic purposes, investigational new drugs, particularly those intended for the treatment of patients with HIV infection.[24,25] In such cases IRBs were offered the option of accepting review by a national committee as fulfilling the regulatory requirement for IRB review. Such practices have caused some commentators to question the strength of the government's commitment to the principle of local review.

The purpose of waiving the requirement for local IRB review was to reduce the inevitable delays that arise when many IRBs review a protocol that is to be conducted at multiple sites. Investigators who conduct studies involving several institutions, such as multi-institutional clinical trials and survey research, may encounter formidable bureaucratic problems. Each IRB interprets the regulations differently and imposes requirements for revision of protocols that may be inconsistent. A dramatic example of the problems presented to investigators by such behavior was published by Kavanagh et al.[26] Their proposal to conduct survey and interview research on genetic counseling services in 51 institutions was reviewed by IRBs in each of these institutions. Securing final authorization to proceed with the research took over a year and involved 384 distinct communications between IRBs and the investigators. Of the 51 institutions, 11 decided that IRB review was not required, 28 approved the protocol as submitted, and 12 approved the protocol after requesting one or more modifications. Rothman calculates that the investigator-hours required to secure all the necessary IRB approvals to initiate a large-scale epidemiologic survey may approximate 3% of an epidemiologist's active professional career.[27]

In the light of the inefficiencies associated with review by multiple IRB reviews, in recent years there has been a movement in the United States to encourage the use of central IRBs rather than local IRBs in the review of multi-institutional research protocols.[28] (CRBs is the name now most commonly used for what earlier were called noninstitutional review boards.) The movement toward central IRBs has been spearheaded by oncologists and seems to have achieved tentative acceptance from OHRP.[24,29] It remains to be seen whether this shift to central IRBs will be accepted widely.

Regulation 45 CFR 46.114—as revised in 1981—was designed to reduce the bureaucratic burdens of IRB approval for research involving multiple institutions. In contrast to the 1974 regulations it replaced, it permitted "reliance upon the review of another qualified IRB, or other similar arrangements aimed at avoidance of duplication of effort." The 1991 revision of the regulations added that such arrangements require the "approval of the (federal) department or agency head" (45 CFR 46.114). The effect of the 1991 revision may be an increased bureaucratic burden, particularly if it is interpreted to require approval of the head of the federal agency or department in advance each time one intends to employ an arrangement designed to avoid wasted effort.

Internationally, there is much less concern about the location of the ethical review committees. The CIOMS *International Ethical Guidelines* recognize the validity of review at a regional, or, "in a highly centralized administration," a national level.[5] Regardless of the locale of the committee, CIOMS requires that it "should have among its members or consultants persons who are thoroughly familiar with the customs and traditions of the...community" in which the research is to be carried out.[5] In many European countries, research ethics committees are regional.[30]

Several commentators have expressed concern that in the United States the local institution has too much power in the field of protection of human research subjects. Fore example, Robertson alerts us to "the danger...that research institutions will use [IRBs] to protect themselves and researchers rather than subjects."[18] Others point to the dominance of investigators in IRB membership, the regulatory requirement for "legally effective informed consent," and close associations between IRBs and risk-management offices in many institutions as evidence that IRBs are being used in this manner.

Given the legal climate in the United States, it is definitely in the interests of the institution to safeguard the rights and welfare of research subjects. The IRB should be highly attentive to the interests of institutions and investigators, as well as those of research subjects. Moreover, it is part of the IRB's function to educate investigators and institutional officials that there are good reasons to see that their interests are not at odds with those of the research subjects. Obtaining legally and ethically valid informed consent is not only responsive to the subject's rights, it also affords the institution and the investigators protection against litigation.

Assuring equitability in the selection of subjects and reasonability in the balance of risks and benefits is not only responsive to the rights and welfare interests of research subjects, it fosters good relations between the institution and the community. What institution wants to see a story in the local newspaper that compares its research activities to the Tuskegee Syphilis Studies? When IRBs are functioning at their best, they harmonize the interests of the institution, the investigators and the subjects to the extent that there is little or no conflict.

Multinational Research

Epidemiologists often conduct research in countries other than their own. Of particular concern are research protocols designed by investigators and sponsors in wealthy industrialized countries and then carried out in low-resource countries or communities. What if there are differences in ethical values in the two cultures? In such cases whose ethical standards should be followed? How are review committees in the external sponsoring country to know what kind of information is considered private in the host country or what kinds of material inducements would be considered undue inducements? There is an extensive body of literature on the differing perceptions in various cultures of the world on issues such as the nature of personhood, gift exchange traditions, the nature and causation of disease, medical ethics, and other matters pertinent to assessing the ethical propriety of proposals to conduct research involving human subjects. (Interested readers may find their way into this literature by consulting Ohnuki-Tierney,[31] De Craemer,[32] Christakis,[33] Christakis and Levine,[34] Baker,[35] Levine,[36,37] Levine and Gorovitz,[38] and Koenig and Marshall.[39])

At the root of the debates over the legitimacy of differing ethical perspectives and standards across cultures is the age-old tension between ethical universalism and ethical pluralism. Universalists, as I am using this term in this chapter, hold that ethical standards are or ought to be the same in all places and in all times. Variations across cultures indicate that some societies are behind others in the degree of moral perceptiveness or the moral progress they have accomplished.[40] Those who most closely approximate the universalist position in arguing for uniform standards for the conduct of research involving human subjects include Macklin,[35] Lurie and Wolfe,[41] and Angell.[42] Ethical pluralists, by contrast, contend that there are no such universal standards, only moral norms relative to cultures. Since ethics are constructed in the course of debates held in particular societies, they will necessarily reflect the histories and traditions of the particular cultures. They regard variations across cultures in ethical standards as both inevitable and legitimate. Among the leading proponents of ethical pluralism in the development of guidelines for research involving human subjects are Christakis,[33,34] Kleinman,[43] and Koenig and Marshall.[39]

Among the leading international codes of research ethics, The *Nuremberg Code* and the *Declaration of Helsinki* seem to reflect their authors' vision that they are universally applicable.[37] The CIOMS *International Ethical Guidelines* aspire to "global applicability."[37] "Global applicability" means that the authors of the guidelines are satisfied that, to the best of their knowledge, the guidelines are currently applicable in all of the world's nations and cultures. It presupposes that the guidelines will require revision from time to time in order to maintain currency with evolving cultural standards and technological developments.[44] Guidelines that are globally applicable necessarily differ from those that apply to more homogeneous constituencies in that they contain relatively fewer substantive standards and more numerous procedural standards. A substantive standard is one that prescribes (or proscribes) specific actions because they are morally right (or wrong). Procedural standards establish procedures to determine which action would be most ethically acceptable in a specific context, such as the requirement for IRB review. (Another type of procedural standard establishes procedures which facilitate accomplishment of the requirements of a substantive standard; e.g., a consent form is a procedural requirement that facilitates accomplishment of the substantive requirement for informed consent.)

The CIOMS *International Ethical Guidelines* set forth procedures to be followed when research is initiated and financed in one country (the external sponsoring country) and carried out by investigators from the external sponsoring country in another country (the host country) involving as subjects residents of the host country:[5]

Committees in both the country of the sponsor and the host country have responsibility for conducting both scientific and ethical review, as well as the authority to withhold approval of research protocols that fail to meet their...standards....

Committees in the external sponsoring country...have a special responsibility to determine whether the scientific methods are sound and suitable to the aims of the research; whether the drugs, vaccines, devices, or procedures to be studied meet adequate standards of safety; whether there is sound justification for conducting the research in the host country rather than in the country of the external sponsoring agency or in another country; and whether the proposed research is in compliance with the ethical standards of the external sponsoring country.

Committees in the host country have a special responsibility to determine whether the objectives of the research are responsive to the health needs and priorities of that country. The ability to judge the ethical acceptability of various aspects of a research proposal requires a thorough understanding of a community's customs and traditions. The ethical review committee in the host country must have as either members or consultants persons with such understanding; it will then be in a favorable position to determine the acceptability of the proposed means of obtaining informed consent and otherwise respecting the rights of prospective subjects as well as of the means proposed to protect [their] welfare....

[T]he ethical review committees in the two countries may, by agreement, undertake to review different aspects of the research protocol. In short, in respect of host countries either with developed capacity for independent ethical review or in which external sponsors and investigators are contributing substantially to such capacity, ethical review in the external sponsoring country may be limited to ensuring compliance with broadly stated ethical standards. The ethical review committee in the host country can be expected to have greater competence for reviewing the detailed plans for compliance, in view of its better understanding of the cultural and moral values of the population in which it is proposed to conduct the research.

Criticisms of IRBs

Before 1962, "a general skepticism toward the development of ethical guidelines, codes, or sets of procedures concerning the conduct of research" prevailed in the medical research community.[10] In the 1970s several biomedical scientists were harshly critical of the IRB system, claiming that it tended to stifle creativity and impede progress.[2] However, survey research showed that only 25% of biomedical researchers agreed with the statement that: "The review . . . is an unwarranted intrusion on the investigator's autonomy—at least to some extent."[21] Behavioral and social scientists were considerably less accepting of review, claiming that their research activities were less likely than those of the biomedical scientist to harm subjects. Some argued that since they only talked with subjects, review was an unconstitutional constraint on their freedom of speech.[2] As a consequence of such arguments, several classes of research involving human subjects are exempt from coverage by federal regulations. Among such classes of research employed by epidemiologists are (45 CFR 46.101b):

(2) Research involving the use of . . . survey procedures, interview procedures or observation of public behavior unless: (i) Information obtained is recorded in such a manner that human subjects can be identified directly or through identifiers linked to the subjects; and (ii) any disclosure of the human subjects' responses outside the research could reasonably place the subjects at risk of criminal or civil liability or be damaging to the subjects' financial standing, employability, or reputation.

(4) Research involving the collection or study of existing data, documents, records, pathological specimens, or diagnostic specimens, if these sources are publicly available or if the information is recorded by the investigator in such a manner that the subjects cannot be identified, directly or through identifiers linked to the subjects.

OHRP requires that investigators not have the authority to make an independent determination that their research proposal is exempt. Such authority resides with an institutional official who is well acquainted with interpretation of the regulations and the exemptions. Although the specified activities are exempt from coverage by U.S. federal regulations, the investigators who engage in such activities are not exempt from relevant ethical obligations. For example, they may not engage in survey research without first securing the knowledgeable agreements of the respondents. Finally, these exemptions are not recognized by the international codes of research ethics.

In many institutions, review of research protocols in the categories exempted from coverage by the federal regulations is conducted by use of an expedited review procedure (45 CFR 46.110b). Expedited review entails review by "the IRB chairperson or by one or more experienced reviewers designated by the chairperson from among members of the IRB." Apart from review of exempt categories of research, use of expedited review procedures is limited by the regulations to (1) a list published in the *Federal Register* of "categories of research" when they present no more than minimal risk and (2) "minor changes in previously approved research during the period... for which approval is authorized."[45]

According to Peter Williams, IRBs do an inadequate job of assuring that risks will be reasonable in relation to anticipated benefits.[46] He argues that this defect is inevitable for three reasons: (1) Federal regulations on this standard are written in vague language in contrast to the more clear direction provided for protecting subjects' rights. Moreover, since the regulations permit consideration of the long-range effects of applying knowledge as benefits but not as risks, they create a bias in favor of approval. (2) The membership of the committee, dominated as it is by professionals, is likely to place a higher value than laypersons would on the benefit of developing new knowledge. (3) Groups confronted with choices involving risks may be either more or less cautious or "risk aversive" than the average of individuals within the group. This is known as the "risky shift" or "group polarization phenomenon." Williams and Veatch[11] maintain that in the context of IRBs, the groups are likely to be more tolerant of higher levels of risk than they would be as individuals.

Several commentators have proposed that IRBs could enhance their effectiveness by sending members to the sites of the actual conduct of research to verify compliance with protocol requirements or to supervise consent negotiations.[47] Others respond that while such activities should be done when there are reasons to suspect problems in specific protocols, routine monitoring activities might be detrimental to the successful functioning of the committee by eroding its support within the institution.[2]

Evaluation of IRBs

Critics of the IRB system claim that little or no objective evidence exists that IRB review prevents the conduct of inadequate research. A national survey of IRBs revealed that the rate of rejection of protocols is less than one in one thousand.[21] Supporters of the system respond that the actual rejection rate is much higher if one includes protocols withdrawn because investigators refuse to modify them as required by IRBs. Moreover, rejection rates may be a poor indicator of the IRB's quality. Protocols may be improved in anticipation of the IRB's requirements and investigators, who may decide not to submit proposals they think might be rejected by the committee.

It is difficult to evaluate the IRB's performance objectively, and satisfactory subjective evaluations can be made only by experienced IRB members and administrators.[2] Jerry Mashaw concludes in his theoretical analysis of IRBs that "If [the IRB] is to do its core job well, we must live with its inevitable incompetence at other tasks. Moreover, we must also live with the rather vague regulatory standards and with the continuing inability of the federal funding agencies to know for sure whether [IRBs] are functioning effectively. If we would have wise judges and...professionals [who are skilled in protecting subjects' rights and welfare interests], we can neither specifically direct nor objectively evaluate their behavior."[48]

In recent years there has been what I call a crisis in confidence in the IRB system.[49] Among those who are losing confidence that the IRB can accomplish its primary mission of protecting the rights and welfare of human research subjects are the public, researchers, governmental officials, and corporations that develop and distribute health-care related products.[49] The origins of this crisis can be traced to certain activities of governmental agencies, the reporting of these and other activities in media addressed to the public, and the response to these events by the administrators of institutions in which research involving human subjects is carried out.[50]

In October 1998, the Office for Protection from Research Risks began its practice restricting or suspending the multiple project assurances of institutions when it found them in substantial noncompliance with its policies for protection of human research subjects.[51] Such restriction or suspension had the effect of completely shutting down research involving human subjects at these institutions. This practice continued until December 2001. In 1998, the DHHS Office of the Inspector General published a report in which it characterized IRBs as a "system in jeopardy." The primary problem was, in the view of the inspector general, that the IRBs were overwhelmed by an enormous and increasing work load.[52]

The foregoing events were given great visibility in the media addressed to the public. At the same time, the media presented dramatic accounts of several unfortunate outcomes of research including, inter alia, the deaths in celebrated cases of Jesse Gelsinger and other normal volunteer subjects.[50] These reports increased the pressure on officials in the legislative and executive branches of the federal government to take action to remedy these problems.

University administrators, fearful of closure by OPRR or its successor, OHRP, reacted by greatly increasing their attention to meticulous compliance with federal regulations and guidance by regulatory bodies such as OHRP and FDA.

The report of the inspector general was correct in observing that IRBs are overwhelmed by an enormous work load, but because much of this is work that need not be done by the IRB, I have called for empirical research to evaluate the utility of relatively pointless practices. Two that I selected for prompt attention are (1) the conduct of continuing review at convened meetings of the IRB (rather than by expedited review) and (2) review of all adverse event reports by the local IRB (rather than by a central data and safety monitoring board).[53] To help put this in perspective, Sugarman et al. have estimated that 9% of the IRB's staff time is spent processing adverse event reports,[54] an activity that should be delegated almost entirely to data and safety monitoring boards.[53]

Further discussion of this topic is beyond the scope of this chapter, and it remains to be seen how this set of problems will be characterized and resolved.

Conclusion

Institutional Review Boards originated in isolated American institutions in the 1950s, became legally mandated in the United States in the 1970s, and in the 1980s became required by international ethical guidelines. They are the most important social control mechanism to assure the ethical conduct of research involving human subjects by contributing to the education of researchers in matters related to research ethics in general and by guiding researchers to comply with ethical and legal expectations. From the 1940s through the 1960s great reliance was placed on the investigators to safeguard the rights and welfare of research subjects and on informed consent to authorize the involvement of any particular individual as a research subject. Subsequently, there has been a partial shift in these responsibilities. The IRB is now relied on to help decide whether the relation of risks to benefits is such that any individual should be invited to enroll as subject and what kinds of individuals or groups should be considered eligible to receive such invitations.

There are some limits to the IRB's capability to assure the ethical conduct of research involving human subjects. For example, although it is generally agreed that the ethical justification of such research requires that it be scientifically sound, the IRB usually cannot render authoritative judgments about scientific merit. In such cases, the IRB has the responsibility to assure that scientific validity has been evaluated and approved by some competent agency.

It is widely assumed that IRBs are most effective when located in the institutions where the research is to be carried out. This point notwithstanding, there are many cases in which research is conducted in institutions far removed from the IRB that has reviewed and approved it, apparently without serious repercussions. The greatest challenge to the principle of local review is presented when research is designed in one country (external sponsoring country) to be carried out by investigators from that country in another country (host country). For such contingencies, the CIOMS *International Ethical Guidelines* specify divisions of responsibility and authority for ethical review committees in each of the two countries.

When IRBs were introduced for the review of biomedical research, there were many angry and resentful criticisms from biomedical researchers about unnecessary and unwarranted stifling of creativity and obstruction of progress. Subsequently, when the scope of IRB authority was extended to include social and behavioral research, such researchers protested that this was an unconstitutional restraint on their freedom of speech. Although some criticisms remain, they are now focused on details of the IRB's performance and how it might be improved rather than on the legitimacy of the entire concept of IRB review.

Finally, it is difficult, and perhaps impossible to evaluate the IRB's performance objectively. Even satisfactory subjective evaluations can be made only by experienced IRB members and administrators. This is an inevitable consequence of the fact that satisfactory performance of the IRB's essential tasks entails the exercise of professional judgment rather than conformity to a regulatory algorithm.

Note

Some passages in this chapter are adapted from *Ethics and Regulation of Clinical Research* (Reference 2).

References

1. World Medical Association. *Declaration of Helsinki* (as amended by the 29th World Medical Assembly). Tokyo, Japan, October, 1975.
2. Levine, R. J. *Ethics and Regulation of Clinical Research.* 2nd ed. New Haven, CT: Yale University Press, 1988.
3. Robertson, J. A. "The Law of Institutional Review Boards," *UCLA Law Review* 26 (1979): 484–49.
4. Medical Research Council of Canada. *Guidelines on Research Involving Human Subjects.* Ottawa: Medical Research Council of Canada, 1987.
5. Council for International Organizations of Medical Sciences. *International Ethical Guidelines for Biomedical Research Involving Human Subjects.* Geneva, Council for International Organizations of Medical Sciences, 2002. Available at http://www.cioms.ch/index.html, accessed November 17, 2008.
6. Council for International Organizations of Medical Sciences. *International Guidelines for Ethical Review of Epidemiological Studies.* Geneva, Council for International Organizations of Medical Sciences, 1991. Available at http://www.cioms.ch/index.html, accessed November 17, 2008.
7. World Medical Association. Available at http://www.wma.net/e/policy/b3.htm, accessed November 17, 2008.

8. Council for International Organizations of Medical Sciences. *Proposed International Guidelines for Biomedical Research Involving Human Subjects.* Geneva, Council for International Organizations of Medical Sciences, 1982.

9. Lipsett, M. B., Fletcher, J. C., and Secundy, M. "Research Review at NIH," *Hastings Center Report* 9, no. 1 (1979): 18–21.

10. Curran, W. J. "Government Regulation of the Use of Human Subjects in Medical Research: The Approaches of two Federal Agencies." In *Experimentation with Human Subjects*, ed. by P. A. Freund. New York: George Braziller, 1970: 402–54.

11. Veatch, R. M. "Human Experimentation Committees: Professional or Representative?" *Hastings Center Report* 5, no. 5 (October, 1975): 31–40.

12. Levine, C. "Has AIDS Changed the Ethics of Human Subjects Research?" *Law, Medicine & Health Care* 16 (1988): 167–73.

13. Levine, R. J. "The Impact of HIV Infection on Society's Perception of Clinical Trials," *Kennedy Institute of Ethics Journal* 4, no. 2 (1994): 93–98.

14. The National Commission for the Protection of Human Subjects of Biomedical and Behavioral Research. *The Belmont Report: Ethical Principles and Guidelines for the Protection of Human Subjects of Research.* DHEW Publication No. (OS) 78–0012, Washington, 1978.

15. Levine, R. J. "The Nature, Scope and Justification of Clinical Research: What is Research? Who is a Subject?" *Oxford Textbook of Clinical Research Ethics*, ed. E. Emanuel, et al. chapter 21, New York: Oxford University Press, 2008.

16. American College of Epidemiology. "Ethics Guidelines." Available at http://www.acepidemiology2.org/policystmts/EthicsGuide.asp, accessed November 17, 2008.

17. Freedman, B. "Scientific Value and Validity as Ethical Requirements for Research: A Proposed Explication," *IRB: A Review of Human Subjects Research* 9, no. 6 (1987): 7–10.

18. Robertson, J. A. "Ten Ways to Improve IRBs," *Hastings Center Report* 9, no. 1 (1979): 29–33.

19. Levine, C., Dubler, N. N., and Levine, R. J. "Building a New Consensus: Ethical Principles and Policies for Clinical Research on HIV/AIDS," *IRB: A Review of Human Subjects Research* 13, nos. 1 & 2 (1991): 1–17.

20. Institute of Medicine Committee on Assessing the System for Protecting Human Research Participants. *Responsible Research: A Systems Approach to Protecting Research Participants.* Washington: National Academy Press, 2003.

21. The National Commission for the Protection of Human Subjects of Biomedical and Behavioral Research. *Institutional Review Boards: Report and Recommendations.* Washington, 1978, DHEW Publication No. (OS) 78–0008.

22. Herman, S. S. "A Noninstitutional Review Board Comes of Age," *IRB: A Review of Human Subjects Research* 11, no. 2 (1989) 1–6.

23. Office for Human Research Protections, Association of American Medical Colleges, and American Society for Clinical Oncology. *Alternative Models of IRB Review: Workshop Summary Report*, November 17–18, 2005. Available at *http://www.hhs.gov/ohrp/sachrp/documents/AltModIRB.pdf, accessed November 17, 2008.*

24. Food and Drug Administration. "Waiver of Institutional Review Board Review of Certain Clinical Studies of Azidothymidine (AZT)." Unsigned memorandum, September 30, 1986.

25. Department of Health and Human Services. "Expanded Availability of Investigational New Drugs Through a Parallel Track Mechanism for People with AIDS and other HIV-related Disease," *Federal Register* 57, no. 73: 13244–13259, April 15, 1992.

26. Kavanagh, C., Matthews, D., Sorenson, J. R., and Swazey, J. P. "We Shall Overcome: Multi-institutional Review of a Genetic Counseling Study," *IRB: A Review of Human Subjects Research* 1, no. 2 (April, 1979): 1–3 and 12.

27. Rothman, K. J. "The Rise and Fall of Epidemiology, 1950-2000 A.D.," *New England Journal of Medicine* 304 (1981): 600-02.

28. Levine, R. J. and Lasagna, L. "Demystifying Central Review Boards: Current Options and Future Directions," *IRB: A Review of Human Subjects Research* 22, no.6 (2000): 1–4.

29. Christian, M. C., Goldberg, J. L., Killen, J., Abrams, J. S., McCabe, M. S., Mauer, J. K., and Wittes, R. E. "A Central Institutional Review Board For Multi-Institutional Trials," *New England Journal of Medicine* 346 (2002): 1405–08.

30. McNeill, P. M. "Research Ethics Committees in Australia, Europe, and North America," *IRB: A Review of Human Subjects Research* 11, no. 3 (1989): 4–7.

31. Ohnuki-Tierney, E. *Illness and Culture in Contemporary Japan: An Anthropological View.* New York: Cambridge University Press, 1984.

32. De Craemer, W. "Cross-cultural Perspective on Personhood," *Milbank Memorial Fund Quarterly* 61 (Winter, 1983): 19–34.

33. Christakis, N. A. "The Distinction between Ethical Pluralism and Ethical Relativism: Implications for the Conduct of Transcultural Research." In *The Ethics of Research Involving Human Subjects: Facing the 21st Century*, ed. H. Y. Vanderpool. Frederick, MD: University Publishing Group, 1996: 261–80.

34. Christakis, N. A. and Levine, R. J. "Multinational Research." In *Encyclopedia of Bioethics*, revised edition, ed. W. T. Reich. New York: Macmillan, 1995: 1780–87.

35. Baker, R. "A Theory of International Bioethics: The Negotiable and the Non-negotiable," *Kennedy Institute of Ethics Journal* 8, no. 3 (1998) 233–74.

36. Levine, R. J. "Informed Consent: Some Challenges to the Universal Validity of the Western Model," *Law, Medicine & Health Care.*19 (1991): 207–13.

37. Levine, R. J. "International Codes and Guidelines For Research Ethics: A Critical Appraisal." In *The Ethics of Research Involving Human Subjects: Facing the 21st Century*, ed. H.Y. Vanderpool. Frederick, MD: University Publishing Group, 1996: 235–59.

38. Levine, R. J. and Gorovitz, S. with the assistance of Gallagher, J. eds. *Biomedical Research Ethics: Updating International Guidelines.* Geneva: Council of International Organizations of Medical Sciences (CIOMS), 2000.

39. Koenig, B. and Marshall, P. "Anthropology and Bioethics." In *Encyclopedia of Bioethics*, 3rd edition, ed. S. G. Post. New York: Macmillan Reference, 2003: 215–24.

40. Macklin, R. "Universality of the Nuremberg Code." In *The Nazi Doctors and the Nuremberg Code: Human Rights and Human Experimentation*, ed. G. J. Annas and M. A. Grodin. New York: Oxford University Press, 1992: 240–57.

41. Lurie, P. and Wolfe, S. M. "Unethical Trials of Interventions to Reduce Perinatal Transmission of the Human Immunodeficiency Virus in Developing Countries," *New England Journal of Medicine* 337 (1997): 853–56.

42. Angell, M. "The Ethics of Clinical Research in the Third World," *New England Journal of Medicine* 337 (1997): 847–49.

43. Kleinman, A. "Moral Experience and Ethical Reflection: Can Ethnography Reconcile Them? A Quandry for the 'New Bioethics'," *Deadalus* 128, no.4 (1999): 69–97.

44. Levine, R. J. "Revision of the CIOMS International Ethical Guidelines: A Progress Report," In *Biomedical Research Ethics: Updating International Guidelines: A*

Consultation, ed. R. J. Levine and S. Gorovitz, with the assistance of J. Gallagher. Geneva: Council for International Organizations of Medical Sciences (CIOMS), 2000: 4–15.

45. Office for Human Research Protection. Available at *http://www.hhs.gov/ohrp/human-subjects/guidance/exprev.htm, accessed november 17, 2008.*

46. Williams, P. C. "Success in Spite of Failure: Why IRBs Falter in Reviewing Risks and Benefits," *IRB: A Review of Human Subjects Research* 6, no. 3 (1984): 1–4.

47. Robertson, J. A., "Taking Consent Seriously: IRB Intervention in the Consent Process," *IRB: A Review of Human Subjects Research* 4, no. 5 (1982): 1–5.

48. Mashaw, J. L. "Thinking about Institutional Review Boards. In The President's Commission for the Study of Ethical Problems in Medicine and Biomedical and Behavioral Research." *Whistleblowing in Biomedical Research: Policies and Procedures for Responding to Reports of Misconduct.* Washington, 1982: 3–22.

49. Levine, R. J. "Institutional Review Boards: A Crisis in Confidence," *Annals of Internal Medicine* 134 (2001): 161–63.

50. Fost, N. and Levine, R. J. "The Dysregulation of Human Subjects Research," *Journal of the American Medical Association* 298 (2007): 2196–98.

51. Burman, W. J., Reves, R. R., Cohn, D. L., and Schooley, R. T., "Breaking the Camel's Back: Multicenter Clinical Trials and Local Institutional Review Boards," *Annals of Internal Medicine* 134 (2001): 152–57.

52. Office of the Inspector General, U.S. Department of Health and Human Services. *Institutional Review Boards: A Time for Reform.* Report NO. OEI-01–97-00193. Washington, 1998.

53. Levine, R. J. "Empirical Research to Evaluate IRB's Burdensome and, Perhaps, Unproductive Policies and Practices: A Proposal," *Journal of Empirical Research on Human Research Ethics* 1, no. 3 (2006): 1–4.

54. Sugarman, J., Getz, H., Speckman, J. L., Byrne, M. M., Gerson, J., and Emanuel, E. J. "The Cost of Institutional Review Boards in Academic Medical Centers," *New England Journal of Medicine* 352 (2005): 1825–27.

13

Good Conduct and Integrity in Epidemiologic Research

COLIN L. SOSKOLNE, PETER H. ABBRECHT,
NANCY M. DAVIDIAN, AND ALAN R. PRICE

Many people believe that those following a career in the health sciences are virtuous, can be trusted to protect the public interest, and are scrupulous in their pursuit of truth.[1,2] This belief, however, is not always reflected in reality. The theft of intellectual property, the creation or fabrication of data, and even the alteration (i.e., falsification) of data to better support certain forms of bias are known to occur in science. Indeed, such cases have garnered media attention.[3-9] These harmful practices demonstrate anything but "good conduct and integrity," and they fall under the general rubric of scientific misconduct. They are contrary to the scientific ethic whose fundamental value is the pursuit of truth in the public interest.

"Scientific or research misconduct" is the term that has been adopted as the North American rubric for the failure to maintain honesty and integrity in science. The Danes, on the other hand, have preferred the term "scientific dishonesty" as the general rubric for those behaviors that are inconsistent with ensuring and promoting good conduct among those engaged in science.[10,11] The United States Public Health Service, which includes the National Institutes of Health, defines misconduct (or, misconduct in science) as "fabrication, falsification, plagiarism, or other practices that seriously deviate from those that are commonly accepted within the scientific community for proposing, conducting, or reporting research. It does not include honest error or honest differences in interpretations or judgments of data."[12,13] Much debate has focused on "honest error" in this definition which can be found in successive U.S. Federal Regulations.

Surveys have attempted to estimate the occurrence and impact of scientific misconduct.[14] Because of poor response rates in these surveys,[15-20] estimates of the incidence of scientific misconduct have been difficult to ascertain,[15-18] despite improved methods for assessing misconduct.[19,20] Nonetheless, it is apparent that misconduct has existed in the past[21-25] and continues into the present across the sciences,[26-29] including epidemiology.[30,31] Consequently, professional scientific organizations have adopted ethics guidelines, codes, or best practices that proscribe what constitutes unethical behavior on the part of its members.[32-35]

In this chapter, we first address the scope of misconduct, including integrity in science. We examine how vested interests can undermine the course of science. Then, we present some recent analytical work from the United States' Office of Research Integrity to demonstrate the nature of both the harms and costs associated with misconduct. The need to protect the public interest over any other interest is emphasized through mechanisms for ensuring accountability and professional self-regulation.

The Public Nature of Science

The focus in defining scientific (or research) misconduct tends to be on ensuring that the scientific pursuit of truth is neither consciously nor subconsciously compromised. A further facet of scientific misconduct relates to the public nature of science. Because science is often publicly funded, there is an implicit public trust in the integrity of the scientific enterprise, especially in its protection of the public interest. The latter provides substantial motivation for science to be both publicly accountable and self-regulating to keep its house in order.[22,29,36]

Besides the pursuit of truth and protection of the public interest, there is a further dimension to good conduct and integrity in science. It relates to the interpersonal conduct not only among researchers, but also among scientists and the various constituency groups with whom epidemiologists (and other scientists) work. Two moral foundations upon which good collegial relationships rest are those of integrity and mutual trust, which, when eroded, severely damage relationships among colleagues. In addition, the work intended to serve the public interest itself could be harmed.[29] Overzealousness may also drive misconduct. Zealots are, by definition, not dispassionate and hence objectivity is likely to suffer.

While the theft of intellectual property—a form of plagiarism—falls within the scope of scientific misconduct, charges of plagiarism are often difficult to prove and can be controversial.[37] Equally pressing are concerns about the accurate attribution of both intellectual contribution and effort found in collegial relationships, mentor–student relationships, and employer–employee relationships. To address this problem, in part, journal editors require of authors that they disclose what part of their article they are intellectually responsible for at the time of submission for publication.

Good science rests on the (moral) integrity of the scientist. Thus, in the mandate of the Office of Research Integrity we see the focus on both the personal integrity of the individual researcher (and also on the scientist's institutional support for maintaining integrity in scientific research) and on scientific research misconduct as defined above. When the integrity of the scientist is undermined by a biasing influence, the integrity of that scientist's research must be questioned. These influences, however, are not included under the formal definition of scientific misconduct, even though they can result in scientific misconduct.

Other forms of scientific misconduct derive from conflicting interests that can, depending on the circumstances, arise from vested interests,[31] or can manifest when one's self-interest is allowed to interfere with one's objectivity.[38,39] Any bias, consciously or subconsciously driven, must be exposed if science is to remain objective. The former derives from external pressure (explicit or implicit) that can influence objectivity. The natural predisposition to please one's sponsor can result in bias, from the very nature of the question that a scientist pursues, through the design, conduct, interpretation, reporting and dissemination of a study's findings. Thus, when sponsorship of research is from a source with a vested (e.g., a financial, religious, or political) interest in the outcome, additional concern about the integrity of the research is warranted. Self-interest, on the other hand, arises, for example, when questions of financial rewards override the very nature of the scientific question being posed and when professional advancement takes precedence over personal relationships among peers motivated by professional jealousies or the like.

Essential to the message of this chapter is the need to recognize that the personal integrity of the researcher, each member of the team of researchers, and institutional support staff maintain the highest standards of integrity in science.[32] Bias and the lack of objectivity, witting or unwitting, are contrary to the conduct of good science and need to be carefully controlled.

How Vested Interests Can Foment Uncertainty

Epidemiology provides the bridge from animal to human studies and therefore has the potential to influence not only medical care, but also national health and social policies. The extent of epidemiology's impact on society can be substantial.

Out of concern for the impact that fraud, deception, or delusion could have on policy, Feinstein[40] drew attention to these concerns insofar as they relate to judgments reached in consensus conferences designed to achieve agreement based on the evidence a hand at the time; such judgments can, however, be influenced by political and nonscientific forces. Instead of consensus conferences, Feinstein urged the exclusive use of "unequivocally valid scientific methods, evidence, and interpretations" when seeking scientific truths. Despite his recommendations, many consensus conferences have taken place since 1988, and whether "unequivocally valid scientific methods, evidence, and interpretations" are attainable remains arguable.

Constituencies that epidemiologists work with include government agencies, universities, labor unions, corporations, the media, private foundations, statutory granting agencies, nongovernmental organizations, and activist groups. Each of these groups has its own agenda and hence promotes its own interests, though most groups are also deeply committed to the pursuit of "good science."

There are instances in which interest groups hire consultant epidemiologists to support a particular argument that could, for instance, arise through an interpretation stemming from the publication of primary research. Such consultants have been accused of being in the pocket of the interest group that has employed their services, giving rise to questions about the work they have critiqued, and causing possible harm to the public interest when the science is thrown into question.[36,41–42]

Tobacco is one example where a global industry has been shown to have worked tirelessly, making prostitutes of scientists who conduct biased research in support of the industry's relentless pursuit of greater markets for their products.[43] Davis has exposed how bias in interpretation for the purpose of protecting vested interests is either explicitly discussed, or is implicit through the nature of the way funding has been channeled. The intent behind such work is to protect the short-term business interests of the particular industry.

By casting doubt on research that negatively implicates a commercial product, business-as-usual is maintained. By raising doubt, not only is science derailed, but the work of the policy-maker is made more challenging. This is so because formulating policy under uncertainty is less attainable.[44] Uncertainty or doubt results in the focus of concern being shifted from the need for a change in policy to the need for more research. This shift in focus then serves to support the *status quo* of business-as-usual by deferring the discussion about a change in policy to a later date.

To protect the public interest, scientists have sometimes been known to alert the media to pressures on themselves to withhold information about harms from products about which they hold evidence. Such scientists are said to "blow the whistle" on their employer by virtue of access to evidence suggesting that a product of concern is causing either *direct* harm to people, or *indirect* harm to people through environmental damage from pollution and the like. These scientists have often been fired by their employers, whether in industry or government. The most celebrated case is that of Dr. Jeffrey Wigand who emerged as a tobacco corporate insider to serve as a central witness in the lawsuits filed by Mississippi and 49 other states in the United States against the tobacco industry and which were eventually settled for $246 billion to $368 billion. This case resulted in the single biggest public health reform in U.S. history (see http://www.jeffreywigand. com/60minutes.php)

Whistleblowing usually involves a concern for fear of job loss or other type of retaliation by those who are in positions of authority over the person blowing the whistle (i.e., the person making the allegations of questionable scientific conduct or of malpractice).[45-48] Whistleblowing has some form of justification in many recent codes of ethics and ethics guidelines that encourage professionals to serve the public interest over any other interest. In support of this guideline, the International Society for Environmental Epidemiology (ISEE) introduced a procedure to provide at least moral support to beleaguered colleagues who were feeling threatened for pursuing their science in the public interest.[49] Guidelines for the handling of allegations of misconduct in a fair way have been difficult to manage, and the issue of due process has become preeminent in such investigations.

Concerns about justice—especially procedural justice—are often present in reporting misconduct. Because allegations do not always prove to be true, the reputation of the accused should be protected unless guilt is established. The process for investigating allegations of misconduct has had to be developed and administered with care and respect for due process.[39,50-53] Consequently, the U.S. Public Health Service (PHS) established its existing Office of Research Integrity (ORI), designed to handle allegations of misconduct in science through any PHS-supported research.

The Office of Research Integrity (ORI)

The Office of Research Integrity (ORI) was created in 1992 as part of the Office of Public Health and Science (OPHS) to investigate allegations of scientific misconduct. The ORI is a component of the United States (U.S.) Public Health Service (PHS) in the Department of Health and Human Services (HHS), preceded for 3 years by the Office of Scientific Integrity (OSI) within the National Institutes of Health (NIH). OSI and ORI worked for 16 years under the initial HHS regulation on scientific misconduct (42 C.F.R. Part 50, Subpart D), until June 2005, when an updated and more detailed HHS regulation (42 C.F.R. Part 93)[54] was promulgated.

For the biomedical research community, the changes in the regulation were small, but significant in the following ways: First, the definition of scientific misconduct was clarified and renamed in the new regulation as "research misconduct," to include falsification, fabrication, and plagiarism (each of which is defined in the regulation) in proposing, conducting, reporting and reviewing research. The latter category applies to applications or proposals for research support made by other independent scientists to NIH or other PHS agencies, or publications and reports of research supported by PHS research funds, which may be plagiarized by someone else.

Institutions are required to conduct the relevant investigations (seldom done by HHS itself), and thus bear the burden of proving, by a preponderance of the evidence, that the respondent committed misconduct intentionally, knowingly, or recklessly, as a significant departure from community standards. The HHS definition continues to exclude honest errors and differences in judgment or interpretation of data, but it specifies that the respondent bears the burden of proof (the standard is the preponderance of evidence) in such a defense.

ORI policy also continues to exclude authorship and credit disputes between former or current collaborators. Part 93 includes a statute of limitations, which applies to research misconduct that occurs within 6 years of the date ORI or the institution receives an allegation, with some exceptions. Institutions must inform researchers in their employ and involved in applying for or receiving PHS support (for biomedical or behavioral research and research training) about the institution's policies and procedures for responding to allegations of research misconduct and its commitment to compliance with them. Part 93 includes a new process to request a hearing before the HHS Departmental Appeals Board, wherein an HHS Administrative Law Judge will conduct a *de novo* (i.e., argued anew from the evidence, independent of prior findings of misconduct) review of the ORI findings, using expert advisors if desired by the judge or the parties; the HHS Assistant Secretary for Health and the HHS Debarring Official are the deciding officials after such hearings. The HHS hearing process is available for those respondents whom ORI has found to have committed research misconduct. Through 2006, ORI had made 175 findings of scientific or research misconduct in 14 years, and had published the findings and the names of the respondents in the *Federal Register*, the *NIH Guide to Grants and Contracts*, and in various ORI publications and online bulletin boards.

Of the 175 findings of scientific/research misconduct made by ORI from 1992 to 2006, about 27 dealt with research related to epidemiology and similar behavioral research. These ORI findings were made against five professors, four research scientists, one postdoctoral fellow, six graduate and undergraduate students, and eleven technicians. Several high-profile cases of scientific misconduct have been revealed through the press over the past few years. Some examples are briefly mentioned with quotes of newspaper headlines. These show how damaging such cases can be to the credibility of science.

1. "$12M worth of research compromised"[9]
2. "Researcher, fraudulent studies evade detection in Canada"[6]
3. "Stem cell fraud casts pall over science world"[4]
4. "Plagiarism allegation symptom of pressure to 'publish or perish'"[8]
5. "For Science's Gatekeepers, a Credibility Gap"[5]

A recent example of a major case of scientific misconduct in epidemiology-related research, handled by the U.S. Office of Research Integrity (ORI), is described below. This analysis reveals several dimensions of misconduct. It also reveals the degree of rigor needed to demonstrate breaches in research integrity.

A Case Study: the ORI Oversight Review of Eric Poehlman

By far the most extensive ORI misconduct case, in terms of scope of fabrication/falsification of data, involved misconduct in epidemiologically related research at the University of Vermont (UVM) from 1992 to 2001 by Eric Poehlman, Ph.D., formerly a tenured professor in the School of Medicine. Dr. Poehlman's research included extensive epidemiologic studies (such as his purported collection of data on the changes in multiple physiological variables in women before and after menopause), as well as research attempting to identify physiological mechanisms for some of his reported findings such as an increase in resting metabolic rate (RMR) with endurance training (ET).

The initial allegations were brought to the attention of UVM officials by a complainant who had been working as Dr. Poehlman's research assistant for several years. We describe here two of the allegations in the case, with emphasis on how the allegations were proved to be valid using databases in the UVM General Clinical Research Center (GCRC), the existence of some of which Dr. Poehlman was not aware.

ALLEGATION I: FALSIFICATION AND FABRICATION OF DATA IN A LONGITUDINAL STUDY OF MENOPAUSE Dr. Poehlman reported making baseline measurements of multiple physiological variables in 35 premenopausal women 44 to 48 years old.[55,56] He also reported that the same variables were remeasured in the same women at an average follow-up time of 6 years, when about half of the group were postmenopausal. All testing was done at the UVM General Clinical Research Center (GCRC).

According to the complainant, Dr. Poehlman described the study to him as being derived from repeated measurements on a subset of women who were studied at UVM as a part of the research reported in 1993 in the *American Journal of Physiology*.[57] The allegation raised in January 2001 was that, because Dr. Poehlman had arrived at UVM in 1987, left in fall 1993 for the University of Maryland and was gathering the first group of subjects over several years, it would have been difficult for him to have obtained 6-year follow-ups on any of these subjects. In November 2001, during UVM's investigation of other allegations of scientific misconduct against Dr. Poehlman, Dr. Poehlman responded that even after he went to Maryland, subjects continued to be followed up at Vermont. Dr. Poehlman also claimed that he no longer had the data for the study and that by university policy he was not required to retain data for more than 5 years.

This study and its allegations have a number of unique aspects, including the resolution of the allegation even though there were no primary data to analyze. Review of the UVM's GCRC administrative records for Dr. Poehlman's studies between 1986 and 1993 identified only 24 women 44 to 48 years old, of whom only 5 might have had a second visit (but less than 1 year after the first visit), in contrast to the 35 women seen with an average of 6 years between visits as claimed in the *Annals of Internal Medicine* paper.[55] In March 2002, Dr. Poehlman provided the UVM investigation committee with copies of limited research records for 35 subjects that he claimed were contacted for follow-up in the study. However, review of GCRC administrative records found that 5 of the 35 subjects had no records of participation in any GCRC protocol. Of the remaining 30 subjects who had been seen in the GCRC between February 1989 and July 1992, 21 were outside the age range of 44 to 48 years at the first visit. Of the remaining nine who were in the appropriate age range, none visited the GCRC again between their first visit and 1995 when the *Annals* article[55] was published. ORI's review of these research records demonstrated that Dr. Poehlman had falsified the age of one of the "participants," and had fabricated a written note to a research assistant to contact a subject for follow-up long after that research assistant left employment at the university, as part of his cover-up.

Dr. Poehlman then submitted an additional 43 names—taken from a computer file—of women. The data in the file documented that, for women 44 to 48 years old at the time of their first visit, that visit occurred too late (after 1989) to allow a 6-year follow-up by the 1995 *Annals* paper. For those "first visits" that did occur in 1989, all women were either underage or overage, except for one whose visit was too late to have allowed a 6-year follow-up. The complainant stated that Dr. Poehlman had told him that the data in the 1995 *Annals* paper were derived from repeated studies on a subset of women whose data were reported in 1993 in the *American Journal of Physiology*.[57] Further, according to the complainant, the 1993 paper reflected the sum total of all the women ever tested in the Poehlman laboratory, whose data were contained in Dr. Poehlman's "reliability" file on the GCRC computer. However, Dr. Poehlman later stated that the *Annals* paper[55] used an overlapping but different set of subjects from the *American Journal of Physiology* paper,[57] and that the GCRC computer that contained his reliability file was not fully functional from December 1992 through November 1993, so that the file could not account properly for all of the subjects he had tested.

In making the above statements, Dr. Poehlman did not know that the GCRC administrative database captured all subjects entered on any GCRC protocol, a database accessible only by GCRC personnel. His claimed "overlapping but different" set of subjects from the 1993 *American Journal of Physiology* paper could not be identified in the GCRC administrative database, proving that his claims were false. For resolving this case, it was fortunate that Dr. Poehlman was unaware that the GCRC collected its own census data on all subjects seen in the GCRC on an inpatient or outpatient basis.

Dr. Poehlman also submitted these fabricated longitudinal menopause data as preliminary data in a grant application (which was subsequently funded) to NIH. In March 2005, the U.S. District Attorney's Office filed a statement of charges against Dr. Poehlman in the U.S. District Court for the District of Vermont. In the plea agreement with the U.S., Dr. Poehlman pleaded guilty to one felony charge under 18 U.S.C. §1001 with mandatory criminal restitution and agreed to civil judgment against him and the imposition of a civil fine.

The PHS settled its findings of scientific misconduct by permanently excluding Dr. Poehlman from receipt of federal funds, and from service on PHS advisory groups or as a consultant, and requiring retraction or correction of 10 papers published between 1992 and 2002.[58] On June 28, 2006, Dr. Poehlman was sentenced to 1 year and a day in federal prison.[59,60] This was the first lifetime exclusion and prison sentence imposed in a case of HHS scientific misconduct.

ALLEGATION 2: FALSIFICATION OF DATA ON VISCERAL FAT LOSS AND HORMONE REPLACEMENT THERAPY (HRT) Dr. Poehlman presented a PowerPoint slide presentation at a meeting of the North American Association for the Study of Obesity (NAASO) in October, 2000. One slide showed a statistically significant relationship between visceral fat loss in women undergoing a weight loss program (restricted calories) and their use of estrogen (HRT) ($P < 0.01$) compared to the weight loss program alone. The complainant, who attended the presentation, recognized the study as Protocol 646, for which he had managed the database at the UVM. His data did not show a significant difference in visceral fat loss between women who reported taking estrogen and those who did not.

Based primarily on the testimony of the complainant and Dr. Poehlman's failure to rebut that testimony, the UVM Investigation Committee concluded that the data presented by Dr. Poehlman at NAASO were false and fabricated. Dr. Poehlman then submitted to that committee a set of data of unknown provenance containing names of seven women who were labeled in handwriting as HRT "users" and eight women who were labeled as "nonusers." Dr. Poehlman claimed that these women constituted a subset matched for weight loss. However, ORI determined that given (1) the "n" for each group, (2) the values for the weight loss in each group, and (3) the amounts of visceral abdominal fat lost by each group, the data in the partial set that Dr. Poehlman provided were not a subset of the data that were presented at NAASO.

To further investigate this allegation, ORI requested that UVM obtain for ORI the data set from the complainant that was the basis for the allegation. In that data set, ORI found the women who were named in the list of 15 that Dr. Poehlman had submitted, with weight losses and losses of visceral abdominal fat as claimed by Dr. Poehlman. However, ORI found marginal significance of the differences between HRT users and nonusers ($P = 0.098$ by paired t-test and $P = 0.05$ by Z test). ORI concurred with the UVM finding of scientific misconduct against

Dr. Poehlman for his presentation at NAASO, and ORI extended this finding to numerous grant applications submitted by Dr. Poehlman with such data. These findings are specified in the PHS settlement noted above[58] and they contributed to the severity of the PHS administrative actions imposed.

EPILOGUE AND THE CONSEQUENCES OF MISCONDUCT   There are many costs that result from scientific misconduct. Some are easily calculable, such as the costs of salaries that were paid to researchers who produced fabricated or falsified, and thus unusable, data. However, the incalculable costs of misconduct constitute a much greater loss to society. In the Poehlman case, the government summarized the loss due to Dr. Poehlman's actions as follows:[61]

The defendant's fraudulent conduct led to the diversion of millions in research funds, which resulted in a direct loss to NIH. Similar to cases where a defendant's fraud diverted government program benefits, the full amount of the grant application should be assessed as the loss in this case, as those funds should never have been expended on the defendant's research projects. Moreover, the defendant's fraudulent conduct directly harmed NIH, UVM (University of Vermont), and the scientific community by making any research results unreliable and virtually useless for other researchers....

[I]n this case, the defendant made material false statements in grant applications that caused NIH to spend money on research at UVM that should not have been done. Those funds are no longer available to other researchers, and as a result, those funds are a total loss for NIH. The fact that research on human subjects was done at UVM does not ameliorate the loss. NIH expended money based on the defendant's false statements, and the research should not have been funded. But for the defendant's fraudulent conduct, the money should and would have gone to fund an entirely different research project.

The Government has attempted to estimate for the court the financial loss from Dr. Poehlman's misconduct, but one cannot even begin to measure the effect of Dr. Poehlman's dishonesty on the six or seven immediate colleagues to whom he gave falsified and fabricated data, to his numerous coauthors, or to other scientists who were mislead. Sox and Rennie[62] discussed the effort required to "cleanse the medical literature" of the misrepresentations introduced by Dr. Poehlman. They concluded:

This discussion has been about repairing damage. However, *preventing* damage would save careers from ruin and save the time spent investigating allegations and assessing the integrity of articles that become suspect by association with a fraudulent author. Everyone has a responsibility to promote a culture in which research misconduct does not happen.

Science and Public Perception

Democracies usually relegate control of the professions to the professions themselves. The professions are expected to maintain control over members' conduct through peer pressure and the establishment of normative standards of conduct. Because science is supported by public funds, it must be concerned with issues of self-regulation to prevent the very type of problem raised through the Poehlman case. However, regardless of the existence of codes or guidelines for good research practices, inevitably, the miscreant researcher will find ways of circumventing them.

When vigilance at the level of the profession fails, then vigilance at the governmental level is necessary to protect the public interest. And, when allegations of misconduct arise, public trust in the system of "science in the public interest" needs to be ensured and so it is essential for investigations into misconduct to be undertaken. In addition, there is a need for these investigations to take reasonable steps to protect the accuser's confidentiality. For, even if a person charged with misconduct is proven innocent, or if the charges are dismissed, the accuser's name could remain tarnished from the experience. So, it is not legal to discus decisions of "no misconduct" unless the parties or government agencies have made the case public. The Imanishi-Kari case provides a well-documented instance of disclosure and its effects.[63]

The amount of money and resources directed to investigating allegations of misconduct are substantial. Each time a scientist is implicated in a case of misconduct, the scientific enterprise is harmed through the erosion of public trust and diminished public confidence.[64,65] This is why science has to be accountable to the public in whose interest research is conducted and through whose purse it is often funded.

Accountability and Professional Self-Regulation

To ensure the highest possible standards, the professions have obligations to control possible misconduct. In the late 1980s, epidemiologists began formally to consider this responsibility.[36] In part, this new professional endeavor has been encouraged through pressure on research institutions, as a prerequisite to seeking NIH funding, to demonstrate their compliance with NIH stipulations. These requirements include the existence of formally established programs and mechanisms within each research institution that address issues of professional responsibility and accountability. For example, programs must exist within each institution for teaching ethics in graduate training programs supported by the NIH,[66] and procedures must be promulgated for investigating allegations of misconduct[54,67–70] to qualify for funding support from the PHS.

Activities such as symposia and workshops provide a basis for professional education and are essential for ensuring "grass roots" participation in professional guideline development. Issues surrounding "scientific misconduct" in particular were addressed at a symposium on "Ethics and Law in Environmental

Epidemiology" in conjunction with the annual meeting of the International Society for Environmental Epidemiology (ISEE) held in Cuernavaca, Mexico in 1992. The symposium was organized because of highly publicized epidemiologic cases of alleged misconduct and of cases at that time judged as misconduct by the former Office of Scientific Integrity (OSI). The symposium Proceedings[10,38,39,50–52] provide, based on the handling of each of those cases, a useful basis for education by virtue not only of process issues in the United States and Denmark, two countries at that time known to have formally addressed these matters, but also by virtue of the extensive discussion and commentary around specific case studies in these two countries. The proceedings also document situations presented from among international symposium participants, extensively commented upon by symposium panelists.

The above-cited symposium was designed to involve epidemiologists at the grass roots and thereby to extend the guidelines in the hope of preventing future acts of misconduct. Despite the several draft ethics guidelines that have been published,[71–76] each of which to some extent does address the need for integrity in science, the presence of grass roots involvement in the development of the subsequently-adopted ethics guidelines reduces the likelihood of noncompliance.

With growing experience and development, ORI has engaged in extensive efforts in education via sponsored research and conferences. In addition, ORI has proposed policies to require formal training in the Responsible Conduct of Research.[77,78] These ought to be accessed by epidemiologists to broaden their individual and collective understanding of the issues involved and the risks to the advancement of their science through breaches of research integrity. Indeed, epidemiologists need actively to engage in these discussions so that relevant ORI policies might be developed and enjoy ever-widening support from the research community.

A distinction is drawn between scientific misconduct on the one hand and acts of unprofessional conduct, such as medical malpractice, on the other. With the existence of guidelines being relatively recent for epidemiologists, there is now a basis against which normative standards of conduct can begin to be assessed. With the ability to make such assessments, the spectere of "enforcement," as possible with medical malpractice, presents difficult and sensitive dilemmas to epidemiologists because volunteer officers elected to run the professional and subspecialty organizations of epidemiologists have not traditionally seen their role as one of policing the profession.

Advancing Good Conduct and Integrity in Epidemiology

Guidelines relating to scientific integrity and honesty are a means to foster the pursuit of truth and the maintenance of ethics in the public interest. Truth, we posit, is most attainable through stakeholders, including representatives with an interest in the outcome under investigation, and a range of disciplinary experts engaging in an open dialogue of the issues and concerns. Such engagement might serve to prevent instances of misconduct.[33]

The notion of prevention is central to epidemiology. Hence, application of epidemiologic methods to elucidate the determinants of misconduct would seem like a natural area of interest for epidemiologic pursuit; at least it ought to enjoy the support of epidemiologists.[79] In practice, however, such support will manifest only when there are incentives for epidemiologists to engage themselves in such pursuits. Indeed, ORI has a grant program on research integrity, and one to which epidemiologists may apply. Results of ORI-sponsored research on integrity have been published.[18,80]

Institutions and professional organizations could assist in preventing misconduct by not only inculcating good ethical conduct in the organizational culture, but also through their own actions. Management has to support its ethics program, not just give it lip service. This is encouraged also by establishing confidential avenues for discussing suspicions of misconduct. How one responds to questionable conduct sends strong messages throughout any organization.[81] Rot at the top is almost certainly going to see rot at the bottom of any organization, be it a professional society, a corporate office, or a government agency. Good conduct at the top, on the other hand, is likely to see good conduct permeate throughout the organization. In the absence of such a model, disincentives prevail in the form of ignorance and a lack of protection for whistleblowers.

With the reluctance on the part of volunteer officers who run professional organizations of epidemiologists to invoke enforcement mechanisms, peer pressure is tacitly applied. So, when misconduct of any degree is detected, the range of penalty in practice ranges from censure through professional ostracizing and even criminal charges. Clearly, not all forms of misconduct should be responded to. There also may be a need for the scientific community to offer rehabilitation in the form of counseling to those found guilty of misconduct; it may be in the public interest to retain their expertise, instead of dismissing them completely from the practice of their science. After all, the potential for misconduct or dishonest conduct exists in all people. Integration of ethics generally, and of scientific misconduct and dishonesty specifically, into training programs as discussed in Chapter 14 by Kenneth Goodman and Ronald Prineas, adequately supported by case study material, is an essential component for the prevention of scientific misconduct. This process includes sensitizing students to prevailing professional norms and values. There remains, however, a need to evaluate the impact of such programs, which have been required only since 1990.[66]

Various epidemiologic organizations have begun integrating ethics into their professional activities by, for example, providing a forum at their respective annual scientific meetings/conferences for the discussion of ethical issues and concerns.

These ought to be promoted as ongoing activities,[32] recognizing that ethics require the application of values and principles to issues that generate dilemmas and tensions among thoughtful people engaged in professional pursuits.

Conferences do provide a forum for such dialogue because values are subject to change over time, and any appeals to ethical principles may need to be re-evaluated in light of these changes. Forums at scientific meetings provide the opportunity for a fuller discussion of concerns and issues and could provide ideas for their resolution; they also provide reasonable justification to revise existing ethics guidelines and standards of conduct. One method by which ethics could be reinforced at the training level is by establishing an incentive program for students to discuss their particular approach to handling an ethical dilemma and, where applicable, its resolution.

In order for each profession to be self-regulating, it must establish an infrastructure whose purpose is to promote ethical conduct in the public interest among members of the profession.[32] Existing committees include the American College of Epidemiology's Ethics Committee, the International Society for Environmental Epidemiology's Committee on Ethics and Philosophy, and the International Society for Pharmacoepidemiology's Public Policy/Ethics Committee.

Some argue for the mandate of ethics committees in the profession to include resources for mediation in disputes, for counseling (ideally) to prevent the need for charges of alleged misconduct being filed, and for the power to intervene in the public interest in circumstances that so warrant. Furthermore, some suggest the need for professions to have some leverage for debarring a member from practice in the event of proven misconduct. Clearly, ORI makes efforts to ensure that no federal funding be available to persons found guilty of serious scientific misconduct. This perspective needs to be weighed against the benefits derived from voluntary rehabilitation.

With these serious consequences, the professions do need to consider their direct role in minimizing the likelihood of scientific misconduct. Indeed, any type of misconduct, whether poor collegial relations, malpractice, or scientific misconduct that damages the fabric that nurtures science, warrants the serious attention of the profession. The implementation of appropriate mechanisms that will serve to prevent such problems as noted in this chapter are encouraged. Not addressed in this chapter is the proposition that formal auditing of research be undertaken[23,24,29,31] by appropriate public interest agencies to deter scientific dishonesty. The longer the profession waits to act on these matters, the greater the likelihood that governments could intervene and that public support for the profession could erode.

ACKNOWLEDGMENTS

The contributions to this chapter by Drs. Abbrecht, Davidian, and Price express the views of the authors and do not necessarily reflect the positions of the Office of Research Integrity, the U.S. Department of Health and Human Services, or any component thereof. The first edition of this chapter was prepared with the coauthorship of Dorothy K. Macfarlane who has since retired from the HHS Office of Research Integrity. The authors thank Tracy Morgan, Gary Lipshultz, and Dany Gagnon for their excellent technical assistance.

References

1. Pellegrino, E. D., Veatch, R. M., and Langan, J. P., eds. *Ethics, Trust, and the Professions: Philosophical and Cultural Aspects.* Washington, DC: Georgetown University Press, 1991.
2. Pellegrino, E. D. "Character and the Ethical Conduct of Research," *Accountability in Research* 2 (1992): 1–11.
3. Cranor, C. F. "Science with Health Consequences" [Editorial], *International Journal of Occupational and Environmental Health* 12, no. 2 (2006): 177–79.
4. Weiss, R. "Stem Cell Fraud Casts Pall over Science World," *The Edmonton Journal* (December 24, 2005): A6.
5. Altman, L. K. "For Science's Gatekeepers, a Credibility Gap," *The New York Times* (May 2, 2006). Available at http://www.nytimes.com/2006/05/02/health/02docs. html?_r=1&oref=slogin, accessed on October 20, 2008.
6. Researcher. "Fraudulent Studies Evade Detection in Canada," *The Edmonton Journal* (March 17, 2006): A5.
7. Valliantos, E. G., "Toxic Sprays are a Political Issue," *Seattle Post-Intelligencer* (January 5, 2006). Available at: http://seattlepi.nwsource.com/opinion/254457_ epa05.html, accessed on October 20, 2008.
8. Mandel, C. "Plagiarism Allegation Symptom of Pressure to 'publish or perish'," *The Edmonton Journal* (December 29, 2005): A5.
9. Munro, M. "$12M Worth of Research Compromised: National Agencies say U of A among Schools Where Data Faked or Destroyed," *The Edmonton Journal* (March 16, 2006): A5.
10. Grandjean, P. and Andersen, D. "Scientific Dishonesty: A Danish Proposal for Evaluation and Prevention," *Journal of Exposure Analysis and Environmental Epidemiology.* 3, Suppl. 1 (1993): 265–70.
11. Andersen, D., Attrup, L., Axelsen, N., and Riis, P. *Scientific Dishonesty & Good Scientific Practice.* Copenhagen: The Danish Medical Research Council, 1992.
12. *Federal Register,* 54 (August 8, 1989): 32449. 42 CFR 50, Subpart A. Available at http://ori.dhhs.gov/misconduct/reg_subpart_a.shtml, accessed on October 20, 2008.
13. "Research Misconduct," *Federal Register* 70, no. 94 (May 17, 2005): 28369–400. 42 CFR 93, Sec. 93.103. Available at http://ori.hhs.gov/documents/FR_Doc_05– 9643.shtml, accessed on October 20, 2008.
14. Steneck, N. H., "Fostering Integrity in Research: Definitions, Current Knowledge, and Future Directions," *Science and Engineering Ethics* 12, no. 1 (2006): 53–74.
15. Goldberg, L. A. and Greenberg, M. R. "Ethical Issues for Industrial Hygienists: Survey Results and Suggestions," *American Industrial Hygiene Association Journal* 54 (1993): 127–34.
16. Greenberg, M. R. and Martell, J. "Ethical Dilemmas and Solutions for Risk Assessment Scientists," *Journal of Exposure Analysis and Environmental Epidemiology* 2 (1992): 381–89.

17. Frankel, M. S., ed. "In the Societies," *Professional Ethics Report. Newsletter of the American Association for the Advancement of Science* 1 (Winter, 1992): 2–3.

18. Martinson, B. C., Anderson, M. S., and deVries, R. "Scientists Behaving Badly," *Nature* 435 (2005): 737–38.

19. Hallum, J. W. and Hadley, S. W. "Scientific Misconduct: The Evolution of Method," *Professional Ethics Report. Newsletter of the American Association for the Advancement of Science* III, no. 3 (Summer, 1990): 4–5.

20. Broome, M. E., Pryor, E., Habermann, B., Pulley, L., and Kincaid, H. "The Scientific Misconduct Questionnaire – Revised (SMQ-R): Validation and Psychometric Testing," *Accountability in Research* 12, no. 4 (2005): 263–80.

21. Broad, W. and Wade, N. *Betrayers of the Truth: Fraud and Deceit in the Halls of Science.* New York: Simon & Shuster, 1982.

22. Lowy, F. H. and Meslin, E. M. "Fraud in Medical Research." In *Textbook of Ethics in Pediatric Research*, ed. G. Koren. Malabar, FA: Kreiger Publishing Company, 1993: 293–307.

23. Shamoo, A. E. and Annau, Z. "Ensuring Scientific Integrity," *Nature* 327 (June 18, 1987): 550. [Taken from Dr. Shamoo's website: Shamoo, A.E. and Z. Annau (1987). "Ensuring Scientific Integrity", correspondence. Nature 327: 550, 1987.]

24. Shamoo, A. E. and Annau, Z. "Data Audit—Historical Perspective." In *Principles of Research Data Audit*, cd. A. E. Shamoo. London: Gordon & Breach, 1989: 1–11.

25. Dawson, N. J. "Ensuring Scientific Integrity" [Letter]. *Nature* 327 (June 18, 1987): 550. [Taken from the Nature website: Nature, Volume 327, Issue 6123: 550 (1987).

26. Teich, A. H. and Frankel, M. S. *Good Science and Responsible Scientists: Meeting the Challenge of Fraud and Misconduct in Science.* Directorate for Science and Policy Programs, Washington, DC: American Association for the Advancement of Science (AAAS Publication Number 92–13S) (1992).

27. American Association for the Advancement of Science, American Bar Association, National Conference of Lawyers and Scientists, and the Office of Scientific Integrity Review, Public Health Service, U.S. Department of Health and Human Services. *Misconduct in Science: Recurring Issues, Fresh Perspectives.* Conference Executive Summary (November 15–16, 1991), Cambridge, MA.

28. Swazey, J. P., Anderson, M. S., and Seashore, L. K. "Encounters with Ethical Problems in Graduate Education: Highlights from National Surveys of Doctoral Students and Faculty," *Professional Ethics Report. Publication of the American Association for the Advancement of Science, Scientific Freedom, Responsibility and Law Program* VI, no. 4 (Fall, 1993): 1, 7.

29. Glick, J. L. and Shamoo, A. E. "A Call for the Development of 'Good Research Practices' (GRP) Guidelines," *Accountability in Research* 2 (1993): 231–35.

30. Bernier, R., ed. "NIH Actions against Breast Cancer Researcher Raise Issues for Epidemiologists," *The New Epidemiology Monitor* 15 (1994): 1–2.

31. Shamoo, A. E. "Policies and Quality Assurance in the Pharmaceutical Industry," *Accountability in Research* 1 (1991): 273–84.

32. Frankel, M. S. and Bird, S. J. "The Role of Scientific Societies in Promoting Research Integrity," *Science and Engineering Ethics* 9 (2003): 139–40.

33. Soskolne, C. L. and Sieswerda, L. E. "Implementing Ethics in the Professions: Examples from Environmental Epidemiology," *Science and Engineering Ethics* 9 (2003): 181–90.

34. Iverson, M., Frankel, M. S., and Siang, S. "Scientific Societies and Research Integrity: What are They Doing and How Well are They Doing It?" *Science and Engineering Ethics* 9 (2003): 138–41.

35. Levine, F. J. and Iutcovich, J. M. "Challenges in Studying the Effects of Scientific Societies on Research Integrity," *Science and Engineering Ethics* 9 (2003): 257–68.

36. Soskolne, C. L. "Epidemiology: Questions of Science, Ethics, Morality, and Law," *American Journal of Epidemiology* 129 (1989): 1–18.

37. Fields, K. L. and Price, A. R. "Problems in Research Integrity Arising from Misconceptions about Ownership of Research," *Academic Medicine* 68, no. 9 (1993), Suppl.: S60–S64.

38. Soskolne, C. L., ed. "Questions from the Delegates and Answers by the Panellists Concerning 'Ethics and Law in Environmental Epidemiology'," *Journal of Exposure Analysis and Environmental Epidemiology* 3, Suppl. 1 (1993): 297–319.

39. Soskolne, C. L. "Introduction to Misconduct in Science and Scientific Duties," *Journal of Exposure Analysis and Environmental Epidemiology* 3, Suppl.1 (1993): 245–51.

40. Feinstein, A. R. "Fraud, Distortion, Delusion, and Consensus: The Problems of Human and Natural Deception in Epidemiologic Science," *The American Journal of Medicine* 84 (1988): 475–78.

41. Soskolne, C. L. "Epidemiological Research, Interest Groups, and the Review Process," *Journal of Public Health Policy* 6, no. 2 (1985): 173–84.

42. Soskolne, C. L. "Ethical Decision-making in Epidemiology: The Case-study Approach," *Journal of Clinical Epidemiology* 44, Suppl. 1 (1991): 125S–130S.

43. Davis, D. *Secret History of the War on Cancer.* New York: Basic Books, 2007.

44. Michaels, D. *Doubt Is Their Product: How Industry's Assault on Science Threatens Your Health.* New York: Oxford University Press: 2008.

45. Weiss, T. "Too Many Scientists Who 'Blow the Whistle' End Up Losing Their Jobs and Careers," *Chronicle of Higher Education* (June, 1991): A36.

46. Westman, D. P. *Whistleblowing: The Law of Retaliatory Discharge.* Washington, DC: Bureau of National Affairs, 1991.

47. Glazer, M. *The Whistleblowers: Exposing Corruption in Government And Industry.* New York: Basic Books, 1989.

48. Revkin, A. C. "NASA Climate Expert Says Bush Tried to Gag Him: Scientist James Hansen Says He Will Not Be Muzzled on Global Warming," *The Edmonton Journal*, January 29, 2006: A12.

49. International Society for Environmental Epidemiology (ISEE). "ISEE Support for Victimized Colleagues," September, 2000. Available at http://www.iseepi.org/about/ethics.html#victimized, accessed on October 20, 2008.

50. Price, A. R. "The United States Government Scientific Misconduct Regulations and the Handling of Issues Related to Research Integrity," *Journal of Exposure Analysis and Environmental Epidemiology* 3, Suppl. 1 (1993): 253–64.

51. Sharphorn, D. H., "Integrity in Science: Administrative, Civil and Criminal Law in the U.S.A.," *Journal of Exposure Analysis and Environmental Epidemiology* 3, Suppl. 1 (1993): 271–81.

52. Dale, M. L. "Integrity in Science: Misconduct Investigations in a U.S. University," *Journal of Exposure Analysis and Environmental Epidemiology* 3, Suppl. 1 (1993): 283–95.

53. Bird S. J. and Frankel M. S. (eds). "The Role of Scientific Societies in Promoting Research Integrity," *A Special Issue of Science and Engineering Ethics* 9, no. 2 (2003): 139–290.

54. Code of Federal Regulations 42, part 93. "Public Health Service Policies on Research Misconduct," *Federal Register* 70 (May 17, 2005): 28370–99.

55. Poehlman, E. T., Toth, M. J., and Gardner, A. W. M. "Changes in Energy Balance and Body Composition at Menopause: A Controlled Longitudinal Study," *Annals of Internal Medicine* 123 (1995): 673–75.

56. Poehlman, E. T., Toth, M. J., Ades, P. A., and Rosen, C. J. "Menopause-associated Changes in Plasma Lipids, Insulin-like Growth Factor I and Blood Pressure: A Longitudinal Study," *European Journal of Clinical Investigation* 27 (1997): 322–26.

57. Poehlman, E. T., Goran, M. I., Gardner, A. W., Ades, P. A., Arciero, P. J., Katzman-Rooks, S. M., Montgomery, S. M., Toth, M. J., and Sutherland, P. T. "Determinants of Decline in Resting Metabolic Rate in Aging Females," *American Journal of Physiology* 264 (1993): E450–55.

58. Office of Research Integrity (ORI). "Misconduct Finding: Eric T. Poehlman," March 23, 2005. Available at http://ori.dhhs.gov/misconduct/cases/poehlman.shtml. See also *Federal Register*, March 24, 2005, 70, no. 56: 15092–95.

59. Kintisch, E. "Poehlman Sentenced to 1 Year of Prison," *Science NOW Daily News* (June 28, 2006): 1.

60. Silverman, A. "Former UVM Professor Sentenced to Jail for Fraud," *Burlington Free Press* (June 26, 2006). [Full text available at http://info.anu.edu.au/OVC/Committees/060PP_Research/_urcmtg3_2006/fraudcase.pdf]

61. Sentencing Memorandum in the United States District Court for the District of Vermont, June 22, 2006. *United States of America vs. Eric Poehlman.* Criminal No. 05-CR-38-01.

62. Sox, H. C. and Rennie, D. "Research Misconduct, Retraction and Cleansing the Medical Literature: Lessons from the Poehlman Case," *Annals of Internal Medicine* 144 (2006): E7–11.

63. Sarasohn, J. *Science on Trial: The Whistle-Blower, the Accused, and the Nobel Laureate.* New York: St. Martin's Press, 1993.

64. Committee on Government Operations together with Dissenting and Additional Views. *Are Scientific Misconduct and Conflicts of Interest Hazardous to Our Health?* Nineteenth Report. 101st Congress, 2nd Session. Union Calendar No. 430, House Report 101–688, Washington: U.S. Government Printing Office, 1990 .

65. Francis, J. R. "The Credibility and Legitimation Of Science: A Loss of Faith in the Scientific Narrative," *Accountability in Research*, 1 (1989): 5–22.

66. *NIH Guide to Grants and Contracts.* Requirement for Programs on the Responsible Conduct of Research in National Research Service Award Institutional Training Programs. Regional Workshops – Protection of human subjects. 18 no. 45 (December, 1989).

67. "Responsibilities of Awardee and Applicant Institutions for Dealing with and Reporting Misconduct in Science," *Federal Register* 54, no. 151, August 8 Rules and Regulations (1989): 32446–451. DHHS-PHS 42 CFR Part 50.

68. Mishkin, B. "PHS rules on scientific integrity: major progress and some remaining questions," *Professional Ethics Report. Newsletter of the American Association for the Advancement of Science* V no. 1 (1992): 5–6.

69. Medical Research Council of Canada, Natural Sciences and Engineering Research Council of Canada, Social Sciences and Humanities Research Council of Canada. *Integrity in Research and Scholarship: A Tri-Council Policy Statement.* 1994, Cat No. CR22-29/1994; ISBN No. 0–662–60220-X.

70. Tosteson, D. C. *Faculty Policies on Integrity in Science.* Faculty of Medicine, Harvard University, 1992, 27 pages.
71. Beauchamp, T. L., Cook, R. R., Fayerweather, W. E., Raabe, G. K., Thar, W. E., Cowles, S. R., and Spivey, G. H. "Ethical Guidelines for Epidemiologists," *Journal of Clinical Epidemiology* 44, Suppl. I (1991): 151S–169S.
72. Russel, E. and Westrin, C-G. "Ethical Issues in Epidemiological Research: Guidelines Containing the Minimum Common Standards of Practice Recommended for Use by Project Leaders and Participants in the Operation of Future Concerted Actions." In *Commission of the European Communities. Medicine and Health: COMAC Epidemiology,* ed. M. Hallen and K. Vuylsteek, Luxembourg, 1992: 19–22.
73. IEA Workshop on Ethics, Health Policy and Epidemiology. "Proposed Ethics Guidelines for Epidemiologists," ed. J. Last. *American Public Health Association (Epidemiology Section) Newsletter* (Winter, 1990): 4–6.
74. Council for International Organizations of Medical Sciences. *International guidelines for ethical review of epidemiological studies.* Geneva: CIOMS, 1991.
75. Council for International Organizations of Medical Sciences. *International Ethical Guidelines for Biomedical Research Involving Human Subjects.* Geneva: CIOMS, 1993.
76. The Chemical Manufacturers Association's Epidemiology Task Group. "Guidelines For Good Epidemiology Practices for Occupational and Environmental Epidemiologic Research," *Journal of Occupational Medicine* 33, no. 12 (1991): 1221–29.
77. "Final PHS Policy for Instruction in the Responsible Conduct of Research," *Federal Register,* 65, no. 236 (December 7, 2000): 76647.
78. Office of Research Integrity. URL: http://ori.hhs.gov/policies/RCR_Policy.shtml
79. Weed, D. L. "Preventing Scientific Misconduct," *American Journal of Public Health* 1: 88, no 1 (1998): 125–29.
80. DeVries R., Anderson M. S., and Martinson, B. C. "Normal Misbehavior: Scientists Talk about the Ethics of Research," *Journal of Empirical Research on Human Research Ethics* 1, no. 1 (2006): 43–50.
81. Hall, W. D. *Making the Right Decision: Ethics for Managers.* New York: John Wiley & Sons (1993): 182–98.

14

Ethics Curricula in Epidemiology

KENNETH W. GOODMAN AND RONALD J. PRINEAS

Since the mid-1990s epidemiology has joined other sciences and health professions in making ethics education a component of the larger curriculum. The growth of an ethics-and-epidemiology literature, the interest of professional societies in ethics, and the obvious importance of ethics to professional practice have all contributed to the evolution of the epidemiology and public health curriculum.

The change is far from total, however. Many programs and schools continue to include ethics only episodically, if at all. Several reasons for this include the following:

- *Unfamiliarity.* Many epidemiologists and public health researchers assume—sometimes wisely—that they do not have the background or competence to introduce ethics into their courses. They recognize that philosophers and others with pedagogic competence in ethics would never presume to teach biostatistics, research design, or foundations of epidemiology without adequate preparation.
- *Shortage of curricular resources.* Even if epidemiology and public health faculty were able and willing, the task of designing a new curriculum or introducing ethical issues into existing curricula can be daunting without familiarity with previous efforts.
- *Uninterested leadership.* This explanation would be difficult to demonstrate or document, but it is apparent that some leaders do not regard ethics as worthy of inclusion in the curriculum.

Additions to established university curricula are often viewed as avoidable entanglements: the schedule is full, the students are busy, and faculty members are stretched thin. Nevertheless, progress and problems in science and other disciplines inevitably force revisions to existing curricula, and developments in epidemiology and ethics have attained such importance that they continue to merit (1) development of new course materials, (2) training of appropriate faculty members, and (3) integration of new courses into epidemiology, public health, and other curricula. In addition, ongoing efforts to include ethics-and-epidemiology sessions in professional conferences ought to be expanded, and short courses, perhaps on special topics or problems, should be developed for students, practitioners, and university faculty. We argue for these recommendations in this chapter.

On the Core Curriculum: Why Ethics Matters in Epidemiology

There are a number of reasons to broaden the emphasis on ethics and epidemiology: First, epidemiology is a basic discipline, the security and rigor of which are essential for developing an informed health policy. When sloppy research or moral shortcomings weaken scientific conclusions—or public confidence in them—there is a need to instruct students and practitioners in professional practice standards and in the moral foundations of scientific inquiry. If flawed science is used as a basis for public health policy it can have adverse health and economic consequences. To the extent that incompetent science can lead to wasted public resources or, worse, to poorer public health, it can be characterized as a misappropriation of public funds or a threat to public health, as discussed by Colin Soskolne et al. in Chapter 13. Concerns in the United States about the public credibility of the research enterprise led the National Institutes of Health (NIH) to require training in research integrity or the responsible conduct of research (RCR) at all institutions receiving NIH training grants. Institutions can thus make a virtue out of necessity by offering high-quality programs in research integrity. (RCR is discussed later in this chapter.)

Ethics-in-epidemiology courses need to be developed and linked to courses in research design and analysis and health policy. Research issues are already a core component of epidemiology courses offered at universities and colleges in North America, Europe, and elsewhere in the world, although links between epidemiology and health policy are less common. Coherent attempts to wed ethics to such hybrids are essential.

A second motivation for expanded bioethics education is that further development of appropriate curricula will stimulate research in both bioethics and epidemiologic science. Serious and sustained attention to ethical issues in epidemiology is relatively recent. Yet this subfield is rich with opportunities to identify and analyze new issues, to clarify existing problems, and to contribute to decision procedures for practitioners, policy makers, public officials, students, and others. Scientific research education, for instance, could continue to be stimulated by curricular development that includes work on topics in which uncertainty or methodological controversy raise ethical issues (regarding study design, meta-analysis, etc.).

Third, a commitment to epidemiology, public health, or even science itself can lack focus and rigor and is weakened in the absence of a clear understanding of the values that shape inquiry and of the conflicts engendered by competing values. Expanded educational programs offer an opportunity to improve such understanding. The proposition that attention to ethics may improve science becomes clear in the following example: (1) an epidemiologist studies the health effects of exposure to a useful chemical compound, (2) the research identifies a correlation between exposure and a particular malady, (3) the epidemiologist prepares for journal publication a manuscript describing these findings, and (4) a manufacturer of the compound learns of the document and offers the epidemiologist a sum of money to alter, omit, or otherwise falsify some of the data in it. If the epidemiologist accepts the offer, submits the corrupted composition (which now identifies no or little correlation between exposure and the malady), and if the altered manuscript is published, readers of the journal and of news accounts based on it have a reason, the publication, to believe that the compound is safe — when the evidence suggests that it is not. The resulting publication, even if it were not intentionally corrupted, is flawed, inaccurate, andmisleading, as well as poor science. The fact that it was corrupted in this way establishes a clear link between high-quality inquiry and the moral duties of scientists. If expanded educational programs can improve understanding of the "values that shape inquiry," ethics and scientific quality will go hand in hand.

Most scientific misconduct akin to the example is not interesting ethically. It is uncontroversially wrong and blameworthy under any account of morality. Fabrication, falsification, and plagiarism are wrong because they deceive people, can hurt people, waste resources, pollute the scientific literature, and so on. Students should be told that these reasons are *why* such actions are wrong, but a fully fledged ethics education program should surely do more. There is a commonly held misconception that ethics education should comprise lessons in how to avoid doing bad things, or a kind of "virtue training." It is not at all clear that such an approach in isolation is productive. Most scientists who falsify data to please a sponsor, insert themselves as authors of papers without doing any of the work, or use information acquired during research for surreptitious financial gain do not generally do so because they are ignorant of the actions' wrongness or are suffering from lack of clarity about what to do when tempted.

There are arguably many ethical issues and conflicts that are more difficult to analyze and that reasonable people disagree about. This is no less true in epidemiology and public health than in clinical medicine or nursing, genetics, and animal research, for instance. The work of ethics consists in part in getting clear the reasons *why* a particular action is blameworthy or praiseworthy. There is a need, therefore, to provide students with the tools or intellectual wherewithal to assess the kinds of arguments offered in support of different positions. Ethical problems and issues arise in a wide variety of circumstances, and it is not feasible to review or anticipate all possible situations and problems. Introducing tools or a framework for ethical thinking can provide students and others with some of the resources necessary for evaluating different, and even novel, kinds of problems. Critical thinking also prepares students to meet future problems related to scientific misconduct. Although fabricating data is wrong, it is not always clear what one ought to do if a colleague is suspected of doing so. To continue the example introduced earlier, suppose a close and longstanding associate learns her colleague has accepted money to falsify data. She then faces the challenge of remaining silent out of loyalty, or disclosing the misconduct at the price of her associate's career or reputation and perhaps at the risk of being seen as a troublemaker, or worse. Providing students with some of the skills needed to address such challenges should be among the goals of an ethics course or curriculum. Beyond misconduct, ethics and epidemiology is a source of interesting and important issues and cases related to vaccination, surveillance, risk communication, disease prevention, and so on.

Finally, the rise of bioethics as a distinct field has seen the emergence of a wide and rich variety of pedagogic tools, and with an unprecedented attention to ethical issues in medicine, scientific research, and health policy. Many of these issues are at the core of clinical practice and involve problems arising at the beginning and end of life, in obtaining valid consent, when protecting confidentiality, in assessing competence, when allocating resources, and the like. However, bioethics and its curricula have also included issues at the periphery of most medical and nursing practice, including xenographic transplants, cadaveric sperm procurement, and cryonics for life extension. Ethics in epidemiology and public health deserve as much attention as these components of what we call "boutique ethics."

We are not suggesting that rare topics are not worthwhile targets for sustained conceptual analysis and policy debate. There is almost always much to be learned from such analyses and debate—and often much that can be applied in more familiar domains. Rather, we are suggesting that the intersection of ethics and epidemiology is a fundamentally important area of ethical inquiry. The point can be made from another direction: many bioethicists are competent to discuss ethical issues and problems in clinical medicine, nursing, surgery, critical care, and so forth. They are also well acquainted with ethical issues related to HIV and AIDS, resource allocation, human subjects research, and the like. However, few have shown evidence of familiarity with issues in epidemiologic ethics or the growing and substantial literature in this area.

Some empirical evidence indicates support among epidemiologists in academia for broadened ethics curricula. A survey of faculty at U.S. schools of public health suggests that 86% of respondents think ethics should be included in the curriculum; 66% say they had already included discussion of ethical issues in other courses.[1] To learn more about ethics in epidemiology courses currently offered in the United States, in 2006 we mailed a letter requesting a description of such courses to departments of preventive medicine in 53 medical schools and to 43 accredited or associated schools of public health. We received positive replies from only 15% of those contacted. This suggests that ethics education is still lacking in the education of epidemiologists, a gap that has existed for some time. A survey of epidemiologists on membership lists of three major epidemiology professional organizations (The American College of Epidemiology, The American Heart Association Council on Epidemiology and Prevention, and The Society for Epidemiologic Research) was completed in 1995 to 1996. Of the 88% who responded, only 54% were aware that ethics guidelines exist for epidemiologists, and only 58% indicated that there was a need to develop syllabi on ethics in epidemiology.[2] Most outlines of ethics-related courses at schools of public health included some lectures directed to epidemiology or public health research, but none presented courses that were solely in the epidemiology curriculum.

There is overlap in ethics guidelines and issues in medicine, public health, and epidemiology. All of these disciplines deal with individuals singly and in groups, and address ethical issues related to research. Epidemiology has unique perspectives that may be missed in more general formal public health or medical ethics courses. The upshot is (1) that ethical issues in epidemiology and public health should be addressed in epidemiology and public health curricula and (2) that students in other disciplines could benefit from such teaching.

What Epidemiologists Need to Know about Ethics

Epidemiologists and philosophers have for some time recognized that epidemiology raises a number of ethical issues.[3,4] Some of these issues will be familiar to those who are acquainted with or have a background in bioethics and research ethics. These issues include informed or valid consent, confidentiality, risk–benefit assessment, patient-subject (or "participant") rights, conflict of interest, and allocation of resources. Nevertheless, epidemiology often offers—perhaps even requires—a broader set of problems under these headings. For instance, what are a researcher's duties to obtain consent from individuals in cultures in which family or community leaders are by custom expected to provide what we might call "consent by proxy" for kin or community? These questions are addressed by Tom Beauchamp in Chapter 2 and Jeffrey Kahn and Anna Mastroianni in Chapter 4. Such cultural differences in ethical norms pose an ensemble of interesting challenges for epidemiologists.

Many ethical issues of concern to epidemiologists are rarely addressed in general bioethics. These issues include, but are by no means limited to, the notion of "ethical imperialism,"[5,6] the danger of social stigma arising from epidemiological findings,[7] and the tensions surrounding decisions whether, to what extent, and by which means to reveal public health risks to study communities.[8,9] The ethics-and-epidemiology literature has matured considerably in the past decade, and faculty and students can avail themselves of a broad variety of supplementary resources, readings, and topics. Given the increase in (perceived) risk of contagion such as SARS and pandemic influenza, as well as bioterrorism, there is also a burgeoning literature and pedagogic opportunities in "all-hazard" preparedness and response.[10,11,12]

Based on analogy with other bioethics curricula and some experience teaching ethics in epidemiology, we offer as a first approximation the suggestion that a course in ethics and epidemiology should consider the following specific goals:

- To help students identify ethical issues, problems, and conflicts in epidemiology, and public health
- To examine the ways in which ethical issues in epidemiology are like and unlike ethical issues in other health sciences
- To provide a decision procedure for approaching ethical issues, problems, and conflicts
- To make clear the connections between sound science and ethically and socially responsible science

Such a course should cover several specific topics depending on available faculty resources, competence, confidence, and expertise. Some topics below have evolved from courses first offered in the early 1990s at the University of Miami and Tulane University and with the encouragement of the American College of Epidemiology, which in 2007 revived an Ethics Committee with a focus on education and curricular support.

Moral Foundations

Students ought to be introduced to core concepts in moral philosophy and bioethics. Professional ethics curricula are often designed and taught by well-meaning scientists and others who somehow believe that excellence in one domain confers competence in another. Tom Beauchamp's review in Chapter 2 provides a survey of key issues in moral philosophy, with attention to epidemiology. Generally, students should be exposed to utilitarianism, a philosophy that right actions are those that maximize the welfare of all affected parties, and Kantianism, a philosophy that demands that we respect persons as autonomous moral agents and not use or exploit them as means to another end. The longstanding conflict between these two theories is a rich source of moral debate and insight, especially in epidemiology in which the rights of individuals can conflict with the duties of communities to protect public health.

Students should also be exposed to major current approaches to bioethics.[13,14] Key examples emphasize (1) principles such as respect for autonomy, nonmaleficence (do no harm), beneficence (providing benefits that contribute to welfare), and justice;[15,16] (2) moral rules and moral ideals undergirded by rationality and impartiality;[17,18] (3) case-based reasoning;[19,20] and (4) some account of rights that emphasizes human rights.[21] This list is not exhaustive, and those with the inclination might profitably review advances in virtue ethics, feminist ethics, and other approaches.

At least as important is a review of relativism and universalism. Many argue that there are knowable moral principles, rights or truths that are independent of culture, era, and nationality, among other considerations. These universalists are prepared to say that some cultures just have it wrong and that their activities or practices violate human rights. Relativists deny this and identify morality as a more or less local phenomenon that cannot be separated from history, culture, nationality, or the like. They reject the possibility of finding a morally neutral vantage point from which to judge the correctness of other cultures' beliefs. Cultural difference is the source of difficult problems in epidemiological ethics, such as varying stances toward informed or valid consent (see Jeffery Kahn and Anna Mastroianni, Chapter 4) and confidentiality (Ellen Wright Clayton, Chapter 5). Research in cultures different from one's own provides a rich and ready source of examples. Students should be challenged to grapple with the differences between *cultural relativism* (which applies to many customs or practices with little or no moral significance—some dietary practices, for instance) and *moral relativism* (the idea, as above, that concepts of right or wrong action vary by culture or context), and urged to identify and take a stand on the kinds of public health values that are often promoted as universal but which are sometimes disdained by local, religious, or other communities (e.g., some religions' objection to vaccination or some political groups' opposition to fluoridation of drinking water).

Research Integrity

Broadly shared values can and have been transmitted between generations of scientists. The universalist will say they are the best values, or the true ones. The relativist will say that they are simply our values. In either case, it is appropriate to share such values with students. Students should be able to evaluate the relation between science and ethics and to show that poorly wrought or sloppy science is not only an inefficient way to learn about the world; it is also wrong because it squanders resources, can put people at risk, and wastes colleagues' time. Sloppiness is a moral consideration and not merely a related to economic or workflow efficiency. One does well to affirm science's commitment to objective inquiry and not to special interests, to mentors' responsibilities for students, and to the open and unfettered enterprise of scientific inquiry. Here too is an opportunity to address several of the touchstone principles of scientific scholarship related to the responsible conduct of research: the need to give credit where credit is due, the obligation not to fabricate or falsify data, the duty to respect the scientific corpus and not pollute it with unnecessary or spurious publications, and the obligations to maintain coherent records and to share data, among others.

Any fascination with "moral dilemmas" creates the mistaken impression that ethics is chatty and impotent, with its task merely the savoring of problems that cannot be solved. This assessment masks the fact that in case after case of scientific misconduct, what is wanted is not a clearer sense of right and wrong, but rather the mettle to do right. Dilemmas are often difficult or impossible to resolve, but this is not the case with many practical problems in epidemiologic and other scientific practice. Such practical problems include communicating risk to study populations, crafting policies for mandatory vaccination, balancing privacy rights against collective health benefits, and managing scientific data that could stigmatize subpopulation groups, among many others.

Valid Consent and Refusal

One of the most difficult problems facing epidemiologists is that of valid consent for people to participate in research. This course component should address the following points and issues:

- The minimal criteria for valid consent (adequate information, absence of undue coercion, and competence)
- The nature and context of valid refusal (informed refusal to participate)
- Criteria addressing questions such as the nature of competence, the level of detail that is minimally required for informing potential subjects about risks, whether monetary and other inducements are undue because they constitute coercion, manipulation, or other forms of undue influence
- Special problems that attach to informed consent forms and their readability and the relation of readability to the criterion above of "adequate information"
- The role, function, and constitution of institutional review boards and other forms of supervisory review
- The potential need for community consent over and above individual consent

Much epidemiologic research would be impossible if the valid consent of all subjects were required. Analysis of data sources ranging from vital statistics to vaccine registries to newborn genetic screening archives involves potentially vast numbers of people, and obtaining their individual consent is often not possible. However, this would be a poor reason to prohibit such research. Steps taken to address this issue include the anonymization of individual records and appropriate institutional oversight. Observe that research on data from which unique identifiers have been removed makes explicit the link between privacy and confidentiality, on the one hand and valid consent, on the other.

Examples of past abuses of subjects have inspired greater adoption of the term "participants." Instructors therefore have an opportunity to familiarize students with historical milestones and documents that chart the evolution of relevant principles and requirements. Research without consent creates a large class of exceptions to the generally preferred use of the term "participants" instead of "subjects" to describe those people whose data are being analyzed: if one does not know one is being studied, one cannot be said to be a "participant."

Privacy and Confidentiality

People expect that details about their personal lives will not be made public. They generally enjoy the right that such information be protected from inappropriate disclosure. However, as data gathering protocols become more refined and as data storage technology progresses, there are always new challenges to privacy and confidentiality. For example, witness the growing use of geographic information systems and of data mining software to make connections among data where these connections reveal facts about individuals, sometimes facts about which the individuals themselves are ignorant. The following curricular items require consideration in any course on ethics and epidemiology:

- Privacy and the degree to which it must be protected, and circumstances under which privacy may be violated (Compare this to the earlier point about plausible exceptions to rules for valid consent.)
- The right of epidemiologists to use databases for purposes not originally foreseen, such as advancing science and informing policy
- Confidentiality and minimal criteria for keeping linked records from inappropriate publication or other disclosure
- Standards for database security and access, addressing criteria for legitimate requests for access
- The relatively free use of unlinked information (where data and a person's identity are decoupled). The relation of this to contexts in which valid consent is presumed unnecessary
- The need for explicit and rigorous justifications for use or maintenance of linked records

The wedding of biology, genetics, and epidemiology also raises issues. Use of computers and networks to store and retrieve genetic information is a rapidly expanding phenomenon. It is reasonable to be concerned about the use of information retrieval techniques to identify genetic patterns or regularities, or to acquire genetic information about individuals or groups.[22]

Risks, Harms, and Wrongs

The distinction among risks, harms, and wrongs (as well as potential benefits) raises issues regarding human subjects and their protection. The term *risk* refers to a possible future harm, whereas *harm* is defined as a setback to interests, particularly in life, health, and welfare. Expressions such as *minimal risk, reasonable risk*, and *high risk* are often used to refer to the chance of a harm's occurrence or its *probability*, but sometimes they also refer to the severity of the harm if it occurs or its *magnitude*. (We are grateful to Tom Beauchamp for these distinctions.) There are also many kinds of harm, including physical, mental, financial, and social. A participant in a research study is at risk of being harmed. If the risk is disclosed before the participant consents to the study and if the harm later occurs, the outcome is unfortunate, though not unethical. However, if information about the risk is withheld and the participant is thereby deceived, in addition to being harmed she is *wronged*. It is not necessary to endure a harm to be wronged; the same participant might not be harmed but be wronged nonetheless because of the deception.

For these reasons, epidemiologists should be given resources for evaluating the following:

- The notion of "acceptable risk"
- What constitutes a harm and how this may vary by culture, community, or even individual
- What constitutes a wrong and how wronging differs from harming
- The need to eliminate or minimize risks, harms, and wrongs, and steps for accomplishing this
- Success in crafting ethically optimized studies, or those that maximize and justly distribute benefits and minimize risks
- What constitutes a risk, harm, or wrong to a group or community, including the problem of research-related stigma
- The relationship among risks, harms, and wrongs, and their inclusion in informed consent documents and processes
- The need for and the role of truth telling by observers and experimenters, and whether and in what contexts deception can be permitted
- Role of disease prevention and issues in mass screening
- Problems and issues that arise in studies involving special or vulnerable populations, including children, the elderly, indigenous peoples, and mental patients

Research Sponsorship, Conflicts of Interest
and Commitment, and Advocacy

The question of professional allegiance and integrity often finds its most difficult challenges when scientists have a financial, social, or personal interest in the results of their research. If he who pays the piper calls the tune, what are we to make of corporate, foundation, or government research sponsorship, and how can such sponsorship—often a valuable source of research funding—be managed to eliminate or minimize bias and to ensure the validity of results?

In general, the concern is that a scientist might be biased as a result of financial, personal, social, political, or other interests or considerations. In our previous example, the epidemiologist studying toxic exposure was motivated by the payment of money—actually a bribe—to abandon his neutrality regarding the data collected. If instead of being offered a direct payment, his spouse were an employee of the company that manufactured the chemical or he owned a great deal of stock in it, his objectivity and neutrality might have been questioned during the initial collection of the data. Such biases reduce accuracy, erode trust, and damage integrity.

Financial interests, although frequently insidious and the source of no little concern, are not unique in compromising research integrity. Investigators who care deeply about the social or policy implications of research might have what has been termed a "conflict of commitment." For instance, a devoutly religious and socially conservative epidemiologist might be suspected of bias if she were to study condom distribution or needle-exchange programs to reduce HIV transmission, and if she were to find these interventions to be ineffective. For these reasons, the question of what constitutes a conflict of interest and what constitutes a conflict of commitment, should be addressed in any comprehensive course on ethics and epidemiology, along with the following:

- Criteria for identifying appropriate and inappropriate sponsorship
- The nature and role of intellectual property in scientific research
- Obligations, and the limits of obligations, to sponsors and employers; managing conflicts
- The extent to which the *appearance* of a conflict should be avoided and whether an appearance of conflict is actually conflict itself
- Contexts in which potential or actual conflicts should be revealed to research subjects and others

Issues of scientific bias are especially important for institutional compliance and policy because of liability issues, institutional credibility and reputation, and the dangers of permitting or being thought to foster an environment conducive to bias. Although conflicts of commitment are generally more difficult to identify and prevent than conflicts of interest, they are in principle no less worrisome sources of bias. A particularly difficult challenge arises when scientists use their knowledge or expertise in attempts to guide or influence public policy. While there is a case to be made that scientists, because of their expertise, are uniquely positioned to contribute to policy debates, there is no bright line between neutral expert opinion and biased social commentary.

Although the primary goal of epidemiology—the study of health effects and improving public health—may be obvious, less clear is the appropriate stance researchers should take in attempts to use their findings or expertise to effect social change or even corporate or institutional policy. Consider, for instance, the environmental health scientist who has political commitments about the sources of climate change, the occupational health researcher with strong feelings about workplace drug abuse or, as above, the socially conservative epidemiologist studying whether condoms reduce the incidence of sexually transmitted disease. These examples point to a body of questions that have been found to enliven the educational experience of adult learners:

- In what contexts, if any, should epidemiologists become advocates for a particular health policy? Does advocacy inherently introduce bias, or can professionals effectively prevent personal views from influencing their research?
- When does such advocacy constitute a conflict of interest or a conflict of commitment?
- How should epidemiologists *qua* advocates address issues of cultural difference?
- What if sincere health policy advocacy conflicts with values prevalent in a study community?
- To what extent is it realistic and proper to demand of researchers a measure of sympathy and respect for values and customs that they find objectionable? Contrarily, is it appropriate to use study results to advocate change in values, customs, or programs?

These are particularly stimulating sources of classroom discussion and debate because reasonable people have disagreed passionately about whether advocacy is morally required or rather objectionable.

Communication and Publication

Unpublished research cannot easily advance the primary goal of improving public health. But publication of scientific results is sometimes problematic. The nature of unpublished research and sometimes the publication of scientific results fall under the increasingly familiar heading "responsible conduct of research." The following topics should be addressed:

- Duties to communicate and problems in communicating study results to subjects, communities, sponsors, and so forth. Issues of health literacy loom large here
- Difficulties in accurate and balanced communication of risks, harms, and wrongs
- Obligation to publish study results, the effects of publication, and responsibilities to colleagues and "science"

- Issues in publication and authorship, including overpublication and redundant publication
- The role of popular news media in communicating public health information

Each of these bears on scientific communication in a number of ways. These connections afford an instructor opportunities to use scholarly media to foster discussion about responsible communication, as well as the popular media to inform debate about public understanding of science, especially the kinds of probabilistic and sometimes conflicting data that sometimes confound or alarm lay people about health risks.

Issues and Cases

It would therefore be a sad oversight if a course or program in ethics and epidemiology were decoupled from current events. Epidemiology is often in the news, and some of the greatest challenges facing scientists and policymakers are prime candidates for inclusion in an ethics course. If applied ethics is to be of any use at all in solving real-world problems, students should be shown how this works in actual cases. In what follows we offer three examples.

1. *Risk communication and pandemic preparedness.* Health planners and others are concerned about the possibility that the H5N1 avian influenza, an Influenza A virus subtype, will mutate and achieve human-to-human transmission. The results of such transmission, if anything like the 1918 to 1919 influenza pandemic, would be disastrous. In that pandemic, 50 million to 100 million people died—as much as 5% of the human population.

   If such a pandemic were to recur, it would evolve and run its course over an extended period (the 1918 to 1919 pandemic lasted approximately 18 months). As it spread, government and public health officials would need to make difficult decisions regarding (1) isolation and quarantine, (2) triage and rationing, and (3) how best to communicate the risks related to these policy challenges and the policy decisions themselves.

   These decisions will likely be based on incomplete and probabilistic data and so therefore will be the messages communicated to concerned citizens. Pandemic risk communication is shaped by the same factors that influence other threats, the likelihood or severity of which are probabilistic. If an alarm is sounded too early or is too shrill, it can elicit panic and distrust and impede cooperation. If it is sounded too late, those at risk will resent that they were not trusted with probabilistic data in the first place. Pandemic risk communication therefore raises issues of decision making under uncertainty, veracity, and trust. How should epidemiologists contribute to such communication?

Pandemic responses related to quarantine and rationing (perhaps of vaccines, ventilators, or hospital beds) are another source of ethical issues that bear on epidemiology and public health. Instructors or leaders of an ethics and epidemiology course will find these issues ripe for discussion and debate. For instance, there are good reasons to use police powers to accomplish public health objectives. Under what circumstances should mandatory quarantine and isolation be ordered? Applied ethics can help answer such a question by invoking, for example, a utilitarian analysis in which maximizing the welfare of all affected parties is assigned a higher priority than protecting rights of free association and movement. Several high-quality online resources are available to the instructor, including those of the World Health Organization and the U.S. Centers for Disease Control and Prevention.[23]

2. *Public understanding of epidemiology research: The case of screening mammography.* Do regular mammograms reduce breast-cancer mortality? Consider the following sequence (adapted from a book about evidence-based medicine[24]):

1997
- A National Institutes of Health consensus conference concludes that there is insufficient evidence to recommend for or against routine mammograms for women in their 40s.[25]
- Congress condemns the consensus statement and seeks "to refute its conclusions and to give American women 'clearer guidance' about the need for mammograms."[26]

2000
- A Cochrane Collaboration report reviews the quality of mammography trials and two meta-analyses and finds that "screening for breast cancer with mammography is unjustified....[T]here is no reliable evidence that screening decreases breast-cancer mortality."[27]

2001
- A "storm of debate and criticism" follows, including criticism of the quality of the research that produced the findings.[28]
- A formal review of the Cochrane report is said to have "confirmed and strengthened our original conclusion."[29]

One authority is quoted in the popular news media as summing up the tension:

The debate has become so sophisticated from a methodology viewpoint that as a doctor my head is spinning.... [Y]ou read an article in *The Lancet* and you nod your head yes. Then you read the studies by people on the other side and you nod your head yes. We're witnessing this fight between the pro- and anti-mammography forces and they're both arguing that "my data are better and we're right and they're wrong."[30]

The issue is rich with opportunities to address the values and goals of research and their implications for public policy; the appropriate use and application of a standard, albeit controversial, technique for data analysis (meta-analysis); and the lay public's (mis-) understanding of the growth of knowledge. Ethical issues include that of the potential personal or financial bias of partisans with commitments to or against a public health initiative and the duty of scientists to communicate data to clarify its scope and limitations.

3. *Planning for bioterrorism—epidemiology and health informatics.* Epidemiologists and other scientists rely on information technology to collect, store, analyze, and propagate information. The growth of computational "early warning systems" to identify sudden and evolving threats to public health raises an ensemble of issues fertile for curricular development.

In addition to pandemic preparedness, the intentional introduction of dangerous biological, chemical, or radioactive agents into the air, water, or food provides superb opportunities to introduce students to ethical issues in epidemiology. Since the anthrax attacks of 2001, which killed five people in the weeks after September 11, 2001, it became clear that a more efficient pathogen, introduced more broadly, could be devastating. What is needed, according to some, is a robust and highly sensitive and specific means of detecting such an attack as quickly as possible. With rapid identification and response, deaths and injuries could be reduced. Computational early warning systems, which we will call "emergency public health informatics" (EPHI), raise ethical issues that are interesting both because of the use of new technology and their links to traditional challenges in epidemiology.[31] These issues include:

Privacy and confidentiality. Although epidemiologists encounter these values on a regular basis, the volume of data needed to fuel early warning systems potentially linked to personal identifiers is extraordinary: pharmacy purchases, satellite photos of cars in drug store parking lots, 911 calls, school system absentees, visits to emergency rooms and veterinary clinics, and so forth. The ability to establish baseline levels for these variables and quickly be able to detect increases is an essential component of early warning systems.

Surveillance or research? Citizens rely on scientists and governments to keep track of changes in threats to health and well-being and to intervene when appropriate. In open societies, at least, such monitoring or surveillance is tacitly permitted—that is, epidemiologists do not ask those citizens if they are willing to share news of births, deaths, vaccinations, domestic violence, and so on. It would be irresponsible not to collect and analyze data on these and many other phenomena. Contrarily, those same citizens expect their consent will be sought before health data are collected for research. Because health research must be reviewed by institutional review boards or research ethics committees, the question whether any particular act of data acquisition is part of a surveillance effort or a research project is of great significance. Computational epidemiology, including EPHI systems, presents extensive opportunities for classroom analysis and debate. (The distinction between surveillance and research is discussed by Robert McKeown and Max Learner in Chapter 8.)

Judgments under uncertainty. Although computers are essential for tracking changes in variables that might signal a bioterrorist attack, they are imperfect, meaning that the data they process can be flawed or incomplete. This also means that the analyses themselves might not be accurate or reliable. However, if that is the case, how reliable are the interventions, warnings, or other responses to signs of an emergency threat? Epidemiologists are generally experienced in the management of incomplete and imperfect data. Computer tracking of emergencies provides a new opportunity to review strategies and their consequences for populations in which the stakes are immediate and potentially very high.

Pedagogic Opportunities

There are many resources for those seeking to introduce or broaden the role of ethics in epidemiology curricula. These include codes of ethics, a global increase of interest in research integrity and the responsible conduct of science, and the efforts of others who have succeeded in developing ethics curricula. This section provides a survey of these resources.

In the case of codes of ethics, epidemiology has joined other sciences in reckoning that professionals are linked by values which ought to be articulated in a code or oath. Codes of ethics, despite ancient precedents and antecedents, are notoriously difficult to draft: If they are too general, they provide little or no guidance in particular cases. If too specific, they risk omitting or overlooking issues and actions that can shape professional practice. In either case, they risk sending the message that a list of rules or principles for right conduct, in the absence of ongoing education and the fostering of critical thinking skills that we earlier identified as essential to high-quality ethics education, is somehow adequate to foster such conduct. Moreover, a code of ethics risks irrelevance and stagnation if it is not regularly reviewed and updated.

Nevertheless, when codes exist and are well written by informed professionals, they can profitably be included in ethics curricula as exemplars of the kinds of behavior expected of professionals trained in a particular field. A committee of the American College of Epidemiology, for instance, drafted a set of "Ethics Guidelines" in 2000 after a series of surveys and workshops.[32] After a statement of "core values, duties, and virtues," this document, offered as one of five official "Statements of the College," emphasizes and addresses issues in human subjects protection under headings such as "Elements of informed consent," "Avoidance of manipulation or coercion," and "Conditions under which informed consent requirements may be waived." The contents of any code are mere slogans, unless there is some sort of analysis about the meaning and import of key terms. The American Public Health Association in 2001 published 12 principles under the title "Principles of the Ethical Practice of Public Health" with accompanying rationale and notes.[33] These broad principles include the statements, "Public health programs and policies should be implemented in a manner that most enhances the physical and social environment," and "Public health institutions should protect the confidentiality of information that can bring harm to an individual or community if made public. Exceptions must be justified on the basis of the high likelihood of significant harm to the individual or others."

That a problem or issue is included or excluded is itself an idea that can inspire and inform a teaching moment. Students benefit from being able to reflect on and debate contemporary challenges in the profession.

Research Integrity and the Responsible Conduct of Science

For better or worse, the past three decades have seen unprecedented attention to human subjects protection and the responsible conduct of research (RCR) in large part because of abuses of research participants and dramatic cases of scientific misconduct. Although we might wish that such attention had been fostered by loftier motivations, it is the result of scandal and of public disclosure of wrongdoing.

Epidemiologists have an opportunity to embrace RCR curricula and render ethics education more than a response to bad actors and corner-cutters. If one accepts that the goal of ethics pedagogy is improved critical thinking skills,[34] then instead of seeking to shame evildoers we should emphasize that improved RCR education will help professionals manage conflicts of interest and commitment, address questions related to intellectual property, and educate others about the importance of research integrity in building public trust.

Such pedagogy should not be a mere recitation of rules against wrong acts, such as fabrication, falsification, and plagiarism. There is nothing ethically challenging about such blatant offenses in that they are uncontroversially wrong under any system of or approach to ethics. The growth of interest in RCR curricula, on the other hand, affords an opportunity to confront more difficult cases and issues and foster greater awareness (perhaps especially in epidemiology) of the importance of public trust in communicating the results of professional activities.

There are many resources that can be used to advance RCR education in the classroom, several of which are listed on an NIH-maintained website.[35]

Ethics-and-Epidemiology Courses and Training

Many institutions have successfully established courses in ethics and epidemiology and public health[36] or incorporated questions of ethics and public policy into existing courses. The question as to which approach is preferable is an interesting one, though any attempt to introduce ethics education where there was none is laudable. One might hope that both approaches could be adopted: Create an ethics-and-epidemiology course *and* include ethics in appropriate places in courses in biostatistics, environmental health, toxicology, and the like. Either effort requires the support of leadership and faculty in academic institutions. For professional societies and industry, it also requires that leaders both believe and are willing to devote resources to the idea that ethics education improves professional development. In some cases, the greatest challenge can be the identification of curricular tools and competent faculty.

The American College of Epidemiology has reconstituted an Ethics Committee (formerly the Ethics and Standards of Practice Committee), which has collected ethics syllabi from institutions willing to make such resources available to the epidemiology community.[37] These syllabi and other materials will be made freely available on the College's website.[38] The Association of Schools of Public Health has created an "Ethics and Public Health: Model Curriculum" containing detailed guidance and useful resources on a number of issues.[39]

A commitment to bioethics will also realize the opportunity to teach and use faculty from other schools or departments. For instance, computer scientists will identify issues in database security, physicians and nurses will examine culturally mediated local public health problems, and philosophers will inform discussions about moral foundations and challenges related to causation, risk, and uncertainty. In addition, links to course offerings in philosophy departments (philosophy of science, ethics, bioethics, etc.) and law schools could be especially useful for students with advanced interests.

Conclusions and Recommendations

There is a need to address ethical issues in a more complete and rigorous manner in epidemiology and public health curricula and at the postgraduate and professional levels. There is a concomitant need for high-quality course materials and for them to evolve. Such course development will improve the quality of public health research, stimulate research in science and ethics, clarify the values that guide epidemiologic inquiry, reduce attrition of idealistic students discouraged by unethical mentors, and raise epidemiology and public health ethics to a pedagogical level commensurate with their importance.

We are therefore advocating a change in the "standard of care" in epidemiology education. The arguments here are not intended to support mere curricular niceties, but they are proposed as requirements for training programs in epidemiology and public health. A failure to include some measure of bioethics training in the curriculum is itself both pedagogically and ethically disappointing. Institutions, professional societies, industry, and government should devote appropriate resources and personnel to realizing these goals. Ethics in epidemiology and public health should enjoy a role that reflects their importance, their potential contributions, and their role in science and society.

References

1. Rossignol, A. M., and Goodmonson, S. "Are Ethical Topics in Epidemiology Included in the Graduate Epidemiology Curricula?" *American Journal of Epidemiology* 142 (1995): 1265–68.
2. Prineas, R. J., Goodman, K. W., Soskolne, C. L., Buck, G., Feinleib, M., Last, J., and Andrews, J. S., for the American College of Epidemiology Ethics and Standards of Practice Committee. Findings of the American College of Epidemiology's Survey of Ethics Guidelines. *Annals of Epidemiology* 8 (1998): 482–89.
3. Coughlin, S. S. and Etheredge, G. D. "On the Need for Ethics Curricula in Epidemiology," *Epidemiology* 6 (1995): 566–67.
4. Coughlin, S. S. "Ethics in Epidemiology at the End of the 20th Century: Ethics, Values, and Mission Statements," *Epidemiologic Reviews* 22 (2000): 169–75.
5. Angell, M. "Ethical Imperialism? Ethics in International Collaborative Research," *New England Journal of Medicine* 319 (1988): 1081–83.
6. Levine, R. J. "Informed Consent: Some Challenges to the Universal Validity of the Western Model." In *Ethics and Epidemiology. International Guidelines,* cd. Z. Bankowski, J. H. Bryant, and J. M. Last. Geneva: Council for International Organizations of Medical Sciences (CIOMS) (1991): 47–58.
7. Gostin, L. "Ethical Principles for the Conduct of Human Subject Research: Population-Based Research and Ethics," *Law, Medicine and Health Care* 19 (1991): 175–83.
8. Sandman, P.M. "Emerging Communication Responsibilities of Epidemiologists." In Industrial Epidemiology Forum's Conference on Ethics in Epidemiology, ed. W. E. Fayerweather, J. Higginson, and T. L. Beauchamp. *Journal of Clinical Epidemiology* 44, Suppl. I (1991): 41S–50S.
9. Higginson, J. and Chu, P. "Ethical Considerations and Responsibilities in Communicating Health Risk Information." In Industrial Epidemiology Forum's Conference on Ethics in Epidemiology, ed. W. E. Fayerweather, J. Higginson, and T. L. Beauchamp. *Journal of Clinical Epidemiology* 44, Suppl. I (1991): 51S–56S.
10. Moreno, J. D., ed. *In the Wake of Terror: Medicine and Morality in a Time of Crisis.* Cambridge, MA: MIT Press, 2003.
11. Levy, B. S. and Sidel, V. W., eds. *Terrorism and Public Health: A Balanced Approach to Strengthening Systems and Protecting People.* New York: Oxford University Press, 2003.
12. Siegel, M. *False Alarm: The Truth About the Epidemic of Fear.* Hoboken, NJ: Wiley, 2005.
13. Weed, D. L. and McKeown, R. E. "Ethics in Epidemiology and Public Health I. Technical Terms," *Journal of Epidemiology and Community Health* 55 (2001): 855–57.
14. McKeown, R. E. and Weed, D. L. "Ethics in Epidemiology and Public Health II. Applied Terms," *Journal of Epidemiology and Community Health* 56 (2002): 739–41.

15. Beauchamp, T. L. and Childress, J. F., *Principles of Biomedical Ethics*, 6th ed. New York: Oxford University Press, 2009.

16. Beauchamp, T. L. "Methods and Principles In Biomedical Ethics," *Journal of Medical Ethics* 29 (2003): 269–74.

17. Gert, B. *Morality: Its Nature and Justification*, revised edition, New York: Oxford University Press, 2009.

18. Clouser, K. D. and Gert, B. "Common Morality." In *Handbook of Bioethics: Taking Stock of the Field from a Philosophical Perspective*, ed. G. Khushf. Dordrecht: Kluwer Academic Publishers (2004): 121–41.

19. Jonsen, A. R. and Toulmin, S. E. *The Abuse of Casuistry*. Berkeley, CA: University of California Press, 1988.

20. Arras, J. D. "Getting Down to Cases: The Revival of Casuistry in Bioethics," *Journal of Medicine and Philosophy* 16 (1991): 29–51.

21. Mann, J. M., Gruskin, S., Grodin, M. A., and Annas, G. J., eds. *Health and Human Rights: A Reader*. New York: Routledge, 1999.

22. Goodman, K. W. "Ethics, Genomics, and Information Retrieval," *Computers in Biology and Medicine* 26 (1996): 223–29.

23. Available at www.who.int/ethics/influenza_project/en/index.html and www.cdc.gov/od/science/phec/ respectively, accessed on October 22, 2008.

24. Goodman, K. W. *Ethics and Evidence-Based Medicine: Fallibility and Responsibility in Clinical Science*. Cambridge: Cambridge University Press, 2003.

25. National Institutes of Health Consensus Development Panel, National Institutes of Health Consensus Development Conference Statement: Breast Cancer Screening for Women Ages 40–49, January 21–23, 1997, *Journal of the National Cancer Institute* 89 (1997): 1015–26.

26. Woolf, S. H. and Lawrence, R. S. "Preserving Scientific Debate and Patient Choice: Lessons from the Consensus Panel on Mammography Screening," *Journal of the American Medical Association* 278 (1997): 2105–08.

27. Gøtzsche, P. C. and Olsen, O. "Is Screening for Breast Cancer with Mammography Justifiable?" *The Lancet* 355 (2000): 129–34.

28. Horton, R. "Screening Mammography—An Overview Revisited," *The Lancet* 358 (2001): 1284–85.

29. Olsen, O. and Gøtzsche, P. C. "Cochrane Review on Screening for Breast Cancer with Mammography," *The Lancet* 358 (2001): 1340–42.

30. Kolata, G. "Study Sets off Debate over Mammograms' Value," *The New York Times*, National Edition (December 9, 2001): A1, A32.

31. Szczepaniak, M. C., Goodman, K. W., Wagner, M. W., Hutman, J., and Daswani, S. "Advancing Organizational Integration: Negotiation, Data Use Agreements, Law, and Ethics." In *Handbook of Biosurveillance,* eds. M. W. Wagner, A. W. Moore, and R. M. Aryel. Boston, MA: Academic Press (2006): 465–80.

32. Available at http://www.acepidemiology2.org/policystmts/EthicsGuide.asp, accessed October 22, 2008.

33. Thomas, J. C., Sage, M., Dillenberg, J., and Guillory, V. J. "A Code of Ethics for Public Health," *American Journal of Public Health* 92 (2002): 1057–59.

34. De Melo-Martin, I. and Intemann, K. K. "Can Ethical Reasoning Contribute to Better Epidemiology? A Case Study in Research on Racial Health Disparities," *European Journal of Epidemiology* 22 (2007): 215–21.

35. http://bioethics.od.nih.gov/casestudies.html, accessed October 22, 2008.

36. Thomas, J. C. "Teaching Ethics in Schools of Public Health," *Public Health Reports* 118 (2003): 279–86.

37. This committee is at this writing chaired by one of the authors of this chapter (KWG).

38. http://www.acepidemiology.org/, accessed October 22, 2008.

39. Available at http://www.asph.org/document.cfm?page=782, accessed October 22, 2008.

Index